Neuropharmacology of Ethanol

New Approaches

Editors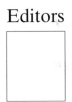

Roger E. Meyer,
George F. Koob,
Michael J. Lewis,
Steven M. Paul

1991

Birkhäuser
Boston · Basel · Berlin

Roger E. Meyer, M.D.
Department of Psychiatry
School of Medicine
University of Connecticut Health Center
Farmington, CT 06032

Michael J. Lewis, Ph.D.
Department of Psychology
Howard University and
O.S.A., N.I.A.A.A.
Rockville, MD 20857

George F. Koob, Ph.D.
Research Institute of the Scripps Clinic
La Jolla, CA 92037

Steven M. Paul, M.D.
N.I.H., N.I.M.H.
Bethesda, MD 20892

Library of Congress Cataloging-in-Publication Data

Neuropharmacology of ethanol : new approaches / Roger E. Meyer ... [et al.], editors. p. cm.
Based on a panel symposium of the American College of Neuropsychopharmacology, held
Dec. 1988, in San Juan, Puerto Rico.
Includes bibliographical references and index.
ISBN 0-8176-3463-0 (hard : alk. paper). – ISBN 3-7643-3463-0 (alk. paper)
1. Alcoholism–Etiology–Congresses. 2. Alcohol–Physiological effect–Congresses. 3. Brain–
Effect of drugs on–Congresses.
I. Meyer, Roger E.   II. American College of Neuropsychopharmacology. [DNLM: 1. Alcohol.
Ethyl.–pharmacology–Congresses. 2. Alcoholism–etiology–Congresses. 3. Brain–drug–effects–
Congresses. OV 84 N494 1988]
RC564.N475 1991
616.85 1071–dc20
DNLM/DLC
for Library of Congress
91–11447
CIP
Printed on acid-free paper.

Typeset by ARK Publications, Newton Centre, MA using TeX.
Printed and bound in Germany

9 8 7 6 5 4 3 2 1

ISBN 0-8176-3463-0
ISBN 3-7643-3463-0

The editors, in association with the American College of Neuropharmacology, have brought together the papers in this volume. The work highlights the progress that has been made in recent years in understanding the effects of ethyl alcohol on brain and behavior. That ethanol, the oldest of psychopharmacological agents, should be the subject of this volume sponsored by ACNP seems both symbolic and timely.

The American College of Neuropsychopharmacology

CONTENTS

List of Contributors ix

Alcohol and Anesthetic Actions: Are They Mediated
by Lipid or Protein?
Floyd E. Bloom 1

Probing Molecular Sites of Action for Alcohol's Acute
and Chronic Effects on Synaptoneurosome Membranes:
A Potential Tool for Studying Drug-Receptor Interactions
R. Preston Mason, Jill Moring, Leo G. Herbette,
Roger E. Meyer and William J. Shoemaker 21

Ethanol and the GABA$_A$ Receptor-Gated Chloride Ion Channel
A. Leslie Morrow, Pascale Montpied and Steven M. Paul 49

The GABA$_A$ Receptor Complex: Is it a Locus of Action
for Inhalation Anesthetics?
Eric J. Moody, Herman J.C. Yeh and Phil Skolnick 77

Ethanol and the NMDA Receptor: Insights Into
Ethanol Pharmacology
Boris Tabakoff, Carolyn S. Rabe, Kathleen A. Grant,
Peter Valverius, Michael Hudspith and Paula L. Hoffman 93

Molecular and Genetic Approaches to Understanding
Alcohol-Seeking Behavior
Ting-Kai Li, David W. Crabb and Lawrence Lumeng 107

The Neuropharmacology of Ethanol Self-Administration
F. Weiss and G.F. Koob 125

Alcohol Effects on Brain-Stimulation Reward:
Blood Alcohol Concentration and Site Specificity
Michael J. Lewis 163

Ethanol and Rewarding Brain Simulation
Conan Kornetsky, Marjorie Moolten and George Bain 179

Electrophysiologic Correlates of Ethanol Reinforcement
Scott E. Lukas, Jack H. Mendelson, Leslie Amass,
Richard A. Benedikt, John N. Henry, Jr. and Elena M. Kouri . . 201

Neuroendocrine Concomitants of Alcohol Reinforcement
Jack H. Mendelson, Nancy K. Mello, Scott E. Lukas,
Siew K. Teoh, William R. Phipps, James Ellingboe,
Isaac Schiff and Susan Palmieri 233

Alcohol Reinforcement: Biobehavioral
and Clinical Considerations
Roger E. Meyer and Zelig Dolinsky 251

Index   265

Contributors

Leslie Amass, PhD   The Alcohol and Drug Abuse Research Center, Harvard Medical School and McLean Hospital, 115 Mill Street, Belmont, MA 02178

George Bain, PhD   Boston University School of Medicine, 80 East Concord Street, Boston, MA 02118

Richard A. Benedikt, PhD   The Alcohol and Drug Abuse Research Center, Harvard Medical School and McLean Hospital, 115 Mill Street, Belmont, MA 02178

Floyd E. Bloom, MD   Department of Neuropharmacology, Scripps Clinic and Research Foundation, 10666 North Torrey Pines Road, La Jolla, CA 92037

David W. Crabb, PhD   Department of Medicine and Biochemistry, Indiana University School of Medicine and VA Medical Center, Indianapolis, IN 46202

Zelig Dolinsky, PhD   University of Connecticut Health Center, 263 Farmington Avenue, Farmington, CT 06032

James Ellingboe, PhD   The Alcohol and Drug Abuse Research Center, Harvard Medical School and McLean Hospital, 115 Mill Street, Belmont, MA 02178

Kathleen A. Grant, PhD   Laboratory of Physiologic and Pharmacologic Studies, National Institute on Alcohol Abuse and Alcoholism, 12501 Washington Avenue, Rockville, MD 20852

John N. Henry Jr., PhD   The Alcohol and Drug Abuse Research Center, Harvard Medical School and McLean Hospital, 115 Mill Street, Belmont, MA 02178

Leo G. Herbette, PhD   Department of Radiology and Biochemistry, and Biomolecular Structure Analysis Center, CSM-011 University of Connecticut Health Center, Farmington, CT 06032

Paula L. Hoffman, PhD   Laboratory of Physiologic and Pharmacologic Studies, National Institute on Alcohol Abuse and Alcoholism, 12501 Washington Avenue, Rockville, MD 20852

Michael Hudspith, PhD   Laboratory of Physiologic and Pharmacologic Studies, National Institute on Alcohol Abuse and Alcoholism, 12501 Washington Avenue, Rockville, MD 20852

George F. Koob, PhD   Department of Neuropharmacology, Scripps Clinic and Research Foundation, 10666 North Torrey Pines Road, La Jolla, CA 92037

Conan Kornetsky, PhD   Boston University School of Medicine, 80 East Concord Street, Boston, MA 02118

Elena M. Kouri, PhD   The Alcohol and Drug Abuse Research Center, Harvard Medical School and McLean Hospital, 115 Mill Street, Belmont, MA 02178

Michael J. Lewis, PhD   Department of Psychology, Howard University, Washington, D.C. 20059 and Office of Scientific Affairs, National Institute of Alcohol Abuse and Alcoholism, 16-C-26 Parklawn Bldg, 5600 Fishers Lane, Rockville, MD 20857

Ting-Kai Li, MD Department of Medicine and Biochemistry, Indiana University School of Medicine and VA Medical Center, Indianapolis, IN 46202

Scott E. Lukas, PhD   The Alcohol and Drug Abuse Research Center, Harvard Medical School and McLean Hospital, 115 Mill Street, Belmont, MA 02178

Lawrence Lumeng, PhD   Department of Medicine and Biochemistry, Indiana University School of Medicine and VA Medical Center, Indianapolis, IN 46202

R. Preston Mason, PhD   Biomolecular Structure Analysis Center, CSM-011 University of Connecticut Health Center, Farmington, CT 06032

Nancy K. Mello, PhD   The Alcohol and Drug Abuse Research Center, Harvard Medical School and McLean Hospital, 115 Mill Street, Belmont, MA 02178

Jack H. Mendelson, PhD   The Alcohol and Drug Abuse Research Center, Harvard Medical School and McLean Hospital, 115 Mill Street, Belmont, MA 02178

Roger E. Meyer, MD   Department of Psychiatry and Alcohol Research Center, University of Connecticut Health Center, 10 Talcott Notch Road, Farmington, CT 06032

Pascale Montpied, PhD   Clinical Neuroscience Branch, National Institute of Mental Health, Bldg. 10, Rm 4N-214, 9000 Rockville Pike, Bethesda, MD 20892

E.J. Moody, PhD   Department of Anesthesiology, Massachusetts General Hospital, Boston, MA 02114

Marjorie Moolten, PhD   Boston University School of Medicine, 80 East Concord Street, Boston, MA 02118

Jill Moring, PhD   Department of Medicine, University of Connecticut Health Center, Farmington, CT 06032

A. Leslie Morrow, MD   Clinical Neuroscience Branch, National Institute of Mental Health, Bldg. 10, Rm 4N-214, 9000 Rockville Pike, Bethesda, MD 20892

Susan Palmieri, PhD   The Alcohol and Drug Abuse Research Center, Harvard Medical School and McLean Hospital, 115 Mill Street, Belmont, MA 02178

Steven M. Paul, MD   Clinical Neuroscience Branch, National Institute of Mental Health, Bldg. 10, Rm 4N-214, 9000 Rockville Pike, Bethesda, MD 20892

William R. Phipps, PhD   The Alcohol and Drug Abuse Research Center, Harvard Medical School and McLean Hospital, 115 Mill Street, Belmont, MA 02178

Carolyn S. Rabe, PhD   Laboratory of Physiologic and Pharmacologic Studies, National Institute on Alcohol Abuse and Alcoholism, 12501 Washington Avenue, Rockville, MD 20852

Isaac Schiff, PhD   The Alcohol and Drug Abuse Research Center, Harvard Medical School and McLean Hospital, 115 Mill Street, Belmont, MA 02178

William J. Shoemaker, PhD   Department of Psychiatry and Alcohol Research Center, University of Connecticut Health Center, Farmington, CT 06032

Phil Skolnick, PhD   Laboratory of Neuroscience, National Institutes of Health, Bldg. 8, Rm 103, Bethsesda, MD 20892

Boris Tabakoff, PhD   Laboratory of Physiologic and Pharmacologic Studies, National Institute on Alcohol Abuse and Alcoholism, 12501 Washington Avenue, Rockville, MD 20852

Siew Koon Teoh, PhD   The Alcohol and Drug Abuse Research Center, Harvard Medical School and McLean Hospital, 115 Mill Street, Belmont, MA 02178

Friedbert Weiss, PhD Department of Neuropharmacology, Scripps Clinic and Research Foundation, 10666 North Torrey Pines Road, La Jolla, CA 92037

Peter Valverius, PhD   Laboratory of Physiologic and Pharmacologic Studies, National Institute on Alcohol Abuse and Alcoholism, 12501 Washington Avenue, Rockville, MD 20852

Herman J.C. Yeh, MD   Laboratory of Analytical Chemistry, National Institutes of Health, Bldg. 8, Rm 103, Bethesda, MD 20892

Alcohol and Anesthetic Actions:
Are They Mediated by Lipid or Protein?

Floyd E. Bloom

INTRODUCTION

Attempts to explain the effects of ethanol and other alcohols on the
central nervous system have historically emphasized similarities between
this class of drug and general anesthetics. Thus, a recent textbook of
pharmacology summarizes the matter as "Despite popular belief in its
stimulant properties, ethanol is entirely depressant in its actions on neurones of the central nervous system. In fact, its actions are qualitatively
similar to those of a general anesthetic" (Bowman and Rand, 1980). Thus,
when considered under the Meyer-Overton "rule," the pharmacological
potency of an alcohol, like some general anesthetics, is proportional to
its lipophilicity, and lipophilicity is in turn directly related to the chain
length and other physicochemical properties of the alcohol. Furthermore,
in contrast to almost all other classes of central nervous system (CNS)
drugs, neither for alcohols nor general anesthetics has it been possible to
identify any membrane receptor responsible for ethanol actions on release,
response to or metabolism of any specific neurotransmitters. Although no
consensus mechanisms have yet emerged for how these physicochemical
properties of alcohols and anesthetics actually "explain" their effects on
cellular and organismic function, the inference has been that the primary
sites of action of these substances takes place within the lipid matrix
of the plasma membranes. It should also be noted, however, that the
pharmacological endpoint on which the lipophilic nature of ethanol was
assessed quantitatively was the blockade of action potentials in isolated
frog sciatic nerves (Seeman, 1972).

This general "lipid perturbation" interpretation was further supported
through observations made *in vitro* on the physical properties of brain
and erythrocyte membrane fragments indicating that acute exposures to

relatively high concentrations of ethanol and lower concentrations of more liposoluble alcohols led to changes in the "ordering" of the membrane lipids. Observers using such methods further inferred that the disordering effects on membrane lipids led to alterations in membrane molecular structure and function, such as had been reported for certain membrane-mounted enzymes (Tabakoff et al., 1987). In addition, examination of membranes from animals exposed chronically to intoxicating doses of ethanol showed consistent changes in membrane lipid composition that could be interpreted as reducing the disordering of lipids, and thus restoring the membrane to a more ordered and presumably functional state (Goldstein, 1987; Hoek and Taraschi, 1988).

Recently, however, data have emerged that question whether the lipid perturbation hypothesis can satisfactorily explain the mechanisms underlying the cellular effects of alcohols and general anesthetics. The first line of evidence suggesting the need for alternative explanations emerges from newer physicochemical methods that have reinterpreted the classical studies of lipophilic interactions based on partition coefficients (see Mason et al., this volume and other references cited below). For example, application of these newer strategies (Mason et al., this volume) and to drug-dielectric interactions in model membrane bilayers (Mason et al., this volume) emphasize a growing trend toward the interpretation that actions based exclusively on drug-lipid permeation are inadequate to explain the experimental observations and that the composition of neurons offers selective sites for presumptive protein lipid interactions that are not detectable in non-neuronal membranes. These revisionist views of the importance of membrane lipids for acute ethanol intoxication are further supported by data indicating that the changes in membrane properties after longer term exposure to intoxicating levels of ethanol are restricted to only a minor class of membrane lipids, namely the phosphatidylinositol fraction (Hoek and Taraschi, 1988; Taraschi et al., 1987).

The second line of evidence is based on analysis of the molecular mechanisms that have been shown to be modified by doses of acutely administered alcohols that are pharmacologically relevant to the time course and dose-response course of alcohol intoxication. These data, reviewed recently elsewhere (Bloom, 1989; Harris and Allan, 1989; Koob and Bloom, 1988; Shefner, 1989; Siggins et al., 1989) emphasize that the sensitivity of specific mammalian neurons to ethanol varies over a wide dose spectrum and that those neurons most sensitive to ethanol (whose threshold doses fall within the minimum human intoxicating dose range) show specific changes in selected intramembranous mechanisms mediating responses to neurotransmitters. Several transmitter-selective effects of ethanol on neuronal function, as well as selected alterations in transmitter biochemistry in animals bred for preference for alcohol consumption, have now been reported (see below). The degree to which the data support a pharmacology of ethanol based on neuronal effects of selected bodies of neurotransmitters would seem to be generally incompatible with the predictions of uniform widespread interference with membranes through disordering of the bulk phase lipids. This chapter will briefly examine the recent data comprising these two lines of evidence.

MOLECULAR INTERACTIONS OF ETHANOL

At first glance, there would seem to be two alternative concepts of how alcohols, and ethanol the drug, affect cells, and more specifically neurons, to produce the biologic effects that eventuate in the forms of altered behavior recognized as intoxication, dependence and tolerance. Either ethanol interacts with selected proteins, such as enzymes, transmitter receptors or structural proteins in or on the membrane of neurons, or ethanol interacts with the lipids of the membrane.

However, a third alternative does exist, which in overview creates many, many alternatives and will therefore be presented as a brief digression from the main theme: rather than viewing ethanol per se as the agent causing the effects that emerge upon consumption of ethanol, an "active catabolite" could be formed in the body in the presence of ethanol, and this active catabolite could then interact with a host of receptive target systems. In the most notorious hypothesis of this sort, the so-called tetrahydroisquinoline hypothesis, either a condensation product of a brain amine with acetaldehyde or other hypothetical condensation products of monoamine catabolism resulting from ethanol effects on brain re-dox systems could generate an active intermediate agent that is responsible for the pharmacology of ethanol and thus not constrained by the physical properties of ethanol (Davis and Walsh, 1970; Myers, 1989; see Bloom et al., 1981 and Smith and Amit, 1987 for nonsupporting evidence). To the degree that such an intermediate could be documented, the greater specificity of its receptor interactions would tend to support a protein site of action.

A more recent iteration of this same general concept would be based on the recognition that a class of steroidal substances is formed in the brain (Hu et al., 1987; Jung-Testas et al., 1989; Le Goascogne et al., 1987) and varies in concentration with behavioral manipulations but not peripheral sources of gonadal or adrenal steroids (Corpechot et al., 1985). The known endproduct of the brain neurosteroid pathway, dehydroepiandrosterone (DHA), is rapidly depleted by intoxicating doses of parenteral ethanol, but not by other CNS depressants (Corpechot et al., 1983, 1985; Vatier and Bloom, 1988). Since the concentrations of delta-5 pregnenalone, the precursor neurosteroid to DHA, are not affected by ethanol, (Vatier and Bloom, 1988), it is reasonable to conjecture that an alternative metabolic pathway (Andersson et al., 1986) has been utilized in the presence of ethanol. A by-product of such an alternative pathway could be a natural version of synthetic steroids known to cause central nervous system depression (Harrison et al., 1987; Majewska and Schwartz, 1987; Majewska et al., 1988; Turner et al., 1989), and again pointing to a specific, presumably protein, receptor for such effects.

ETHANOL AND "THE" MEMBRANE

Several recent reviews have examined whether the neuronal events underlying the intoxication, dependence and tolerance responses to ethanol are mediated through changes in the properties of plasma membrane lipids or membrane-mounted proteins. As scientific concepts of "the membrane" have matured (Gallagher, 1989) the bilayer arrangement of membrane lipids, with their longer hydrophobic tails apposed within the membrane interior and their polar head groups exposed to the extracellular space and the inner cytoplasmic surface, is now conceived of as a "sea" in which heterogeneous membrane proteins float. The physical property of membrane "fluidity"–namely the ease of motion through this lipid sea–is now taken to infer the separable properties of viscosity of membrane lipid molecules and their relative ordered arrangements within the plane of the membrane. The conclusions reached by Harris et al. (1987; also see Wood and Schroeder, 1988) were that at concentrations up to lethal levels, ethanol does not in fact alter the microviscosity of membrane lipids nor can it be viewed as affecting membrane function during intoxication through alterations in membrane lipid order.

ETHANOL AND OTHER ALCOHOLS

Seeman (1972) examined the membrane biophysical effects of ethanol and the more powerful anesthetic drugs and solidified the view that the Meyer-Overton relationships strongly supported the general bulk lipid action sites, and that erythrocyte membranes were as useful a model of this effect as were neuronal membranes. The intramembrane binding of general anesthetics requires a protein-like binding site that neurons possess but erythrocytes do not. Nevertheless, there have been many pharmacological tests of alcohol series, in general showing potency to increase with chain length, especially when the effective concentrations of a given alcohol are expressed in terms of the volume of the membrane displaced by the alcohol.

While such data continue to appear (see below; Lovinger et al., 1989; Treistman and Wilson, 1987), their interpretation has become less lipid oriented. For example, when Rabin et al. (1986) compared the effects of ethanol, butanol and ketamine on the activity of a critical signalling enzyme (adenylate cyclase; see below for additional studies on this second messenger system) in the membrane of L6 lymphocytes, they found that although butanol was more potent than ethanol in activating this enzyme and in "disordering" the membrane lipids, the maximum activation achievable with butanol was considerably less than the maximum activation attainable by ethanol. Furthermore, there was more enzyme activation than lipid disordering for ethanol than there was for butanol. Moreover, while ketamine also decreased membrane lipid order, it depressed enzyme activity. Thus, there seemed in this study to be no predictable relationship between cellular effects and membrane ordering effects either within a series of aliphatic alcohols or across alcohols and anesthetics. As an example of the sorts of rethinking being engaged, Gruber (1988) has recently proposed a "buffering-membrane partitioning" concept for the interaction of amphiphilic substances with membrane proteins, in which the well documented increases in potency of lipophilic substances with longer chain length are interpreted as a "competition" in which bulk phase binding to the lipids of the membrane allows for greater specificity of the interaction with proteins in selected domains of the membrane.

ETHANOL AND HYPERTHERMIA

One of the observations that has been taken as critical in this series of re-examinations is that whereas modest changes in lipid order can be observed after first exposures to very large doses of alcohol, similar changes in membrane fluidity can also be produced by raising body temperature approximately 2°C, yet this elevation does not produce the neurological and behavioral signs of ethanol intoxication (Goldstein, 1987; Harris et al., 1987; Hunt, 1985). These authors concluded that although the membrane fluidity changes of ethanol and modest hyperthermia are to some degree similar, the functional effects of these differed. Such differences may also point up differences in the cellular sources of the membranes and the indices used to assess them, suggesting to Wood and Gibson (1988) that the similarity of ethanol and hyperthermia on the membrane fluidity index should not be accepted as a total refutation of the view that some effects of ethanol are lipid mediated.

On the other hand, after chronic exposure to alcohol, similar studies of membrane properties support the concept of a physicochemical adaptation that results in membranes that resist the actions of alcohol. Harris et al. (1987) noted that there was a correlation between sensitivity of membrane lipids, particularly the most external surface of the membrane and ethanol sensitivity of an individual animal, whether due to genetic differences or recent pharmacological exposure and tolerance. Bode and Molinoff (1988) studied the effects of chronic exposure to ethanol on the physical and functional properties of the plasma membrane in cultured S49 lymphoma cells. Chronic exposure of S49 cells to 50 mM ethanol or growth of cells at elevated temperature both resulted in a decrease in adenylate cyclase activity. Those correlations suggest, without conclusive proof, that the lipid changes, although minor, can influence membrane function (Goldstein, 1987; Hoek and Taraschi, 1988).

ALCOHOL AND NEURONAL PROTEINS

Alcohol can influence neuronal function through membrane actions on the proteins within the membrane, such as the receptors for neurotransmitters or the macromolecular intermediates that allow the activated receptors to regulate ion movement through the membrane. Recent exploitations of molecular biology have led to the isolation, cloning and amino acid sequence determinations of several classes of neurotransmitter receptors. These studies permit the conclusion that such transmitter signal receptors may be divided into two categories. In one category are receptors in which the receptor molecule is a multimeric collection of membrane-spanning glycoproteins that create a dual-function macromolecule containing the receptor for the specific transmitter and the ion channel whose openings and closings are regulated by receptor occupancy. This receptor-ionophore complex is represented by the cholinergic nicotinic receptor and the receptors for the amino acids, gamma-aminobutyric acid (GABA) (Pritchett et al., 1989) and glycine.

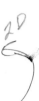

The second category of receptors exhibits a distinctly different molecular configuration, in being large monomeric proteins, containing exactly seven membrane-spanning sequences separated by both cytoplasmic and extracellular loops of variable lengths. The initial series of receptors with this configuration all mediate signal transductions that involved intracellular second messengers. Receptors for extracellular signals that are mediated by intracellular second mesengers are themselves engaged in a multimeric intramembranous cascade in which the occupied receptor activates the synthesis of the second messenger through association with a class of guanine nucleotide binding proteins (G-proteins). Three types of G-protein interactions have been reported: those in which the second messenger synthesizing enzyme is stimulated (G_s), those in which it is inhibited (G_i), and those in which the qualitative outcome of the interaction remains uncertain (G_o). The extracellular sequences of the receptor molecule are viewed as sites for the interaction of the receptor with the ligand, while the intracellular loops offer opportunities for interaction with the second messenger synthetic enzymes. It has also been suggested that some such receptors may influence ion channel properties through G-proteins directly without the necessity for intracellular second messenger systems. Because the multimeric, receptor-G-protein-second messenger systems offer the opportunity to examine membrane protein interactions, they have been a frequent target in studies of the nature of ethanol actions, and their alterations in the lymphocytes of alcoholic patients have recently been reported to be consititutively altered beyond that of the general population regardless of recent ethanol exposure (Mueller et al., 1988; Nagy et al., 1988).

ETHANOL AND THE SECOND MESSENGER REGULATION

Although early results on the effects of ethanol on cyclic nucleotide synthesis *in vivo* indicated inhibitions (Volicer and Gold, 1973), Rabin and Molinoff (1983) established that very high doses of of alcohol (far above levels attained during intoxication) can enhance basal activity of the enzyme adenylate cyclase *in vitro*, and that these same high doses enhance the ability of the transmitter dopamine to activate this second messenger response. Subsequently, similar effects were reported for norepinephrine-mediated activation of mouse brain adenylate cyclase (Saito et al., 1985; Hoffman et al., 1987).

Although the mechanisms of this effect remain unclear, the progress in this area has been extensive. Bode and Molinoff (1988) examined this question *in vitro* using membranes prepared from S49 lymphoma cells, in which selective mutations allow for the evaluation of the receptor G-protein interactions on the cyclase. Ethanol caused a dose-dependent increase in adenylate cyclase activity in membranes prepared from wild-type cells in the presence of guanosine triphosphate (GTP). Ethanol also shifted the dose-response curve for stimulation of the enzyme by isoproterenol to the right, by decreasing the affinity of the β-adrenergic receptor for isoproterenol. Dose-response curves for NaF and guanosine-5'-O-(3-thiotriphosphate), agents that stimulate adenylate cyclase activity through the guanine nucleotide-binding protein G_s, were shifted to the left by ethanol. However, with CYC-variant of S49 cells, lacking the α-subunit of G_s, ethanol effects were not seen.

Saito et al. (1987) have also directed similar studies at the α_2-receptor-coupled adenylate cyclase (AC) of the human platelet and reported that ethanol increased "basal" activity with a linear dose-response effect. However, when G-protein effects were controlled, the slope of the dose-response curve for ethanol stimulation became biphasic, with doses of ethanol below 100 mM producing much sharper effects than the increases produced by higher concentrations. These authors also implicated the G_s-protein enzyme interaction as the most likely site of the ethanol effect. Although Saito et al. (1987) concluded that ethanol did not affect the G_i regulation of adenylate cyclase, Bauche et al. (1987) suggested that this protein interaction is in fact inhibited by ethanol when the G_i-mediated adenylate cyclase inhibition caused by the adenosine analog N6-phenylisopropyladenosine (N6-PIA) was examined in brain cortical membranes. If ethanol may also impair G_i-mediated adenylate cyclase responses in brain as well as enhancing the activation of the cyclase, the net effect would be even more strongly in the direction of cyclase activation, with both basal activity and transmitter activation enhanced. Interestingly, the brain-specific protein IIIb, identified by Greengard and colleagues as a substrate for cyclic adenosine monophosphate (AMP)-induced protein phosphorylation, appears to be diminished in content in postmortem assays on abstinent alcoholics compared to alcoholics of comparable intensity who died while intoxicated (Browning et al., 1987; Perdahl et al., 1984).

ETHANOL EFFECTS ON DIRECTLY REGULATED ION CHANNEL RECEPTORS

At the cholinergic nicotinic receptor, in an *in vitro* purified model system, the effects of alcohol, like those of general anesthetics, have also been linked to effects on the protein itself rather than on the surrounding lipids (Miller et al., 1987). No significant acute alterations in other receptor or ion channel functions have been reproducibly observed at pharmacologic- ally relevant alcohol concentrations, although effects on tracer fluxes of both calcium and chloride "channels" have been reported. The reservations associated with these *in vitro* assessments of ion tracer movements are that comparable channels do not appear to be altered by pharmacologically pertinent doses of ethanol when assessed by electrophysiological measurements (Siggins et al., 1987b; see below).

ETHANOL AND OTHER TRANSMITTER EFFECTS

Despite multiple studies, no consistent relationship has been established between the content, synthesis or catabolism of any neurotransmitter and the doses of alcohol required to produce intoxication. Most such efforts have focused on the catecholamines (Weiner, 1987). More promising data on alterations in content, but not reuptake of serotonin, may underlie the neurochemical differences between alcohol-preferring rat lines relative to nonpreferring controls (Gatto et al., 1987a,b; Murphy et al., 1985, 1987). We have recently reviewed the cellular actions of alcohol on pontine and midbrain catecholamine neurons Koob and Bloom, 1988; Siggins et al., 1987a; 1989) for their relevance to the reinforcing and tolerance adaptational effects of ethanol and the possible role of learning mechanisms in this process (see Foote et al., 1983, Robbins et al., 1985, for more global views of the functions of these systems and Shefner, 1989 for a review of the effects of ethanol on other cellular systems). However, for this discussion two sets of neurons offer additional insights into the objective of defining the molecular sites at which ethanol interferes with neuronal function.

ETHANOL AND CEREBELLAR FUNCTION

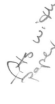

Halothane-anesthetized rats given modest to low doses of ethanol (local tissue concentrations of 25-100 mM) exhibit significant alterations in the distinctive firing pattern of the Purkinje neuron, revealing an increased frequency of the climbing fiber bursts with modest increases in modal intervals of single-spike firing (Rogers et al., 1980). However, the effects of known transmitters within the cerebellum are not altered under these conditions (Bloom et al., 1984; Siggins et al., 1987a). Climbing fiber bursts reflect the activity of the neurons from which climbing fibers arise, namely neurons of the inferior olivary nucleus. Thus, the apparent activation of olivary neurons by systemic ethanol, as well as the evidence of resistance to direct effects of ethanol on Purkinje neurons, favors the interpretation that the known acute intoxicating effects of ethanol on cerebellar and vestibular function do not arise through actions at the synaptic level within the cerebellar cortex.

The extracellular electrical activity of single neurons of the inferior olivary nucleus, recorded by standard methods in alcohol-naive rats, confirmed that there were significant increases in olivary unit activity (70-80% over baseline) as inferred from recordings in the cerebellum. Recovery occurred approximately 80 minutes or more after the ethanol injection (Rogers et al., 1986). Since the rodent inferior olivary complex is heavily innervated with serotonin (5-HT)-containing fibers (Steinbusch, 1984), we (Madamba et al., 1987) investigated their role in the effects of ethanol by treating rats intracisternally or intracerebroventricularly with the 5-HT specific toxin, 5,7 dihydroxytryptamine (Daly et al., 1974). This treatment greatly reduces the number of 5-HT immunoreactive terminals within the inferior olive, leaving mainly a few grossly distorted preterminals. Animals given this treatment fail to exhibit the consistent and dramatic activation of olivary neuronal firing seen after alcohol dosing in the normal rats. The indirect mediation of the ethanol effect on inferior olive could thus be attributed to a hypothetical metabolite of ethanol, such as a harmaline-like β-carboline (formed by condensation of acetaldehyde and serotonin), whose effects would be presumed to derive from more typical transmitter receptor actions.

ETHANOL AND HIPPOCAMPAL FUNCTION

The hippocampal pyramidal cell (HPC) has also provided much information on ethanol effects. Extracellular recordings *in vivo* indicate that systemically administered ethanol can alter hippocampal electroencephalograms (EEGs) and multi- and single-unit firing rates, as well as field potential and single unit responses evoked by stimulation of afferent inputs (Siggins et al., 1987a,b). Although most of these studies found depressant effects (usually at high supraintoxicating doses of ethanol), Newlin et al. (1981) noted that systemic ethanol also can facilitate both excitatory and inhibitory responses to certain afferent stimulation. Local application to HPCs of ethanol by microelectro-osmosis or pressure can produce an early excitatory response, sometimes followed by a depression at higher doses, although depression alone is also seen (Siggins et al., 1987a).

To determine the transmitters involved in the enhancement by ethanol of the excitatory and inhibitory responses of pyramidal cells to stimulation of afferent pathways, Mancillas et al. (1986a) tested the effect of ethanol (blood levels of 80-150 mg%) on the responses of identified pyramidal cells to iontophoretically applied transmitters in the halothane-anesthetized rat. Systemic ethanol markedly enhanced excitatory responses to iontophoresis of acetylcholine (ACh) in CA1 or CA3 pyramidal cells within 15 to 30 minutes, and recovered by about 60 minutes after injection. No comparable effect was observed on glutamate-induced excitation in cells tested alternatively with both transmitters. Systemic ethanol also significantly increased the amplitude and duration of inhibitory responses to iontophoretically applied neuropeptide somatostatin (somatostatin-14; SS-14). This enhancement was evident by 10 to 15 minutes after ethanol injection, and recovered at 60 to 80 minutes. Ethanol had no statistically significant effect on inhibitory responses to serotonin or norepinephrine. It is perhaps relevant that SS-14 also potentiates responses to ACh in the hippocampus (Mancillas et al., 1986b). Thus, it is possible that ethanol-induced enhancement of responses to ACh may be secondary to an enhancement of the effects of endogenously released somatostatin, which in turn enhance postsynaptic responses to iontophoretically applied ACh. The ethanol-induced alteration of ACh and SS-14 responses may underly the enhancement by ethanol of inhibitory and excitatory synaptic transmission previously described in hippocampus (Newlin et al., 1981).

More recent findings suggest that other transmitter receptor mechanisms operating within the hippocampus may also be selectively altered by modest doses of ethanol. Two groups (Lima-Landman and Albuquerque, 1989; Lovinger et al., 1989) have thus reported that the N-Methyl D-Aspartic Acid (NMDA) receptor, one of the subtypes of the glutamatergic receptor family (see Siggins and Gruol, 1986 for review) is uniquely sensitive to ethanol when studied electrophysiologically in acutely isolated hippocampal neurons *in vitro*. Lima-Landman and Albuquerque (1989) noted that very low concentrations of ethanol (1.7-8.6 mM) tended to increase the probability of opening of the NMDA-activated cation channels, and both groups found that at higher concentrations of ethanol (5-50 mM) the opening of this channel by NMDA was diminished. Lovinger et al. (1989) further noted that whereas the other two main types of glutamate receptors (i.e., the quisqualate and kainate receptor subtypes) were also affected by ethanol, the latter effects were far less potent. Lovinger et al. (1989) also noted that the inhibitory effects of ethanol on the NMDA receptor were replicated with other aliphatic alcohols according to a potency related to their chain length and their intoxicating potency in behaving rodents. Although the authors have not yet been able to identify the precise mode of action of this selective effect on NMDA receptors, it seems unlikely that such effects could be mediated "merely" through actions on bulk membrane lipids. Whether the NMDA receptor complex could be uniquely embedded in a selective lipid domain of the membrane or in some other way is a protein whose lipid environment is critical to its function, remain opportunities to be pursued.

ETHANOL AND GABA TRANSMISSION

One of the earliest results of a cellular pharmacological analysis of ethanol were reports that GABA responses are enhanced by very low doses of ethanol (Nesteros 1980; Ticku and Burch, 1980; Ticku et al., 1983). In our tests (Siggins et al., 1987a, 1989; Mancillas et al., 1986 a,b) ethanol initially seemed to cause a small (average, 25%) but consistent potentiation of inhibitory responses to GABA, but most of these "potentiations" did not recover for up to 3 hours after ethanol administration. Furthermore, in our control experiments cortical and hippocampal neurons tested with GABA repeatedly for comparable periods of observation without ethanol showed a similar apparent potentiation. These and other control experiments (Mancillas et al., 1986a) suggest that the apparent potentiation of GABA was an artifact of the repetitive iontophoretic application under these experimental conditions rather than a true pharmacological interaction. In contrast, changes in responses to ACh and SS-14 (see above) were observed only after ethanol injections and all recovered within 1 to 2 hours.

Siggins and colleagues (1987a,b) have also examined the effects of ethanol superfusion on the responses of CA1 pyramidal cells to GABA as determined by intracellular recordings *in vitro* to evaluate further whether ethanol potentiated GABAergic transmission and to determine the pre- or postsynaptic locus of action for their finding that ethanol (see above, and 1987a,b) reduces inhibitory postsynaptic potential (IPSP) size. GABA was applied locally by micropipette and uniform responses were obtained by repetitive testing. In all cells GABA produced hyperpolarizations of 5 to 10 mV accompanied by cessation of discharge, but ethanol had little effect on the responses to GABA.

These results thus do not support the conclusion that ethanol enhances GABAergic IPSPs, although it is clear that results at the behavioral level (Ticku et al., 1983) and the *in vitro* biochemical level (Suzdak et al., 1987) strongly suggest that ethanol in some fashion not detected by cellular electrophysiology enhances GABAergic synaptic transmission sites. Ethanol produces effects similar to benzodiazepines and can be synergistic with benzodiazepines in the anticonflict test, and both drug effects are antagonized by FG 7142, an antagonist of the benzodiazepine receptor (Koob et al., 1986) (a carboline "inverse benzodiazepine agonist") as well as by naloxone (Koob et al., 1980). Since a benzodiazepine binding site has recently been attributed to a specific protein monomer of the GABA receptor complex (Pritchett et al., 1989), these results would seem to reinforce the expectation of a significant interaction of ethanol with GABA transmission sites, as has been seen with the anesthetic steroids (Majewska et al., 1988; Turner et al., 1989). Nevertheless, as noted above, direct tests of GABA responsiveness (i.e., iontophoretic dose-response curves before and after ethanol (E)) failed to confirm GABA potentiation in cerebellum (Bloom et al., 1983), as have more recent tests in hippocampus (Siggins et al., 1987a; Mancillas et al., 1986a).

Clearly, there are insufficient data to conclude whether GABAergic mechanisms per se account for any, many or all of the intoxicating effects of ethanol, although the degree of open-mindedness on this issue varies considerably throughout the research community. It thus remains to be determined whether the apparent mimicry of ethanol and GABA effects at both behavioral and biochemical levels may derive from similar but distinct mechanisms or from effects on selected populations of neurons and their synapses, which have thus far escaped detection with microelectrodes in studies of the intact nervous system.

CONCLUSIONS

Until the molecular mechanisms responsible for any of the cellular responses to ethanol have been definitely established, it will be impossible to reject totally the hypothesis that some aspect of lipophilic interaction is more important for the observed responses than is any hypothesized effects of ethanol or a chemical surrogate on specific intramembranous protein transductions. Nevertheless, substantial conceptual movement has occurred with the presentation of a wide variety of observations that place the lipid perturbation hypothesis in a far less central position. This movement is based both on the lack of extensive cause and effect relationships among the biophysical actions attributed to the lipophilic and other functional effects of ethanol and by the cumulative bodies of evidence suggesting that neurons differ in their sensitivity to ethanol according to the selective effects of ethanol on their neurotransmitter receptors. If the bulk lipids of the neuronal membrane have lost in their mediative participation in the emerging neuropsychopharmacology of ethanol, it remains possible that selective lipid domains surrounding selective membrane proteins may well become a focus in future studies.

ACKNOWLEDGMENTS

I wish to acknowledge our Alcohol Research Center Grant AA 06420. This is RISC publication NP # 5990.

REFERENCES

Andersson S, Cronholm T, Sjovall J (1986): Redox effects of ethanol on steroid metabolism. *Alcoholism: Clin Exp Res* 10:55S-63S

Bauche F, Bourdeaux-Jaubert AM, Giudicelli Y, Nordmann R (1987): Ethanol alters the adenosine receptor-Ni-mediated adenylate cyclase inhibitory response in rat brain cortex *in vitro*. *FEBS Lett* 219:296-300

Bloom FE (1989): Neurobiology of alcohol action and alcoholism. In: *Review of Psychiatry, Vol. 8.* Meyer RG, ed. Washington, DC: American Psychiatry Press, pp 309-322

Bloom FE, Siggins GR, Foote SL, Gruol D, Aston-Jones G, Rogers J, Pittman Q, Staunton D (1984): Noradrenergic involvement in the cellular actions of ethanol. In: *Catecholamines, Neuropharmacology and Central Nervous System—Theoretical Aspects* Usdin E, ed. New York: Alan R Liss Inc, pp 159-167

Bode DC, Molinoff PB (1988): Effects of ethanol *in vitro* on the beta adrenergic receptor-coupled adenylate cyclase system. *J Pharmacol Exp Ther* 246:1040-1047

Bowman WC, Rand MJ (1980): *Textbook of Pharmacology,* 2nd ed. Oxford: Blackwell Scientific Publications, pp 8.12-8.13

Browning MD, Huang CK, Greengard P (1987): Similarities between protein IIIa and protein IIIb, two prominent synaptic vesicle-associated phosphoproteins. *J Neurosci* 7(3):847-853

Corpechot C, Leclerc P, Baulieu EE, Brazeau P (1985): Neurosteroids: regulatory mechanisms in male rat brain during heterosexual exposure. *Steroids* 45:229-234

Corpechot C, Shoemaker WJ, Bloom FE (1983): Endogenous brain steroids: effect of acute ethanol ingestion. *Soc Neurosci Abstr* 13:1237

Daly J, Fuxe K, Jonsson G (1974): 5,7-dihydroxytryptamine as a tool for the morphological and functional analysis of central 5-hydroxytryptamine neurons. *Res Comm Chem Pathol Pharmacol* 7:175-187

Davis VE, Walsh MJ (1970): Alcohol, amines and alkaloids: a possible basis for alcohol addiction. *Science* 167:1005-1007

Fargin A, Raymond JR, Lohse MJ, Kobilka BK, Caron MG, Lefkowitz RJ (1988): The genomic clone G-21 which resembles a β-adrenergic receptor sequence encodes the 5-HT1 α receptor. *Nature* 335:358-360

Foote SL, Bloom FE, Aston-Jones G (1983): Nucleus locus ceruleus: new evidence of anatomical and physiological specificity. *Physiol Rev* 63:844-914

Gallagher GL (1989): Evolutions: The plasma membrane. *J NIH Res* 1:131-132

Gatto GJ, Murphy JM, Waller MB, McBride WJ, Lumeng L, Li TK (1987a): Chronic ethanol tolerance through free-choice drinking in the P line of alcohol-preferring rats. *Pharmacol Biochem Behav* 28(1):111-115

Gatto GJ, Murphy JM, Waller MB, McBride WJ, Lumeng L, Li TK (1987b): Persistence of tolerance to a single dose of ethanol in the selectively-bred alcohol-preferring P rat. *Pharmacol Biochem Behav* 28(1):105-110

Goldstein DB (1987): Ethanol-induced adaptation in biological membranes. *Ann NY Acad Sci* 492:103-111

Gruber HJ (1988): Interaction of amphiphiles with integral membrane proteins. II. A simple, minimal model for the nonspecific interaction of amphiphiles with the anion exchanger of the erythrocyte membrane. *Biochim Biophys Acta* 944:425-436

Harris RA, Allan AM (1989): Alcohol intoxication: ion channels and genetics. *FASEB Journal* 3:1689-1695

Harris AR, Burnett R, McQuilkin S, McClard A, Simon FR (1987): Effects of ethanol on membrane order: fluorescence studies. *Ann NY Acad Sci* 492:125-135

Harrison NL, Vicini S, Barker JL (1987): A steroid anesthetic prolongs inhibitory postsynaptic currents in cultured rat hippocampal neurons. *J Neurosci* 7:604-609

Hoek JB, Taraschi TF (1988): Cellular adaptation to ethanol. *Trends Biochem Sci* 13:269-274

Hoffman PL, Saito T, Tabakoff B (1987): Selective effects of ethanol on neurotransmitter receptor-effector coupling systems in different brain areas. *Ann NY Acad Sci* 492:396-397

Hu ZY, Bourreau E, Jung-Testas I, Robel P, Baulieu EE (1987): Neurosteroids: oligodendrocyte mitochondria convert cholesterol to pregnenolone. *Proc Natl Acad Sci (USA)* 84:8215-8219

Hunt WA (1985): *Alcohol and Biological Membranes*. New York: Guilford Press

Jung-Testas I, Alliot F, Pessac B, Robel P, Baulieu EE (1989): Immunocytochemical localization of cytochrome P-450scc in cultured rat oligodendrocytes *CR Acad Sci* 308:165-70

Koob GF, Bloom FE (1988): Cellular and molecular mechanisms of drug dependence. *Science* 242:715-723

Koob GF, Braestrup C, Thatcher-Britton K (1986): The effects of FG 7142 and RO 15-1788 on the release of punished responding produced by chlordiazepoxide and ethanol in the rat. *Psychopharmacol* 90:173-178

Koob GF, Strecker RE, Bloom FE (1980): Effects of naloxone on the anticonflict properties of alcohol and chlordiazepoxide. *Substance Alcohol Actions/Misuse* 1:447-457

Lambert JJ, Peters JA, Cottrell GA (1987): Actions of synthetic and endogenous steroids on the GABA receptor. *TIPS* 8:224-227

Le Goascogne C, Robel P, Gouezou M, Sananes N, Baulieu EE, Waterman M (1987): Neurosteroids: cytochrome P-450scc in rat brain. *Science* 237:1212-1215

Lima-Landman MTR, Albuquerque EX (1989): Ethanol potentiates and blocks NMDA-activated single-channel currents in rat hippocampal pyramidal cells. *Fed Eur Biochem Soc* 247:61-67

Lovinger DM, White G, Weight FF (1989): Ethanol inhibits NMDA-activated ion current in hippocampal neurons. *Science* 243:1721-1724

Madamba SG, Siggins GR, Battenberg EL, Bloom FE (1987): Depletion of brain-stem 5-hydroxytrypamine (5HT) suppresses the excitatory effect of systemic ethanol on inferior olivary neurons (ION). *Soc Neurosci Abstr* 13:501

Majewska MD, Schwartz RD (1987): Pregnenolone-sulfate: an endogenous antagonist of the gamma-aminobutyric acid receptor complex in brain? *Brain Res* 404:355-60

Majewska MD, Mienville JM, Vicini S (1988): Neurosteroid pregnenolone sulfate antagonizes electrophysiological responses to GABA in neurons. *Neurosci Lett* 90:279-284

Mancillas J, Siggins GR, Bloom FE (1986a): Systemic ethanol: selective enhancement of responses to acetylcholine and somatostatin in the rat hippocampus. *Science* 231:161-163

Mancillas J, Siggins GR, Bloom FE (1986b): Somatostatin-selectively enhances acetylcholine-induced excitations in rat hippocampus and cortex. *Proc Natl Acad Sci USA* 83:7518-7521

Miller KW, Firestone LL, Forman SA (1987): General anesthetic and specific effects of ethanol on acetylcholine receptors. *Ann NY Acad Sci* 492:71-85

Mueller GC, Fleming MF, LeMahieu MA, Lybrand GS, Barry KJ (1988): Synthesis of phosphatidylethanol—a potential marker for adult males at risk for alcoholism. *Proc Nat Acad Sci (USA)* 85:9778-9782

Murphy JM, McBride WJ, Lumeng L, Li T-K (1987): Contents of monoamines in forebrain regions of alcohol-preferring (P) and nonpreferring (NP) lines of rats. *Pharmacol Biochem Behav* 26(2):389-392

Murphy JM, Waller MB, Gatto WJ, Li T-K (1985): Monoamine uptake inhibitors attenuate ethanol intake in alcohol-preferring (P) rats. *Alcohol* 2(2):349-352

Myers RD (1989): Isoquinolines, beta-carbolines and alcohol drinking: involvement of opioid and dopaminergic mechanisms. *Experientia* 45:436

Nagy LE, Diamond I, Gordon A (1988): Cultured lymphocytes from alcoholic subjects have altered cAMP signal transduction. *Proc Nat Acad Sci (USA)* 85:6973-6976

Nestoros JN (1980): Ethanol specifically potentiates GABA-mediated neurotransmission in feline cerebral cortex. *Science* 209:708-710

Newlin SA, Mancillas-Trevino J, Bloom FE (1981): Ethanol causes increase in excitation and inhibition in area CA3 of the dorsal hippocampus. *Brain Res* 209:113-128

Perdahl E, Wu WC, Browning MD, Winblad B, Greengard P (1984): Protein III, a neuron-specific phosphoprotein: variant forms found in human brain. *Neurobehav Toxicol Teratol* 6:425-431

Pritchett DB, Sontheimer H, Shivers BD, Ymer S, Kettenman H, Schofield PR, Seburg PH (1989): Importance of a novel GABA$_A$ receptor subunit for benzodiazepine pharmacology. *Nature* 338:582-585

Rabin RA, Bode DC, Molinoff PB (1986): Relationship between ethanol-induced alterations in fluorescence anisotropy and adenylate cyclase activity. *Biochem Pharmacol* 35:2331-2335

Rabin RA, Molinoff PB (1983): Multiple sites of action of ethanol on adenylate cyclase. *J Pharmacol Exp Ther* 227:551-556

Rogers J, Madamba SG, Staunton DA, Siggins GR (1986): Ethanol increases single unit activity in the inferior olivary nucleus. *Brain Res* 385:253-262

Rogers J, Siggins JR, Schulman JR, Bloom, FE (1980): Physiological correlates of ethanol intoxication, tolerance, and dependence in rat cerebellar purkinje cells. *Brain Res* 196:183-198

Saito T, Lee JM, Tabakoff B (1985): Ethanol's effects on cortical adenylate cyclase activity. *J Neurochem* 44:1037-1044

Seeman P (1972): The membrane actions of anesthetics and tranquilizers. *Pharmacol Rev* 24:583-655

Shefner SA (1989): Electrophysiological effects of ethanol on brain neurons. In: *Focus on Biochemistry and Physiology of Substance Abuse*. CRC Press, Watson RR, ed. Boca Raton, Florida, pp 25-53

Siggins GR, Bloom FE, French ED, Madamba SG, Mancillas J, Pittman QJ, Rogers J (1987a): Electrophysiology of ethanol on central neurons. *Ann NY Acad Sci* 492:350-366

Siggins GR, French E (1979): Central neurons are depressed by iontophoretic and micro-pressure applications of ethanol and tetrahydropapaveroline. *Drug Alcohol Depend* 4:239-243

Siggins GR, Gruol DL (1986): Synaptic mechanisms in the vertebrate central nervous system. In: *Handbook of Physiology, Volume on Intrinsic Regulatory Systems of the Brain*, Bloom FE, ed. Bethesda, Maryland: The American Physiological Association, pp 1-114

Siggins GR, Madamba SG, Moore S (1990): Electrophysiological evaluation of acute ethanol effects on transmitter responses in central neurons. In: *NIAAA Research Monograph: Initial sensitivity to ethanol*. Deitrich R, Pawlowski A, eds. Keystone, Colorado, pp 197-232

Siggins GR, Pittman QJ, French ED (1987b): Effects of ethanol on CA1 and CA3 pyramidal cells in the hippocampal slice preparation: an intracellular study. *Brain Res* 414:22-34

Smith BR, Amit Z (1987): False neurotransmitters and the effects of ethanol on the brain. *Ann NY Acad Sci* 492:384-389

Steinbusch HWM (1984): Serotonin-immunoreactive neurons and their projections in the CNS. In: *Handbook of Chemical Neuroanatomy, Vol. 3: Classical Transmitters and Transmitter Receptors in the CNS, Part II*. Aökfelt T, Björklund A, Kuhar M, eds. Elsevier Science Pub. New York, pp 68-125

Tabakoff B, Hoffman PL, Liljequist S (1987): Effects of ethanol on the activity of brain enzymes. *Enzyme* 37:70-86

Ticku MK, Burch T (1980): Alterations in GABA receptor sensitivity following acute and chronic ethanol treatments. *J Neurochem* 34:417-423

Ticku MK, Burch TP, Davis WC (1983): The interactions of ethanol with the benzodiazepine GABA receptor ionophore complex. *Pharmacol Biochem Behav* 18:(Suppl)15-18

Treistman SN, Wilson A (1987): Alkanol effects on early potassium currents in Aplysia neurons depend on chain length. *Proc Natl Acad Sci (USA)* 84:9299-9303

Turner DM, Ransom RW, Yang JS, Olsen RW (1989): Steroid anesthetics and naturally occurring analogs modulate the gamma-aminobutyric acid receptor complex at a site distinct from barbiturates. *J Pharmacol Exp Ther* 248:960-966

Vatier OC, Bloom FE (1988): Effect of ethanol on the nerosteroids concentrations in the rat brain. *Soc Neurosci Abstr* 14: 195

Volicer L, Gold BI (1973): Effect of ethanol on cylic AMP levels in rat brain. *Life Sci* 13:269-280

Wada K, Ballivet M, Boulter J, Connolly J, Wade E, Deneris ES, Swanson LW, Heinemann S, Patrick J (1988): Functional expression of a new pharmacological subtype of brain nicotinic acetylcholine receptor. *Science* 240:330-332

Weiner H (1987): Subcellular localization of acetaldehyde oxidation in liver. *Ann NY Acad Sci* 492:25-34

Wood WG, Schroeder F (1988): Membrane effects of ethanol: bulk lipid versus lipid domains. *Life Sci* 43:467-475

Probing Molecular Sites of Action for Alcohol's Acute and Chronic Effects on Synaptoneurosome Membranes: A Potential Tool for Studying Drug-Receptor Interactions

R. Preston Mason, Jill Moring, Leo G. Herbette,
Roger E. Meyer and William J. Shoemaker

INTRODUCTION

Ethanol's Molecular Interactions with the Membrane Bilayer

Ethanol is active in the central nervous system (CNS), producing a variety of effects when administered acutely. Long-term administration of ethanol produces tolerance and physical dependence. The study of alcohol's effects on the CNS has been complicated by the absence of a specific binding site that would indicate the primary locus of action for this molecule on the cells of the CNS. Unlike other drugs of abuse such as opiates, psychomotor stimulants and hallucinogens, there is no receptor molecule, reuptake site or ion channel that possesses high affinity binding for ethanol. Historically, Meyer (1906) and Overton (1901) described the solubility of ethanol and its ability to reach rapid equilibrium between the intra- and extracellular environment to explain some of ethanol's actions on cellular processes and the biophysical state of cells and cellular organelles. The seemingly diverse effects of ethanol on the CNS were explained by a common underlying mechanism: through the distribution of ethanol within the matrix of biological membranes and subsequent alterations in the structure and function of these membranes.

The literature on the effects of ethanol and membrane structure/function demonstrates little consensus. Using electron spin resonance of probes, several laboratories have defined an order parameter that indicated membrane disordering effects of ethanol (Goldstein et al., 1982; Lyon and Goldstein, 1983). Harris and his colleagues (Polokoff et al., 1985) have found increased fluidity in liver plasma membranes exposed to chronic ethanol and indicate changes in membrane polar lipid composition and ethanol oxidation. Rottenberg et al. (Waring et al., 1981, 1982) have published their findings suggesting that membranes from chronic alcoholic rats were resistant to the membrane disordering by alcohol, perhaps caused by changes in membrane composition. However, this hypothesis was challenged by Gordon et al. (1982) who found no correlation in membrane structure and function in ethanol-fed rats. At this juncture the difficulty in associating membrane functional indices with chronic alcohol administration remains, as a recent well-designed study on human subjects has demonstrated (Puddey et al., 1986).

Biophysical techniques that include electron paramagnetic resonance, nuclear magnetic resonance, differential scanning calorimetry, freeze fracture and fluorescence polarization have been used in membrane research in recent years. The general finding that has emerged from the various studies employing these techniques suggests that ethanol and other alcohols increase the molecular motion within the bilayer of biological membranes, particularly if these alcohols are in high concentrations in the surrounding extramembraneous environment. Since membrane function can be influenced by the physical condition of the membrane lipid environment in relation to important proteins, e.g., receptors and/or ion channels, this may be the unifying mechanism of ethanol's action at the membrane level. Even slight alterations produced by physiologically relevant levels of ethanol could alter neurotransmission, especially for those neurotransmitter or neuromodulator substances whose receptor target lies in the hydrophobic, transmembrane domain.

In this chapter we review the molecular mechanisms for drug-receptor interactions and summarize data that suggest that a "membrane bilayer pathway" may mediate small molecule interactions with specific receptors within neuronal membranes. This two-step "membrane bilayer pathway" (Fig. 1) involves nonspecific drug partitioning into the membrane's bulk lipid phase to an energetically favorable location, orientation and conformation followed by rapid lateral diffusion to a hydrophobic, intrabilayer receptor site. This pathway has been proposed to explain the binding mechanism of local anesthetics in neural tissue (Blanton et al., 1988; Hille, 1977) and 1,4-dihydropyridine (DHP) calcium channel agonists and antagonists' binding to L-type voltage-sensitive calcium channels in the cardiac sarcolemma (Rhodes et al., 1985). In the case of DHPs, x-ray and neutron diffraction have shown that these drugs occupy a well-defined, time-averaged location in the membrane bilayer while fluorescence redistribution after photobleaching (FRAP) experiments demonstrated that DHP membrane lateral diffusion was as rapid as that of phospholipid analogs ($3.8 \times 10^{-8} \mathrm{cm}^2/\mathrm{sec}$) (Chester et al., 1987; Mason and Chester, 1989). In experimentally testing this pathway and extending it to ethanol's effects on neuronal membranes we describe our experience using a variety of biophysical techniques, including small angle x-ray and neutron diffraction. We also summarize recent evidence suggesting that some of ethanol's functional actions may be mediated by changes in ion channels, e.g., chloride and calcium flux. Thus, the acute and chronic effects of ethanol on membrane structure and function may be studied by examining the effect of other drug-receptor interactions in the paradigms described.

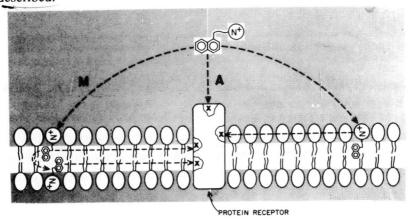

PROTEIN RECEPTOR

Figure 1. Schematic diagram of molecular pathways by which an amphiphilic or lipophilic drug could reach its membrane bound receptor site: a single-step aqueous pathway (A) or a two-step membrane pathway (M) as described in the text. According to the membrane pathway, a drug may enter the bulk lipid phase on the side of the membrane to which it was added and diffuse laterally to a hydrophobic (left side) or hydrophilic (right side) binding site. Alternatively, a drug could diffuse or flip-flop across the bilayer to gain access to the opposite side of the membrane. Reprinted with permission of the American Society for Pharmacology and Experimental Therapeutics from Rhodes et al. (1985): Kinetics of binding of membrane-active drugs to receptor sites; diffusion limited rates for a membrane bilayer approach of 1,4-dihydopyridine calcium channel antagonists to their active site. *Mol Pharmacol* 27:612-623.

STUDIES ON THE EFFECTS OF ETHANOL ON CHLORIDE AND CALCIUM CHANNEL FLUX

Chloride Channel

Several laboratories have described significant ethanol effects at the γ-aminobutyric acid $(GABA)_A$/benzodiazepine receptor-modulated chloride channel. For example, some recent publications from the laboratory of Dr. Steven Paul at NIH (see also this volume) have demonstrated that Ro15-4513, an imidazobenzodiazepine, can selectively antagonize several ethanol-induced behavioral and physiological effects (Suzdak et al., 1986b). Ro15-4513 is of interest but does not have an electron-dense halogen, which serves as a strong scattering source for the x-ray scattering methods; Ro15-1788 has the halogen fluorine as part of its covalent structure (Fig. 2) and blocks Ro15-4513 but has no direct effect on alcohol. Thus, we have begun our work using x-ray diffraction on Ro 15-1788 using x-ray diffraction and will study deuterated analogs of Ro15-4513 using neutron diffraction in subsequent studies.

At the $(GABA)_A$ receptor-modulated chloride channel, pharmacologically relevant concentrations of ethanol (20 to 100 mM) stimulated chloride transport directly and potentiated muscimol-stimulated chloride uptake (Suzdak et al., 1986a). The imidazobenzodiazepine Ro15-4513 antagonized the effects of ethanol on the channel; the closely related drug Ro15-1788 antagonized the effects of Ro15-4513 (Suzdak et al., 1986b). Ro15-4513 also blocked the anticonflict and behavioral intoxication effects of ethanol in rats; given alone, Ro15-4513 had no behavioral effects (Suzdak et al., 1986b). Suzdak et al. concluded that the action of ethanol on the Cl^- channel may be responsible for some of ethanol's behavioral effects. Although there is some disagreement on this point (Britton et al., 1988), Suzdak et al. (1988) have shown that Ro 15-4513 was a selective antagonist of both ethanol-stimulated Cl^- uptake into rat cerebral cortical synaptoneurosomes and some behavioral effects of ethanol. It does not antagonize pentobarbital- or muscimol-stimulated Cl^- uptake. However, other investigators have found that ethanol had no effect or had a stimulatory effect on phenomena known to be inhibited by GABA (Gage and Robertson, 1985; Mancillas et al., 1986). These investigators used tissue other than cerebral cortex and probed with other techniques; Mancillas et al. (1986) measured inhibitory responses to GABA in rat hippocampal pyramidal cells in situ; Gage and Robertson (1985) measured spontaneous inhibitory postsynaptic currents in rat hippocampal slices. Neither group found any effect of ethanol. Harris and Sinclair (1984), however, found that ethanol antagonized the GABA-mediated inhibition of cerebellar Purkinje cells of anesthetized rats.

The binding characteristics, distribution and average densities of the $(GABA)_A$/benzodiazepine receptor are similar in rat brain and human brain (Sieghart et al., 1985). $(GABA)_A$/benzodiazepine receptors in rat and human cerebellum have been shown to have some regions of structural homology as well (Sweetnam et al., 1987). The cerebral cortex

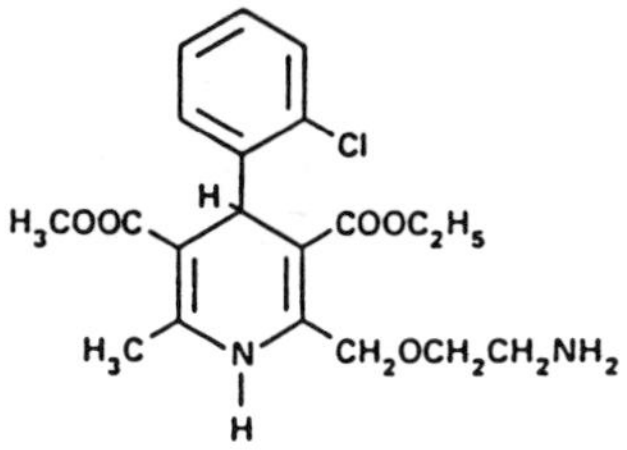

Amlodipine

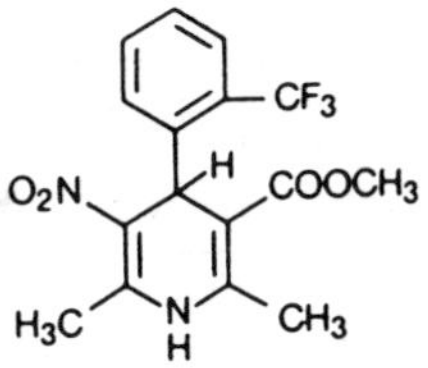

Bay K 8644

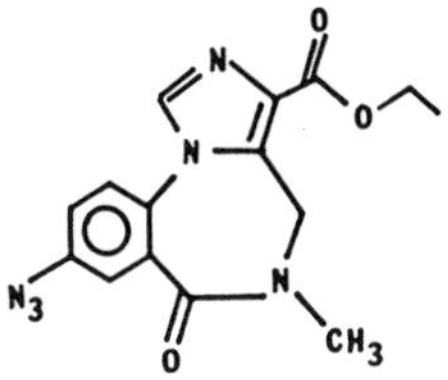

Ro15-4513

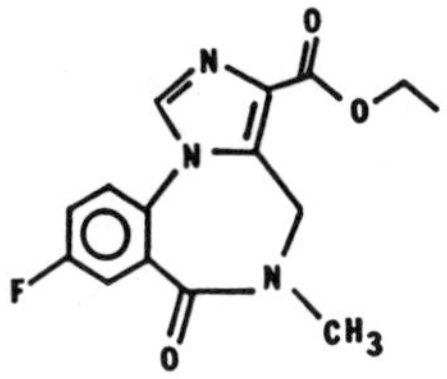

Ro15-1788

Figure 2. This figure shows the chemical structure for the 1,4 dihydropyridines amlodipine and Bay K 8644 as well as the imidazobenzodiazepines Ro15-4513 and Ro15-1788. The higher electron density of the halogen substituents for the 1,4 dihydropyridines and Ro15-1788, in contrast to the lipid bilayer, allowed the time-averaged position of the ligand in the membrane bilayer to be determined by small-angle x-ray diffraction.

is a region of high receptor density (Braestrup et al., 1977; Mohler and Okada, 1977). The receptor itself is a complex protein comprising several sites: a GABA binding site, a benzodiazepine binding site, a picrotoxin binding site and a chloride channel (Muller, 1987).

We expect the benzodiazepine binding site on the $(GABA)_A$/benzodiazepine receptor complex to be located at approximately the same depth in the membrane bilayer as the sites of nonspecific binding of Ro15-1788 and Ro15-4513, so that the drugs diffusing through the membrane can approach the binding site efficiently. This is consistent with a consensus view of the molecular "picture" of the $(GABA)_A$/benzodiazepine receptor now emerging from molecular biology studies.

Calcium Channel Studies

Acute ethanol administration appears to inhibit the uptake of calcium in rat synaptosomes (Harris and Hood, 1980; Leslie et al., 1983). Recent work indicates that the DHP-sensitive voltage-dependent (L-type) calcium channel is involved in the development of the ethanol withdrawal syndrome and the development of tolerance to ethanol. It was demonstrated that the calcium channel agonist Bay K 8644 was able to mimic the ethanol withdrawal syndrome in the rat (Dolin et al., 1987; Littleton and Little, 1988), and that DHP calcium antagonists were effective in preventing withdrawal symptoms in rats that had been made physically dependent on ethanol (Little et al., 1986).

Concurrent administration of the DHP calcium channel antagonist nitrendipine with ethanol prevented development of tolerance, but the behavioral effect of a dose of ethanol was not altered by 10 days' treatment with nitrendipine alone (Little and Dolin, 1987). Chronic treatment with nitrendipine has been shown to reduce the apparent number of DHP binding sites in mice (Panza et al., 1985). It has been suggested that increased inositol phospholipid breakdown, possibly due to greater influx of calcium through DHP-sensitive channels, is the cause of the calcium hypersensitivity in ethanol-dependent rats (Hudspith et al., 1987; Hudspith and Littleton, 1986). The acute and chronic effects of ethanol on DHP-sensitive voltage-dependent calcium channel function in PC12 cells, a cell line of neural origin, have been investigated by Messing et al. (1986). Acute ethanol exposure was found to decrease calcium flux, whereas longer exposure produced an increase in calcium uptake and the apparent number of binding sites for nitrendipine. Increased sensitivity due to an increased number of binding sites is a well-known phenomenon.

Other investigators have found that calcium uptake in synaptosomes was inhibited by addition of ethanol *in vitro* (Harris and Hood, 1980; Leslie et al., 1983). Using crude synaptosomal membrane preparations from rats given a single dose of ethanol, Rius et al. (1987) found that the number of nitrendipine binding sites (Bmax) increased very shortly after ethanol administration, but soon decreased to normal as the binding affinity (Kd) increased. Ethanol administered *in vitro* had no effect on nitrendipine binding (Rius et al., 1987). Davidson et al. (1988) found that acute ethanol exposure increases synaptosomal free calcium concentration although uptake was decreased. The investigators believed that this increase was due to an effect on intracellular calcium storage. Greenberg and coworkers (1987) showed that calcium channel agonist and antagonist drugs of four types (1,4-dihydropyridine, diphenylalkylamine, phenylalkylamine and benzothiazepine) were at least as effective at modulating K^+-depolarization-invoked $^{45}Ca^{+2}$ uptake in PC12 cells cultured in 200 mM ethanol as in control media. Verapamil, a phenylalkylamine calcium channel antagonist, was significantly more effective in ethanol-cultured cells than in control cells. The IC_{50} of verapamil (concentration that produced half maximal inhibition of $^{45}Ca^{+2}$ uptake) decreased to half its original value in the ethanol-cultured cells.

MOLECULAR MECHANISMS FOR DRUG-RECEPTOR INTERACTIONS

Historically, the mechanism for exogenous small molecule interaction with a plasma membrane receptor has been considered to be analogous to that of endogenous ligands such as hormones, growth factors, neurotransmitters, and so forth. These agonists are generally water soluble and thought to bind to an extracellular portion of the receptor. For example, the charged acetylcholine neurotransmitter and its competitive antagonist bind to an extracellular portion of the nicotinic acetylcholine receptor, a subunit near the opening of the ion channel (Changeux et al., 1984).

   In contrast to drug binding directly from the aqueous, extracellular environment, there is experimental support for highly lipophilic drugs to bind within the membrane bilayer (Fig. 1). Hille (1977) suggested that various local anesthetics utilize a membrane bilayer pathway in their interaction with target sodium channels. Although the experiments examined drug binding to sodium channels, it was hypothesized that "a modulated receptor with alternative hydrophobic and hydrophilic pathways [for drug binding] is probably applicable to other cases" (Hille, 1977). For example, local anesthetics that are noncompetitive blockers (NCB) bind to the nicotinic acetylcholine receptor at a site distinct from that of the agonist (Peper et al., 1982). Photoaffinity labeling experiments suggest that the binding site for NCB to the nicotinic acetylcholine receptor is deep in the pore of the channel, in a transmembrane region (Giraudat et al., 1987; Heidmann and Changeux, 1984). Electron spin resonance (ESR) studies (Blanton et al., 1988) examined the binding of reversibly charged forms of an NCB anesthetic to the receptor. Consistent with previous studies, the charged form of the anesthetic binds only when the channel is open. However, when the channel is closed only the uncharged form of the anesthetic (as controlled by pH) can bind to the high-affinity receptor, presumably through the lipid phase. ESR experiments indicate that the uncharged compound is associated with the membrane hydrocarbon core and thereby binds to the receptor protein after diffusion through the membrane (Blanton et al., 1988).

Evidence for an intrabilayer receptor site that must be accessed by diffusion through the lipid phase has also been implicated for the β-adrenergic receptor. The human genes for both the alpha-2 and beta-2 adrenergic receptor have been cloned and expressed in Xenopus oocytes. The receptors are homologous with each other and contain seven hydrophobic domains that have been modeled as seven transmembrane spanning segments (Kobilka et al., 1988). Deletion mutations have indicated that the seventh membrane spanning domain is necessary for drug binding (Kobilka et al., 1988). These mutations give experimental support to a transmembrane, intrabilayer receptor site. Although certain β-adrenergic antagonists are formally charged, as in the case of propranolol, small-angle neutron diffraction experiments (Fig. 7) have observed the drug's time-averaged location to be in the hydrocarbon core near the glycerol backbone of biological membranes (Herbette et al., 1983). Also consistent with a membrane bilayer pathway, the partition coefficient of propranolol into biological membrane was relatively high, $K_p > 10^3$ (Herbette et al., 1989).

To examine the molecular interactions of ethanol and drugs with model and native membranes, small-angle x-ray and neutron diffraction was used. The drugs used for this study have an electron-dense halogen atom as part of its covalent structure, for example, Ro15-1788 and Bay

K 8644, which serves as a strong scattering center for x rays (Fig. 2). In the case of ethanol, hydrogen atoms were substituted with heavy deuterium atoms, which scatter neutrons strongly relative to the background membrane bilayer. These techniques were used to generate electron or neutron density maps of the membranes from which the location of these drugs could be seen after background correction. Thus, using x-ray and neutron diffraction, the molecular interactions of ethanol and drugs that act on voltage-sensitive ion channels (associated with ethanol's possible site of action) can be examined in their native membrane environment.

METHODS FOR EXAMINING DRUG INTERACTIONS WITH MEMBRANES

Small-Angle X-Ray and Neutron Diffraction

To investigate the molecular interactions of drugs with the membrane bilayer, small-angle x-ray diffraction was used with partially dehydrated multibilayers (Figs. 3 and 4). The drugs used for this study were the imidazobenzodiazepine Ro15-1788 and the DHP calcium channel agonist Bay K 8644 (see Fig. 2). For x-ray diffraction studies, these compounds were ideal because they contain an electron-dense halogen as part of their molecular structure. These electron dense "tags" serve as strong scattering centers for the incident x-ray beam relative to the membrane bilayer electron density "background." Ro15-1788 differs from Ro15-4513 by the substitution of a fluorine atom in the place of an azido group (see Fig. 2). Although this single chemical substitution accounts for the functional difference between Ro15-1788 and Ro15-4513, it most likely does not significantly affect these drugs' interaction with the membrane bulk lipid phase. For example, the partition coefficient into synaptoneurosomal membranes was not significantly different for these imidazobenzodiazepine analogs, as will be discussed. Thus, Ro15-1788 serves as a useful experimental drug for probing imidazobenzodiazepine membrane interactions.

For neutron diffraction studies, deuterated analogs of ethanol, propranolol and timolol were used. The deuterated or protonated ethanol was equilibrated with the membrane samples in the vapor phase for several hours after partial dehydration at 88% relative humidity overnight. Dimyristoyllecithin (DML) and propranolol or timolol in a ratio of 1.25:1 (mg/mg) was prepared in chloroform. Alternatively, DML was sonicated

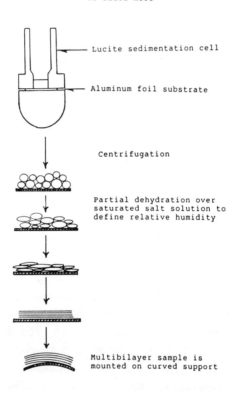

MULTIBILAYER SAMPLE
PREPARATION

Drug solution may
be added here

Lucite sedimentation cell

Aluminum foil substrate

Centrifugation

Partial dehydration over
saturated salt solution to
define relative humidity

Multibilayer sample is
mounted on curved support

Figure 3.   This figure summarizes the multibilayer preparative procedure for small-angle x-ray diffraction experiments. Multilamellar vesicles prepared in the presence and absence of known quantities of drug are added to clear, lucite sedimentation cells (University of Pennsylvania Biomedical Instrumentation Shop; design previously described by Herbette et al., 1977) and spun down on to an aluminum foil substrate. During sedimentation the vesicles are simultaneously dehydrated using the centrifuge's own vacuum (the centrifuge bucket caps have 100 μm holes drilled in them to allow for removal of water from the samples). The membrane vesicles fuse into multibilayers that have been previously characterized for homogeneity using microscopy (Chester et al., 1987). The sample is then placed on a curved glass support for small-angle x-ray diffraction. The samples are kept in sealed brass canisters with saturated salt solutions to control temperature and relative humidity.

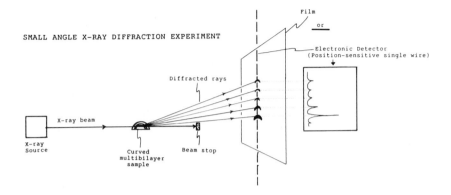

Figure 4. This figure summarizes the conditions for small-angle x-ray diffraction experiments. The experimental method used a single Franks' mirror defining a line source of copper K_α x rays with a wavelength of 1.54 angstroms. The multibilayer sample was placed on a curved glass mount such that the planes of the multibilayers were oriented around an axis perpendicular to the incoming x-ray beam at discrete Bragg's angles. The incident unreflected beam was absorbed by the metal beam stop while the Bragg reflections were collected on film or a one-dimensional position-sensitive electronic detector. The diffraction order intensities were then integrated from the films with a densitometer or directly from digitized computer plots of the electronic detector data.

in a buffer solution of deuterated propranolol at 23°C and used to make multilayers for diffraction. Control samples using fully protonated propranolol were treated in an identical manner. These dispersions were centrifuged onto aluminum foil and glued to a glass slide. Lamellar neutron diffraction data were collected at the high-flux beam reactor using the low-angle diffractometer at the Brookhaven National Laboratory, Upton, NY.

Neural Membrane Preparation for Diffraction Studies

For studying drug interaction with neural membranes, we used the "synaptoneurosome" preparation, a recent refinement of the original Whittaker synaptosome preparation developed by Hollingsworth (Hollingsworth et al., 1985). This preparation treats the tissue in a gentle manner that facilitates "rounding up" of the sheared axon terminals and dendritic processes. The re-annealing of the plasma membrane back onto itself is an important difference in the procedures since synaptoneurosomes are used for the study of ligand-gated ion fluxes (Suzdak et al., 1986a). Thus, the resealed "mini-cells" preserved some of their cellular integrity to the point of maintaining ion gradients and the ability to respond appropriately to agonists and antagonists that control ion flux (Suzdak et al., 1986b). The model and neural membrane vesicles were then centrifuged and partially dehydrated to form multilamellar bilayers by a modification of the procedures of Clark et al. (1980), as previously described by our laboratory (Chester et al., 1987).

The location of the imidazobenzodiazepine drug Ro15-1788 (see Fig. 2 for chemical structure) was examined in native synaptoneurosome membranes and in multibilayers made from lipids extracted from those membranes by the method of Bangham et al. (1965). Synaptoneurosome membrane vesicles from rat cerebral cortex were prepared by the method of Hollingsworth et al. (1985). These native membranes must be treated more gently than model membranes because of their protein content. After osmotic lysis of the synaptoneurosomes to remove extraneous non-membrane material, the preparation was centrifuged at a slow speed (1000 × g) for 15 minutes. The supernatant was discarded and the pellet was partially dehydrated over a saturated salt solution to form a multibilayer sample for x-ray diffraction.

The multibilayers, consisting of regularly stacked membrane bilayers, were placed on a curved glass substrate and mounted in brass canisters for controlled relative humidity and temperature (see Figs. 3 and 4). The multilayers are then exposed to a collimated, monochromatic copper K_α x-ray beam that intersects the sample at grazing incidence (Herbette et al., 1985a). The experimental method used a single Franks' mirror defining a line source where $K_{\alpha 1}$ and $K_{\alpha 2}$ are unresolved. Diffraction occurs when the planes of the multibilayers are oriented around an axis perpendicular to the incoming x-ray beam resulting in the bilayer planes being positioned at specific angles described by Bragg's Law:

$$h\lambda = 2D\sin\Theta$$

in which h is the diffraction order number, λ is the wavelength of the x-ray radiation (1.54 Å), D is the bilayer unit cell repeat distance, and Θ is the Bragg angle equal to one half of the angle between the incident beam and the scattered beam. The coherent scattering from the membrane sample is then recorded on either film or a one-dimensional electronic detector. The undiffracted main beam is absorbed by a metal beam-stop (see Fig. 4).

To determine the phase of the lamellar reflections, a hydration series and swelling analysis was carried out (Moody, 1963). We used at least three sets of data at different relative humidities, each with unique unit cell repeat distances in order to assign an unambiguous phase combination to the experimentally obtained structure factors. Structure factors were plotted as a function of h/D ($\mathring{A}^{-1}$) to determine the phases of the data. An algorithm written by Stamatoff and Krimm (1976) was also used to compute the delta values for all possible phase combinations with the most probable profile structure possessing the least deviation.

The lamellar intensity functions from multilayer samples collected with the electronic detector were corrected by a factor of $s = (2\sin\Theta/\lambda)$ or (h/D). Known as the Lorentz correction factor, the correction arises from the cylindrical curvature of the multilayers and hence is a weighting function for the intersection of the reciprocal lattice of the multilayer with the sphere of reflection, or Ewald's sphere.

Step-function equivalent profiles with step widths constrained by the resolution of the experimental data were fitted to the experimental electron density profile to examine perturbations in the electron-density of the membrane due to the addition of the halogenated drugs. The steps used to model the electron-density profile corresponded to the interbilayer water space, phosphate headgroup region, acyl chains and the methyl trough (King and White, 1985). Step-function equivalents were Fourier transformed once to generate the continuous structure factor function, which was truncated at a resolution equivalent to the experimental intensity data. This continuous structure factor function was then Fourier transformed to provide a calculated continuous electron-density profile function. When the calculated profile structure and its intensity function correlated, within experimental error, with the experimental profile structure and intensity function, the calculations were terminated (King and White, 1985).

Partition Coefficient Measurements

The nonspecific binding of 1,4-dihydropyridines and imidazobenzodiazepines to model and native membranes was determined by centrifugation of various concentrations of drug as explained in detail by Herbette et al. (1989). The membrane partition coefficients were measured by suspending the membrane vesicles in buffer containing a specific drug concentration. The samples were then centrifuged in polyethylene micro-centrifuge tubes (400 μl). Control experiments contained the same reaction mixture but were not centrifuged. The tip of the centrifuge tube containing the membrane pellet was cut off; the excess water above the pellet was blotted dry and placed in scintillation fluid to be counted for ^{3}H radioactivity.

The amount of labeled and nonlabeled drug added to each centrifuge tube was corrected to account for any loss of drug during transfer from the reaction mixtures to the microcentrifuge tubes. The free drug concentration to which the membrane vesicles were exposed during centrifugation was determined by correcting for the total amount of drug added to the tubes, that is, the amount of drug remaining in the supernatant after binding to the walls of the centrifuge tube, calculated using the labeled drug-specific activity (adjusted for counter efficiency).

Membrane partition coefficients were calculated using the following equation: K_p = (grams of drug bound to membrane/grams lipid)/(grams of drug in supernatant/grams buffer). The amount of drug in the pellet (bound to membrane) and in the supernatant were determined as described above. The amount of lipid was adjusted for the recovery of membrane in the pellet after centrifugation.

RESULTS

The Membrane Location of the Imidazobenzodiazepine Ro15-1788 and 1,4-Dihydropyridine Bay K 8644 in Synaptoneurosomal Membranes

To investigate the location of *nonspecific* binding of drugs to the synaptoneurosomal membrane, x-ray diffraction experiments were carried out. We are unlikely to see *specific* binding of a drug to its receptor on a membrane-bound protein in this experiment because of the low concentration of receptors. Either the DHP calcium channel agonist Bay K 8644 or the imidazobenzodiazepine Ro15-1788 was added directly to the synaptoneurosome preparation before the diffraction samples were made. Both of the drugs appeared to be distributed from the upper acyl chain region to the phospholipid headgroup, although Bay K 8644 (Fig. 5) appears to go somewhat deeper into the bilayer than Ro15-1788 (Fig. 6) does (Moring et al., 1990). The distribution of Bay K 8644 in rat synaptoneurosomal membranes differs from its distribution in canine cardiac sarcolemma lipids (CSL) as summarized in Fig. 5. In CSL

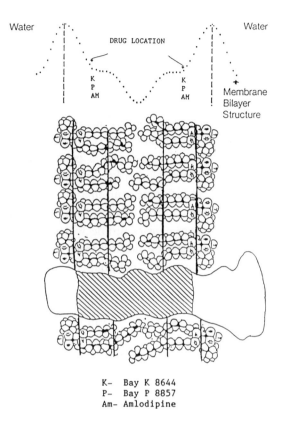

K— Bay K 8644
P— Bay P 8857
Am— Amlodipine

Figure 5.   Summary of location for the DHPs Bay K 8644, Bay P 8857 and amlodipine in multibilayers using native cardiac lipid multibilayers or model DPPC phospholipids in the liquid crystalline state. The electron density profile is correlated with a hypothetical membrane bilayer with a transmembrane protein. This figure illustrates the common center-of-mass location of the DHPs near the hydrocarbon core/water interface compared to amiodarone's center of mass near the bilayer center. This location for the DHPs could in turn define a region or plane for lateral diffusion to an intrabilayer receptor site (hatched portion of the protein).

In synaptoneurosomal membranes, Bay K 8644 and the imidazobenzodiazepine Ro-1788 appeared to be distributed from the upper acyl chain region to the phospholipid headgroup, although Bay K 8644 was somewhat deeper in the bilayer than Ro15-1788. The location for Bay K 8644 in synaptoneurosomal membranes was not as well defined as in canine cardiac sarcolemma lipids due perhaps to fundamental differences in the membrane bilayer composition between the two membrane types.

the location of the drug is better defined, occurring just below the hydro-carbon core/water interface in the upper acyl chain region. The difference in location may be due to a fundamental difference in the composition of the membrane bilayer lipids between the two membrane types (Mason et al., 1989a,b).

The presence of protein in the membrane is a source of some disorder in the membrane bilayer stack; some of the protein also interacts with the drug. Extracted lipids are a simpler system, and the results should be more easily interpretable. The diffraction patterns for the extracted lipid multibilayer samples showed six orders and the electron density profile structure was somewhat different from that of the native membrane. When Ro15-1788 was added to the extracted lipid vesicle preparation, the comparison of the electron density profile with that of lipids without added drug showed excess electron density from the glycerol backbone region of the bilayer through the headgroup and aqueous regions, as shown in Fig. 6. We believe that this electron density represents the non-specific location of the drug in the bilayer. Only a small electron density increase would be expected, since Ro15-1788 has only a single fluorine atom. Because of the low partition coefficient of Ro15-1788, the drug would not be expected to penetrate to the center of the bilayer. A small amount of drug was also found in the water space between bilayers.

Step function models of the lipid electron density profiles help to localize the electron-density increase due to the drug to a certain area of the bilayer. Comparison of the models shows most of the increased electron density in the phospholipid headgroup and glycerol backbone regions of the drug-containing lipids rather than in the acyl chain region.

Drug Partition Coefficients into Neural Membranes from Normal and Ethanol Pretreated Animals

Membrane/buffer partition coefficients of some DHP drugs and the imi-dazobenzodiazepines Ro15-1788 and Ro15-4513 have been determined in rat cerebral cortical synaptoneurosomes and in rabbit light sarcoplas-mic reticulum (LSR); the partition coefficients of the DHP drugs in each membrane system are about 100 times higher than those of the imidazo-benzodiazepines. The partition coefficients for both DHPs and imida-zobenzodiazepines are 2 to 4 times higher in LSR than in synaptoneuro-some membranes; this increase may be due to the low cholesterol content of LSR membranes relative to synaptoneurosome membranes. In rat skeletal muscle sarcoplasmic reticulum, the cholesterol concentration is 54 nmol/mg protein (Fiehn et al., 1971); in rat synaptosomal membranes it is 540 nmol/mg protein (Renau-Piqueras et al., 1987).

Partition coefficients were similarly determined in cerebral cortical synaptoneurosome from rats that had been fed a liquid diet containing 5% ethanol for 6 weeks. The partition coefficients of the DHP drugs were not significantly different from those determined in control membranes. However, the partition coefficients for the imidazobenzodiazepines were

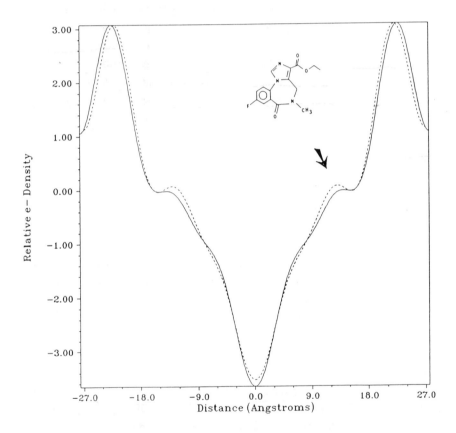

Figure 6. Electron density profiles of membrane bilayers made from lipids extracted from a preparation of synaptoneurosomes. Ro15-1788 is present at an approximate drug:lipid mole ratio of 1:30. The solid line is the electron density profile of the lipid without added drug; the dotted line is the profile of the lipid to which Ro15-1788 has been added. The arrow indicates the location of Ro15-1788 in the lipid bilayer.

increased approximately fivefold in the ethanol-exposed membranes. The reason for the increase is unknown, although it might be related to a change in membrane lipid composition and structure.

DISCUSSION

Previous studies suggest that acute and chronic administration of ethanol substantially affects the function of (GABA)$_A$/benzodiazepine receptor-modulated chloride channel and DHP-sensitive voltage-dependent calcium channels (Messing et al., 1986). The mechanism by which ethanol produces these effects is not understood. Currently, there is no evidence of specific binding of the ethanol to these membrane proteins to induce the necessary conformational change in the ion channel. As an alternative model, the effect of ethanol on these membrane proteins may be the result of perturbation of the ion channel's membrane bilayer environment. Indeed, neutron diffraction studies showed that ethanol was located primarily in the hydrated headgroup region of native membrane bilayers (Fig. 7). The ethanol was shown to remain tightly associated with the membrane bilayer even after the removal of ethanol vapor and equilibration in an ethanol-free environment (Herbette et al., 1985b). Further, at equilibrium the concentration of ethanol in the membrane is threefold higher than in the surrounding aqueous buffer (Herbette et al., 1986). These data suggest significant physical and chemical interactions of ethanol with the membrane bilayer, which may be a clue to understanding its mechanism of action. For example, by perturbing the membrane bilayer at this location the protein conformation of the ion channel may in turn be altered resulting in a reduction in the ion current.

In addition to direct examination of ethanol interaction with native membranes, the results of our studies show that drugs that specifically antagonize or mimic the effects of ethanol had high affinity for the membrane bilayer and occupied specific, time-averaged locations in neural membranes. These drugs were Ro15-1788, an imidazobenzodiazepine structurally very similar to Ro15-4513, and the DHP Bay K 8644 which was able to mimic the ethanol withdrawal syndrome in the rat. Consistent with a "membrane bilayer pathway," these drugs had high partition coefficients that demonstrated that the drugs were present in the membrane bilayer at concentrations two and three orders of magnitude

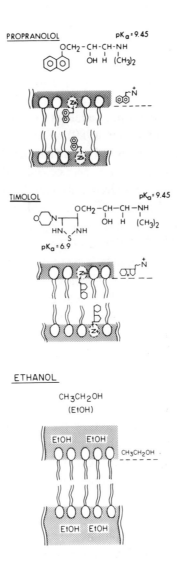

Figure 7. Schematic representation of the location of the β-adrenergic antagonist propranolol, timolol and ethanol in a model membrane system. The naphthalene ring of propranolol anchors the charged amine side chain as shown. Ethanol is seen to associate primarily with the membrane phospholipid-charged headgroup and aqueous layers hydrating the lipid bilayer structure. The Ro15-1788 molecule was also observed to occupy the headgroup region of the bilayer (see Fig. 6.)

greater than that found in the surrounding aqueous buffer. In addition, x-ray diffraction studies indicate that these drugs occupy specific, time-averaged locations in the membrane bilayer. This nonspecific location for these drugs may correspond to a *specific* protein receptor site at this depth in the membrane bilayer. Upon partitioning to this location, DHP analogs were shown to diffuse laterally through the membrane at rates similar to those observed for lipid analogs (3.8×10^{-8} cm^2/sec; Chester et al., 1987; Mason and Chester, 1989).

There is good immunological evidence that the DHP receptor site is buried in the membrane bilayer. Monoclonal antibodies raised against skeletal muscle transverse tubule membranes (a rich source for the slow type, voltage-sensitive calcium channel) to isolate the protein receptor for DHP binding were found to immunoprecipitate a 170 kDa polypeptide that bound the DHP, [3H]PN 200-110 (Vandaele et al., 1987). Antibodies binding to antigenic determinants outside the membrane were unable to displace DHP binding from its receptor. Moreover, the DHP receptor subunit can be heavily labeled by a hydrophobic photoaffinity probe, indicating that the protein consists of multiple transmembrane helices (Takahashi et al., 1987).

The primary structure of the DHP receptor subunit from rabbit skeletal muscle has been deduced from its DNA sequences. The polypeptide is structurally similar to the voltage-dependent sodium channel with four units of homology that putatively comprise six hydrophobic transmembrane alpha helices that may serve as the channel for calcium (Tanabe et al., 1987). In light of the high homology of the hydrophobic domains of calcium channels with sodium channels, it is interesting that DHPs have been shown to bind with high affinity and stereoselectivity to the sarcolemmal sodium channel (Yatani et al., 1988). These data suggest that the specific receptor site for the DHPs common to both the calcium and sodium channel is a hydrophobic, transmembrane domain.

The (GABA)$_A$ receptor has also been sequenced from bovine brain and exhibits homology with other ligand-gated receptor subunits (Blair et al., 1988; Schofield et al., 1987). The subunit to which the benzodiazepine binds possesses both hydrophilic and hydrophobic domains, including four domains that putatively traverse the membrane to partially comprise the channel. The location of the benzodiazepine-specific binding site has not yet been deduced. In light of these drugs' strong interaction with the headgroup region of the membrane bilayer we would expect a corresponding binding site on the receptor at this depth in the membrane.

In light of a membrane bilayer pathway for the binding mechanism of imidazobenzodiazepines and 1,4-dihydropyridines to their membrane receptors, one can propose that perturbation of the membrane bilayer structure would in turn affect, negatively or positively, some aspect of these drugs' binding mechanism. The results of this study demonstrate that ethanol has strong affinity for the membrane bilayer and occupies the charged headgroup region. Thus, it potentially could affect drug-membrane interaction of other drugs that partition into this specific region of the membrane. This hypothesis was tested with the imidazobenzodiazepines and the DHP Bay K 8644. The partition coefficient of these drugs into membranes isolated from rats after chronic alcohol administration was compared to control membranes. The imidazobenzodiazepines that share a similar molecular location in the membrane as the ethanol showed an approximate fivefold increase in the membrane partition coefficient from the alcohol exposed rat when compared with the control. By contrast, DHP partitioning into experimental versus control membranes was unchanged. The DHP Bay K 8644, located deeper in the hydrophobic core of the membrane, was not affected by the ethanol in the headgroup region.

These observations highlight the fact that the membrane bilayer is anisotropic with significantly different physical and chemical properties as a function of membrane bilayer depth. Each structurally distinct class of drugs will differentially exploit these changes in the membrane to arrive at an energetically favorable location, orientation and conformation. Furthermore, altering the membrane structurally should modify these drug-membrane interactions. For example, it was recently demonstrated that the partition coefficient of DHPs was significantly changed by altering the membrane cholesterol content (Mason et al., 1990) or physical structure of model phospholipid membranes (Mason et al., 1989a). Thus, the effects of ethanol may be mediated through changes in the membrane bilayer structure. These membrane changes in turn may functionally affect membrane proteins, for example, ion channels and drug-receptor interactions that require a membrane bilayer pathway binding mechanism.

One of the more interesting aspects emerging from these studies concerns the nature of the "nonspecific binding" that occurs in any ligand-binding study. In the past, efforts were focused on "high-affinity" binding resulting from the physicochemical equilibrium properties between a drug and a receptor that allows very low concentrations of drug to produce a significant biological effect. The paradigm in this regard was acetylcholine's action on muscarinic receptors at the neuromuscular junction. The model derived from those studies has been very fruitful in further studies on ligand-binding phenomena where the receptor is complexed with or closely coupled to an ion channel.

The situation encountered with ethanol, a CNS active compound that lacks affinity for specific receptor molecules, has brought our attention to the nature of nonspecific binding. It could be said that all of ethanol's targets are "nonspecific binding sites." If "nonspecific binding" involves partitioning into the membrane bilayer, our results indicate that this type of interaction is hardly nonspecific and is worthy of continued investigation. It may well be that many psychoactive agents use these nonspecific pathways, perhaps in addition to or in combination with higher affinity binding, to produce their effects. We can take this concept one step further in order to explain why so many psychotropic drugs require long periods of time (days or weeks) to produce their effects. It may require that a certain membrane concentration must be reached, rather than a plasma level, before the biological response is triggered. This concept could be useful in models of action for psychotherapeutic drugs that have a demonstrated high affinity site (e.g., tricyclic antidepressants) as well as those that do not (e.g., lithium).

ACKNOWLEDGMENTS

We would like to thank Dr. R. Janis, Miles Pharmaceuticals, New Haven, CT, for providing Bay K 8644. We are grateful to Dr. P. Sorter of Hoffman-LaRoche, Nuting, NJ, for the gift of Ro15-1788. This work was carried out in the Biomolecular Structure Analysis Center at the University of Connecticut Health Center. We would like to thank the staff of the Structure Center for their dedication in keeping the facilities in optimal running condition. We would also like to thank Yvonne Vant Erve for her technical assistance in determining drug partition coefficients and binding.

This project was supported in part by NIAAA center grant # P50-AA03510 #R01-AA06927 and # T32-AA0720. A research grant was also provided from Pfizer Central Research and Miles Laboratories with additional support from the National Institutes of Health (HL-33026), Americant Heart Association and a grant from the American Health Assistance Foundation. RPM is supported by a Connecticut Affiliate American Heart Association Research Fellowship and the John A. Hardford Foundation. LGH is an Established Investigator of the American Heart Association. The Biomolecular Structure Analysis Center acknowledges support from RJR Nabisco Inc., the Patterson Trust Foundation and the State of Connecticut Department of Higher Education's High Technology Programs.

REFERENCES

Affolter H, Coronado R (1985): Agonists of Bay K 8644 and CGP Z8392 Open channels from skeletal muscle transverse tubules. *Biophys J* 48:341-347

Affolter H, Coronado R (1986): The sidedness of reconstituted calcium channels from muscle transverse tubules as determined by D-600 and D-890 blockade. *Biophys J* 49:197a

Bangham AD, Standish MM, Watkins JC (1965): Diffusion of univalent ions across the lamellae of swollen phospholipids. *J Mol Biol* 13:238-252

Blair LAC, Levitan ES, Marshall J, Dionee VE, Barnard EA (1988): Single subunits of the $GABA_A$ receptor form ion channels with properties of the native receptor. *Science* 242:577-579

Blanton M, McCardy E, Gallaher T, Wang HH (1988): Noncompetitive inhibitors reach their binding site in the acetylcholine receptor by two different paths. *Mol Pharm* 33:634-642

Blaurock AE, King GI (1977): Asymmetric structure of the purple membrane. *Science* 186:1101-1104

Braestrup C, Albrechtsen R, Squires RF (1977): High densities of benzodiazepine receptors in human cortical areas. *Nature* 269:702-704

Brett RS, Dilger JP, Yland KF (1988): Isoflurane causes "flickering" of the acetylcholine receptor channel: observations using the patch clamp. *Anesthesiology* 69:161-170

Britton KT, Ehlers CL, Koob GF (1988): Is ethanol antagonist Ro15-4513 selective for ethanol? *Science* 239:648-649

Carvalho CM, Oliveira CR, Lima MP, Leysen JE, Carvalho AP (1989): Partition of Ca^{+2} antagonists in brain plasma membranes. *Biochem Pharmacol* 38:2121-2127

Changeux J, Devillers-Thiery A, Chemouilli P (1984): Acetylcholine receptor: an allosteric protein. *Science* 225:1335-1345

Chester DW, Herbette LG, Mason RP, Joslyn AF, Triggle DJ, Koppel DE (1987): Diffusion of dihydropyridine calcium channel antagonists in cardiac sarcolemmal lipid multibilayers. *Biophys J* 52:1021-1030

Clark NA, Rothschild KJ, Luipold DA, Simon BA (1980): Surface-induced lamellar orientation of multilayer membrane arrays. Theoretical analysis and a new method with application to purple membrane fragments. *Biophys J* 31:65-96

Colvin RA, Ashavaid TF, Herbette LG (1985): Structure-function studies of canine cardiac sarcolemmal membranes. I. Estimation of receptor site densities. *Biochim Biophys Acta* 812:601-608

Davidson M, Wilce P, Shanley B (1988): Ethanol increases synaptosomal free calcium concentration. *Neurosci Lett* 89:165-169

Dolin S, Little H, Hudspith M, Pagonis C, Littleton J (1987): Increased dihydropyridine-sensitive calcium channels in rat brain may underlie ethanol physical dependence. *Neuropharmacology* 26:275-279

Fiehn W, Peter JB, Mead JF, Gan-Elepano M (1971): Lipids and fatty acids of sarcolemma, sarcoplasmic reticulum, and mitochondria from rat skeletal muscle. *J Biol Chem* 248:5617-5620

Franks NP, Lieb WR (1981): X-ray and neutron diffraction studies of lipid bilayers. In: *Liposomes: From Physical Structure to Therapeutic Applications.* Knight et al., eds. New York: Elsevier/North-Holland Biomedical Press, pp 243-271

Gage PW, Robertson B (1985): Prolongation of inhibitory postsynaptic currents by pentobarbitone, halothane and ketamine in CA1 pyramidal cells in rat hippocampus. *Br J Pharmacol* 85:675-681

Giraudat J, Dennis M, Heidmann T, Haumont PY, Lederer R, Changeux JP (1987): Structure of the high-affinity site for noncompetitive blockers of the acetylcholine receptor. [^{3}H] chlorpromazine labels homologous residues in the beta and delta chains. *Biochemistry* 26:2410-2418

Goldstein DB, Chin JH, Lyon RC (1982): Ethanol disordering of spin-labeled mouse brain membranes: correlation with genetically determined ethanol sensitivity of mice. *Proc Natl Acad Sci* 79:4231-4233

Gordon ER, Rochman J, Arai M, Lieber CS (1982): Lack of correlation between hepatic mitochondria membrane structure and functions in ethanol-fed rats. *Science* 216:1320-1321

Greenberg DA, Carpenter CL, Messing RO (1987): Ethanol-induced component of 45Ca^{2+} uptake in PC12 cells is sensitive to Ca^{2+} channel modulating drugs. *Brain Res* 410:143-146

Harris RA, Hitzemann RJ (1981): Membrane fluidity and alcohol actions. *Curr Alcohol* 8:379-404

Harris RA, Hood WF (1980): Inhibition of synaptosomal calcium uptake by ethanol. *J Pharmacol Exp Ther* 213:562-568

Harris DP, Sinclair JG (1984): Ethanol-GABA interactions at the rat purkinje cell. *Gen Pharmacol* 15:449-454

Heidmann T, Changeux J-P (1984): Time-resolved photolabeling by the noncompetitive blocker chlorpromazine of the acetylcholine receptor in its transiently open and closed ion channel conformation. *PNAS (USA)* 81:1897-1901

Herbette LG, Chester DW, Rhodes DG (1986): Structural analysis of drug molecules in biological membranes. *Biophys J* 49:91-94

Herbette LG, Katz AM, Sturtevant JM (1983): Comparisons of the interactions of proparanol and timolol with model and biological membrane systems. *Mol Pharm* 24:259-269

Herbette LG, MacAlister T, Ashavaid TF, Colvin RA(1985a): Structure-function studies of canine cardiac sarcolemmal membranes. II. Structural organization of the sarcolemmal membrane as determined by electron microscopy and lamellar x-ray diffraction. *Biochim Biophys Acta* 812:609-623

Herbette LG, Marquardt J, Scarpa A, Blasie JK (1977): A direct analysis of lamellar x-ray diffraction from hydrated oriented multilayers of fully functional sarcoplasmic reticulum. *Biophys J* 20:245-272

Herbette LG, Napolitano CA, Messineo FC, Katz AM (1985b): Interaction of amphiphilic molecules with biological membranes. In *Advances in Myocardiology*. Vol. 5. Harris P, Poole-Wilson PA, eds. New York: Plenum Publishing Corp. pp 333-346

Herbette LG, Vant Erve YMH, Rhodes DG (1989): Interaction of 1,4-dihydropyridine calcium channel antagonists with biological membranes: lipid bilayer partitioning could occur before drug binding to receptors. *J Mol Cell Cardiol* 21:187-201

Hille KB (1977): Local anesthetics: hydrophilic and hydrophobic pathways for the drug receptor reaction. *J Gen Physiol* 69:497-515

Hollingsworth EB, McNeal ET, Burton JL, Williams RJ, Daly JW, Creveling CR (1985): Biochemical characterization of a filtered synaptoneurosome preparation from guinea pig cerebral cortex: cyclicadenosine $3':5'$-monophosphate-generating systems, receptors, and enzymes. *J Neurosci* 5:2240-2253

Hudspith MJ, Brennan CH, Charles S, Littleton JM (1987): Dihydropyridine-sensitive Ca^{2+} channels and inositol phospholipid metabolism in ethanol physical dependence. *Ann NY Acad Sci* 492:156-169

Hudspith MJ, Littleton JM (1986): Enhanced effect of Bay K 8644 on inositol phospholipid breakdown in brain slices from ethanol dependent rats. *Br J Pharmacol* 88:623P

King GI, White SH (1985): Molecular packing and area compressibility of lipid bilayers. *Proc Natl Acad Sci (USA)* 82:6532-6536

Kirschner DA, Sidman RL (1976): X-ray diffraction study of myelin structure in immature and mutant mice. *Biochim Biophys Acta* 448:73-87

Kobilka B, Kobilka TS, Daniel K, Regan JW, Caron MG, Lefkowitz RJ (1988): Chimeric alpha$_2$-, beta$_2$-adrenergic receptors: delineation of domains involved in effector coupling and ligand binding specificity. *Science* 240:1310-1316

Kokubun S, Reuter H (1984): Dihydropyridine derivatives prolong the open state of Ca^{++} channel in cultured cardiac cells. *Proc Natl Acad Sci (USA)* 81:4824-4827

Leslie SW, Barr E, Chandler J, Farrar RP (1983): Inhibition of fast- and slow-phase depolarization-dependent synaptosomal calcium uptake by ethanol. *J Pharmacol Exp Ther* 225:571-575

Little HJ, Dolin S, Halsey MJ (1986): Calcium channel antagonists decrease ethanol withdrawal syndrome. *Life Sci* 39:2059-2065

Little HJ, Dolin SJ (1987): Lack of tolerance to ethanol after concurrent administration of nitrendipine. *Brit J Pharmacol* 92:606P

Littleton JM, Little HJ (1988): Dihydropyridine-sensitive Ca^{2+} channels in brain are involved in the central nervous system hyperexcitability associated with alcohol withdrawal states. *Ann NY Acad Sci* 522:199-202

Lyon RC, Goldstein DB (1983): Changes in synaptic membrane order associated with chronic ethanol treatment in mice. *Mol Pharmacol* 23:86-91

Mancillas JR, Siggins GR, Bloom FE (1986): Systemic ethanol: selective enhancement of responses to acetylcholine and somatostatin in hippocampus. *Science* 231:161-163

Mason RP, Gonye GE, Chester DW, Herbette LG (1989a): Partitioning and location of Bay K 8644, 1,4-dihydropyridine calcium channel agonist, in model and biological lipid membranes. *Biophys J* 55:769-778

Mason RP, Campbell SF, Wang S-D, Herbette LG (1989b): Comparison of location and binding for the positively charged 1,4-dihydropyridine calcium channel antagonist amlodine with uncharged drug of this class in cardiac membranes. *Mol Pharmacol* 36:634-640

Mason RP, Chester DW (1989): Diffusional Dynamics of an active rhodamine-labeled 1,4-dihydropyridine in sarcolemmal lipid multibilayers. *Biophys J* 56:1193-1201

Mason RP, Moring J, Herbette LG (1990): A molecular model involving the membrane bilayer in the binding of lipid soluble drugs to their receptors in heart and brain. *Nucl Med Biol* 17:13-33

McCloskey M, Poo M-M (1986): Rates of membrane associated reactions: reduction in demensionality revisited. *J Cell Biol* 102:88-96

Messing RO, Carpenter CL, Diamond I, Greenberg DA (1986): Ethanol regulates calcium channels in clonal neural cells. *Proc Natl Acad Sci (USA)* 83:6213-6215

Meyer HH (1906): *Harvey Lectures.* pp 11-17

Mohler H, Okada T (1977): Benzodiazepine receptor: demonstration in the central nervous system. *Science* 198:849-851

Mohler H, Sieghert W, Richards JG, Hunkeler W (1984): Photoaffinity labeling of benzodiazepine receptors with a partial inverse agonist. *Eur J Pharmacol*

102:191-192

Moody MF (1963): X-ray diffraction pattern of nerve myelin: a method for determining the phases. *Science* 142:1173-1174

Moring J, Shoemaker WJ, Skita V, Mason RP, Hayden HC, Salomon RM, Herbette LG (1990): Rat cerebral cortical synaptoneurosomal membranes. Structure and interactions with imidazobenzodiazepine and 1,4-dihydropyridine calcium channel drugs. *Biophys J* 58:513-531

Muller WE (1987): *The Benzodiazepine Receptor.* Cambridge University Press

Overton E (1901): Studien über die Nar Kose. Jena: Fisher

Panza G, Grebb JA, Sanna E, Wright Jr. AG, Hanbauer I (1985): Evidence for down-regulation of ^{3}H-nitrendipine recognition sites in mouse brain after long-term treatment with nifedipine or verapamil. *Neurophamacology* 24:1113-1117

Peper K, Bradley RJ, Dreyer F (1982): The acetylcholine receptor at the neuromuscular junction. *Physiol Rev* 62:1271-1340

Polokoff MA, Simon TJ, Harris RA, Simon FR, Iwahashi M (1985): Chronic ethanol increases liver plasma membrane fluidity. *Biochemistry* 24:3114-3120

Puddey IB, Beilin LJ, Vandongen R (1986): Lack of effect of acute alcohol ingestion on erythrocyte NA^+, K^+-ATPase activity or passive sodium uptake in vivo in man. *J Stud Alcohol* 47(6)

Renau-Piqueras J, Miragall F, Marques A, Baguena-Cervellera R, Guerri C (1987): Chronic ethanol consumption affects filipin-cholesterol complexes and intramembranous particles of synaptosomes of rat brain cortex. *Alcholism: Clin Exp Res* 11:486-493

Rhodes DG, Sarmiento JG, Herbette LG (1985): Kinetics of binding of membrane-active drugs to receptor sites. Diffusion limited rates for a membrane bilayer approach of 1,4-dihydropyridine calcium channel antagonists to their active site. *Mol Pharmacol* 27:612-623

Rius R, Bergamaschi S, Di Fonso F, Govoni S, Trabucchi M, and Rossi F (1987): Acute ethanol effect on calcium antagonist binding in rat brain. *Brain Res* 402:359-361

Rottenberg H, Waring A, Rubin E, reply by Gordon ER. (1984): Alcohol-induced tolerance in mitochondrial membranes. *Science* 223:193-194,

Schofield PR, Darlison MG, Fujita N, Burt DR, Stephenson FA, Rodriguez H, Rhee LM, Ranachandran J, Reale V, Glencorse TA, Seeburg PH, Barnard EA (1987): Sequence and functional expression of the $GABA_A$ receptor shows a ligand-gated receptor super-family. *Nature* 328:221-227

Sedzik J, Toews AD, Blaurock AE, Morell P (1984): Resistance to disruption of multilamellar fragments of central nervous system myelin. *J Neurochem* 43(5):1415-1420

Sieghart W, Eichinger A, Riederer P, Jellinger K (1985): Comparison of benzodiazepine receptor binding in membranes from human or rat brain. *Neuropharmacology* 24:751-759

Stamatoff JB, Krimm S (1976): Phase determination of x-ray reflections for membrane-type systems with constant fluid density. *Biophys J* 16:503-516

Suzdak PD, Glowa JR, Crawley JN, Skolnick P, and Paul SM (1988): Response. *Science* 239:649-650

Suzdak PD, Glowa JR, Crawley JN, Schwartz RD, Skolnick P, Paul SM (1986b): A selective imidazobenzodiazepine antagonist of ethanol in the rat. *Science* 234:243-1247

Suzdak PD, Schwartz RD, Skolnick P, Paul SM (1986a): Ethanol stimulates γ-aminobutyric acid receptor-mediated chloride transport in rat brain synaptoneurosomes. *Proc Natl Acad Sci (USA)* 83:4071-4075

Sweetnam P, Nestler E, Gallombardo P, Brown S, Duman R, Bracha HS, Tallman J (1987): Comparison of the molecular structure of GABA/benzodiazepine receptors purified from rat and human cerebellum. *Mol Brain Res* 2:223-233

Szabo G, Hoffman PL, Tabakoff B (1988): Forskolin promotes the development of ethanol tolerance in 6-hydroxydopamine-treated mice. *Life Sci* 42:615-621

Tabakoff B, Hoffman PL, Liljequist S (1987): Effects of ethanol on the activity of brain enzymes. *Enzyme* 37:70-86

Takahashi M, Seagar MJ, Jones JF, Reber BFX, Catterall WA (1987): Subunit structure of dihydropyridine-sensitive calcium channels from skeletal muscle. *PNAS (USA)* 84:5478-5482

Valverius P, Hoffman PL, Tabakoff B (1987): Effect of ethanol on mouse cerebral cortical beta-adrenergic receptors. *Mol Pharmacol* 32:217-222

Vandaele S, Fosset M, Galizzi J, Lazdunski M (1987): Monoclonal antibodies that coimmunoprecipitate the 1,4-dihydropyridine and phenylalkylamine receptor and reveal the Ca^{+2} channel structure. *Biochemistry* 26:5-9

Waring AJ, Rottenberg H, Ohnishi T, Rubin E (1981): Membranes and phospholipids of liver mitochondria from chronic alcoholic rats are resistant to membrane disordering by alcohol. *Proc Natl Acad Sci* 78(4):2582-2586

Waring AJ, Rottenberg H, Ohnishi T, Rubin E (1982): The effect of chronic ethanol consumption of temperature-dependent physical properties of liver mitochondria membranes. *Arch Biochem Biophys* 216(1):51-61

Yatani A, Kuntze DL, Brown AM (1988): Effects of dihydropyridine calcium channel modulators on cardiac sodium channels. *Am J Physiol* 254:H140-H147

Ethanol and the GABA$_A$ Receptor-Gated Chloride Ion Channel

A. Leslie Morrow, Pascale Montpied and Steven M. Paul

INTRODUCTION

The cellular (viz., biochemical and neurophysiological) mechanisms underlying the behavioral (e.g., intoxicating, anxiolytic and sedative/hypnotic) actions of ethanol are not well understood. Ethanol has many of the physiochemical properties of other anesthetic agents, conferring nonspecific disordering effects on neuronal membranes, especially at high concentrations. It is generally acknowledged that ethanol shares more specific pharmacologic actions with other sedative/hypnotic drugs such as the barbiturates and benzodiazepines. These include anxiolytic, anticonvulsant and sedative activity (Liljequist and Engel, 1984) and in certain behavioral paradigms, the development of cross tolerance and cross dependence (Boisse and Okamoto, 1980; Le et al., 1986). These findings suggest that ethanol, barbiturates and benzodiazepines may share at least one common mechanism of action.

Many lines of evidence have supported the hypothesis that gamma-aminobutyric acid (GABA)-mediated neurotransmission is involved, at least in part, in the behavioral actions of ethanol (for a detailed review see Hunt, 1983). For example, it has been shown that GABA-mimetic drugs ameliorate the signs and symptoms of ethanol withdrawal, whereas GABA antagonists potentiate these symptoms (Goldstein, 1978). Furthermore, benzodiazepine receptor inverse agonists, such as Ro15-4513 and FG-7142, antagonize many ethanol-induced behaviors in the rat (Koob et al., 1988; Lister, 1987; Lister, 1988; Suzdak et al., 1986a; Suzdak et al., 1988b).

The most direct evidence that ethanol interacts with the GABA$_A$ receptor complex derives from recent studies using subcellular brain preparations and cultured embryonic neurons, where ethanol and other short chain alcohols have been shown either to stimulate directly (Suzdak et al., 1986a; Suzdak et al.,1987) or potentiate $GABA_A$ receptor-mediated $^{36}Cl^-$ uptake (Allan and Harris, 1986; Mehta and Ticku, 1988; Suzdak et al., 1986a; Suzdak et al., 1987; Ticku et al., 1986). The effects of ethanol in stimulating $GABA_A$ receptor-mediated $^{36}Cl^-$ flux are observed at concentrations well within the range of tissue ethanol concentrations observed during acute intoxication (20-60 mM), while subintoxicating concentrations augment muscimol or pentobarbital stimulation of ^{36}Cl-uptake (Allan and Harris, 1986; Suzdak et al., 1986a; Suzdak et al., 1987; Ticku et al., 1986). The actions of ethanol and other short chain alcohols in stimulating $^{36}Cl^-$ uptake *in vitro* appears to be mediated via the GABA-coupled Cl^- channel since it is blocked by the specific $GABA_A$ receptor antagonists bicuculline and picrotoxin (Mehta and Ticku, 1988; Suzdak et al., 1986a).

Electrophysiological evidence supporting alcohol's actions in augmenting GABA-mediated inhibitory responses has been controversial, with some investigators reporting enhancement of GABA-mediated neuronal responses (Celentano et al., 1988; Davidoff, 1973; Mereu and Gessa, 1985; Nestores, 1980), and others finding little or no effect (Harrison et al., 1987; Mancillas et al., 1986). For example, earlier studies have reported that ethanol enhances GABA-mediated recurrent inhibition in spinal cord (Davidoff, 1973), and GABA-mediated inhibition in the cerebral cortex (Nestores, 1980) and substantia nigra pars reticulata (Mereu and Gessa, 1985), suggesting that the lack of effect of ethanol on the excitability of hippocampal neurons *in vivo* (Mancillas et al., 1986) or on embryonic hippocampal neurons *in vitro* (Harrison et al., 1987) may represent a selective regional difference in ethanol responsivity. Nevertheless, several recent studies have reported that ethanol can potentiate both GABA and glycine-induced chloride currents in voltage-clamped spinal cord and cerebral cortical neurons (Aguayo, personal communication; Celentano et al. 1988), suggesting that poorly delineated methodological issues may account for the difficulties in the detection of ethanol's effects on GABA-activated chloride conductance using electrophysiological techniques. Ethanol has also recently been shown to depress single unit activity in cerebellar Purkinje cells (Palmer et al., 1988) and zona reticulata neurons (Marrosu et al., 1989); effects that are reversed by Ro15-4513 and other benzodiazepine receptor inverse agonists. Further studies will be needed to delineate the critical factors involved in the electrophysiological responses of GABAergic neurons to ethanol.

THE GABA$_A$ RECEPTOR

GABA, the most ubiquitous inhibitory neurotransmitter in the brain, interacts with a receptor subtype that contains recognition sites for benzodiazepines and barbiturates. These binding sites are linked allosterically to the GABA recognition site, and each site is involved directly or indirectly in the gating properties of an integral Cl$^-$ channel. GABA receptor-mediated activation of Cl$^-$ conductance results in membrane hyperpolarization and decreased neuronal excitability (Skolnick and Paul, 1982). Barbiturates and benzodiazepines have been shown to augment the activity of GABA via these specific recognition sites on the GABA-receptor complex (Olsen, 1982). By contrast, ethanol interacts very weakly, if at all, with the recognition sites for GABA, benzodiazepines, barbiturates and cage convulsants (Davis and Ticku, 1981; Greenberg et al., 1984). Thus, the exact mechanism(s) underlying ethanol's actions in augmenting GABA$_A$ receptor function is unknown.

In this chapter we review recent pharmacologic evidence supporting a role for the GABA$_A$ receptor chloride channel complex in mediating some of ethanol's acute pharmacological actions. In addition, we present and review data showing that chronic ethanol administration results in functional subsensitivity of GABA$_A$ receptors and that a reduction in the level of GABA$_A$ receptor α_1-subunit mRNAs is associated with this subsensitive response. We hypothesize that alterations in GABA$_A$ receptor structure and function may contribute to the tolerance, altered seizure sensitivity and development of the ethanol withdrawal syndrome observed after repeated ethanol administration.

THE EFFECTS OF ETHANOL AND OTHER SHORT CHAIN ALCOHOLS ON GABA$_A$ RECEPTOR-MEDIATED Cl$^-$ UPTAKE *IN VITRO*

Ethanol has been reported to stimulate dose-dependently ^{36}Cl$^-$uptake into cerebral cortical synaptoneurosomes (Suzdak et al., 1986a; Suzdak et al., 1986b; Suzdak et al., 1987) or into cultured spinal cord neurons (Mehta and Ticku, 1988; Ticku et al., 1986) (Fig. 1). Significant stimulation of ^{36}Cl$^-$ uptake is observed at physiologically relevant concentrations (20-70 mM). These effects are biphasic with higher concentrations of ethanol (>80 mM) resulting in diminished ^{36}Cl$^-$ uptake. The ability of ethanol to increase Cl$^-$ transport is qualitatively similar to that of the barbiturate pentobarbital, which also produces a biphasic concentration response curve (Fig. 1).

The ability of alcohols to induce a behavioral state of intoxication, correlates with their membrane/buffer partition coefficients and membrane disordering properties (McCreery and Hunt, 1978; Seeman, 1972). The ability of various short chain alcohols to stimulate GABA receptor-mediated Cl^- uptake *in vitro* at "intoxicating" concentrations was also highly correlated with their intoxication potencies and membrane buffer partition coefficients (Fig. 2). The stimulatory action of ethanol on Cl^- transport is almost certainly mediated via the GABA receptor complex since the GABA receptor antagonists bicuculline and picrotoxin inhibit ethanol's effects (Suzdak et al., 1986a). These antagonists have similar effects on GABA- and pentobarbital-induced stimulation of Cl^- flux (Suzdak et al., 1986a). By contrast, other neurotransmitter receptor antagonists, such as haloperidol, propranolol, verapamil, strychnine, clonidine and phenoxybenzamine failed to alter ethanol-stimulated chloride ion flux (Suzdak et al., 1986a).

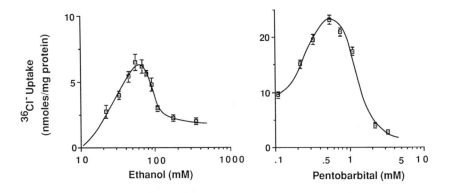

Figure 1. Concentration response curves for ethanol and pentobarbital-stimulated $^{36}Cl^-$ uptake in rat cerebral cortical synaptoneurosomes. Ethanol (20-320 mM), or pentobarbital (0.1-3 mM) was incubated with $0.5\,\mu Ci$ of $^{36}Cl^-$ for 5 sec. Data shown are the mean $\pm$SEM of three experiments, each conducted in quadruplicate. Adapted from Morrow et al. (1988b): Benzodiazepine, barbiturate, ethanol and hypnotic steroid hormone modulation of GABA-mediated chloride ion transport in rat brain synaptoneurosomes. In: *Chloride Channels and Their Modulation by Neurotransmitters and Drugs.* pp 247-261.

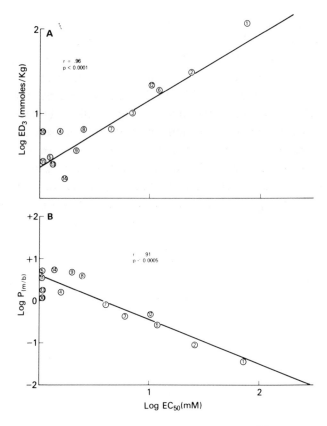

Figure 2. The effect of various short-chain alcohols on ^{36}Cl$^-$ uptake into rat cerebral cortical synaptoneurosomes: correlation with their intoxication potencies (A) and membrane buffer partition coeffients (B). Individual EC$_{50}$ values for alcohol stimulation of ^{36}Cl$^-$ uptake were determined from concentration response curves using a minimum of six concentrations for each alcohol. Each point represents the log of the mean EC$_{50}$ determined in three separate experiments. Alcohols tested were: (1) methanol, (2) ethanol, (3) 1-propanol, (4) 1-butanol, (5)1-pentanol, (6) 2-propanol, (7) 2-butanol, (8) 2-pentanol, (9) 3-pentanol, (10) isobutanol, (11) iso-amyl alcohol, (12) butanol, (13) t-amyl alcohol, (14) 2-methyl-2 pentanol. A: Correlation between the log EC$_{50}$ values for stimulation of ^{36}Cl$^-$ uptake and their potencies in producing behavioral intoxication (r = 0.96, p < .0001, Pearson's product moment). Behavioral intoxication potencies were taken from McCreery and Hunt (1978). B: Correlation between the log EC$_{50}$ values for stimulation of ^{36}Cl$^-$ uptake and their membrane buffer partition coefficients (r = 0.91, p < .0005, Pearson's product moment) obtained from McCreery and Hunt, 1978). Adapted from Suzdak et al. (1987): Alcohols stimulate GABA receptor-mediated chloride uptake in brain vesicles: correlation with intoxication potency. *Brain Res* 444:340-344.

The ability of ethanol to stimulate chloride uptake directly is a relatively weak effect when compared to the magnitude of the response to pentobarbital or GABA itself. Ethanol, like barbiturates, however, has been shown to potentiate the effects of both GABA and pentobarbital at concentrations between 10 and 70 mM (Allan and Harris, 1986; Suzdak et al., 1987). Low concentrations of ethanol (20 mM) have no effect on basal chloride uptake, but markedly potentiate muscimol-stimulated $^{36}Cl^-$ uptake (Fig. 3). The potentiation of muscimol-stimulated $^{36}Cl^-$ uptake by ethanol appears to be the result of an increase in the V_{max} of muscimol-stimulated $^{36}Cl^-$ uptake rather than a change in the apparent K_m (Suzdak et al., 1987). Ethanol (at subthreshold concentrations) had

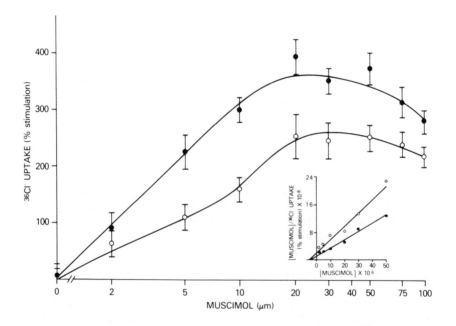

Figure 3. Ethanol potentiation of muscimol-stimulated $^{36}Cl^-$ uptake. Increasing concentrations of muscimol (2-100 mM) alone (o) or in combination with ethanol (20 mM) (•) were incubated with synaptoneurosomes and 0.5 μCi $^{36}Cl^-$ for 5 sec. Inset: A Hanes-Woolf plot of the data indicates that ethanol increased the V_{max} for muscimol-stimulated $^{36}Cl^-$ uptake. The apparent K_m for muscimol was not significantly altered in the presence of ethanol. Adapted from Suzdak et al. (1986b): A selective imidazobenzodiazepine antagonist of ethanol in the rat. *Science* 234:1243-1247.

a similar effect on pentobarbital-induced ^{36}Cl$^-$ flux, except that ethanol altered both the apparent V$_{max}$ and K$_m$ of pentobarbital-stimulated chloride ion flux (Morrow et al., 1988b; Suzdak et al., 1987). The demonstration that relatively low concentrations of alcohol potentiate GABA receptor-mediated chloride ion flux is consistent with previous behavioral studies in which the actions of ethanol are blocked by GABA antagonists such as bicuculline and picrotoxin (Cott et al., 1976; Liljequist and Engel, 1982; Liljequist and Engel, 1984). These data suggest that the anxiolytic and intoxicating properties of ethanol may be mediated, in part, by their interaction with GABA receptors in the central nervous system (CNS).

Ro15-4513 BLOCKS ETHANOL STIMULATION OF GABAERGIC CHLORIDE ION FLUX *IN VITRO*

Benzodiazepine agonists have been shown to dose-dependently, stereo-specifically and reversibly potentiate GABA-mediated Cl$^-$ flux in isolated cerebral cortex vesicles by altering the apparent K$_m$ of muscimol stimulation (Morrow and Paul, 1988). Likewise, benzodiazepine inverse agonists have been shown to inhibit muscimol-stimulated ^{36}Cl$^-$ uptake by decreasing the apparent K$_m$ for muscimol stimulation of Cl$^-$ flux with no significant effect on the V$_{max}$ (Morrow and Paul, 1988). Benzodiazepine inverse agonists were also screened for their ability to alter ethanol-stimulated ^{36}Cl$^-$ uptake. Of the benzodiazepine receptor ligands tested, the partial inverse agonist, Ro15-4513, was found to be a very potent antagonist of ethanol-stimulated ^{36}Cl$^-$ uptake (Suzdak et al. 1986b). At a concentration of 100 nM, Ro15-4513 completely antagonized ethanol-stimulated ^{36}Cl$^-$ uptake *in vitro* (Fig. 4) (Suzdak et al., 1986b). However, Ro15-4513 was ineffective in antagonizing pentobarbital- or muscimol-stimulated ^{36}Cl$^-$ uptake at concentrations as high as 1 μM (Fig. 5). Higher concentrations of Ro15-4513, as expected, inhibit muscimol-stimulated ^{36}Cl$^-$ uptake (unpublished observation). The ability of ethanol to potentiate GABA at subthreshold concentrations was also inhibited by Ro15-4513 (100nM), whereas pentobarbital enhancement of muscimol-stimulated Cl$^-$ flux was unaffected. These effects were not shared by other inverse agonists of the β-carboline series, including FG-7142, DMCM and β-CCE, when tested at concentrations up to 1 μM, suggesting that the inhibitory effects of Ro15-4513 on

THE EFFECT OF Ro15-4513 ON ETHANOL-STIMULATED ³⁶CI⁻UPTAKE

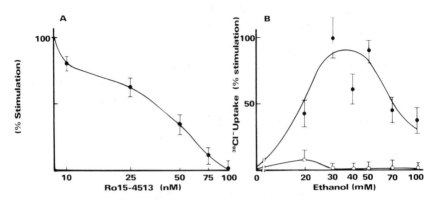

Figure 4.   The effect of the imidazobenzodiazepine Ro15-4513 on ethanol-stimulated $^{36}Cl^-$ uptake into rat cerebral cortical synaptoneurosomes. A: Various concentrations of Ro15-4513 (10-100 nM) were added to synaptoneurosomes 5 min before the addition of ethanol (50 mM) and $^{36}CI^-$. The data shown represent the mean ±SEM of quadruplicate determinations from a typical experiment carried out three times with similar results. B: The effect of various concentrations of ethanol alone (•) or in the presence of Ro15-4513 (100 nM) (o) on $^{36}CI^-$ uptake into synaptoneurosomes. Ro15-4513 significantly decreased ethanol-stimulated $^{36}CI^-$ uptake at all concentrations tested (p < 0.01, ANOVA followed by Newman Keuls test). Adapted from Suzdak et al. (1986): Ethanol stimulates gamma-aminobutyric acid receptor-mediated chloride transport in rat brain synaptoneurosomes. *Proc Natl Acad Sci (USA)* 83:4071.

ethanol-mediated Cl⁻ flux may be distinct from its inverse agonist effects. If the effects of Ro15-4513 in antagonizing the action of both high and low concentrations of ethanol were related to its weak inverse agonist properties, then other inverse agonists should also be effective ethanol antagonists. However, none of the other partial or full benzodiazepine receptor inverse agonists tested blocked ethanol-stimulated $^{36}Cl^-$ uptake. The effect of Ro15-4513 appears to be mediated by central benzodiazepine receptors because its ability to inhibit ethanol-stimulated $^{36}Cl^-$ uptake is blocked by the benzodiazepine receptor antagonists Ro15-1788 and CGS-8216 (Suzdak et al., 1986b). The exact mechanism(s) underlying the specificity of Ro15-4513 in blocking the neurochemical actions of ethanol are unknown, but appear to involve a unique interaction with the benzodiazepine recognition site coupled to the GABA receptor complex. Insofar as the ability of alcohols to stimulate Cl$^-$ flux is correlated with their physiochemical properties, ethanol's effects on chloride ion flux may involve an alteration in the lipid-protein microenvironment of

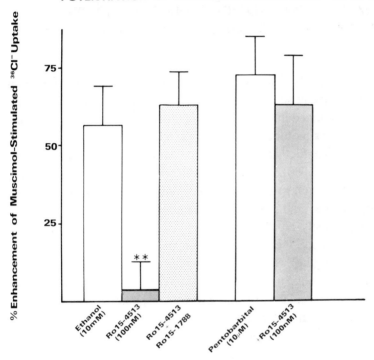

Figure 5. The effect of Ro15-4513 on ethanol- (50 mM), muscimol- (5 μM) and pentobarbital- (500 mM) stimulated ^{36}Cl$^-$ uptake into rat cerebral cortical synaptoneurosomes. Ro15-4513 (100 nM) was added 5 min before the addition of ^{36}Cl$^-$ and ethanol, muscimol or pentobarbital. Ro15-1788 (300 nM) was added simultaneously with ^{36}Cl$^-$ and ethanol. Data represent the mean and SEM of quadruplicate determinations from a typical experiment repeated three times with similiar results. Ro15-4513 significantly blocked ethanol-stimulated ^{36}Cl$^-$ uptake (p < 0.01, ANOVA followed by Newman Keuls test). This effect was antagonized by the benzodiazepine receptor antagonist Ro15-1788. In contrast, Ro15-4513 had no effect on either muscimol- or pentobarbital-stimulated ^{36}Cl$^-$ uptake. Adapted from Suzdak et al. (1986a): Ethanol stimulates γ-aminobutyric acid receptor-mediated chloride transport in rat brain synaptoneurosomes. *Proc Natl Acad Sci (USA)* 83:4071.

the GABA receptor complex. Thus, ethanol and Ro15-4513 may interact at a common hydrophobic domain of this receptor complex in close
proximity to the benzodiazepine recognition site. Further studies will be
necessary to elucidate the exact mechanism(s) responsible for the ability
of Ro15-4513 to antagonize the pharmacological activity of ethanol.

THE BENZODIAZEPINE RECEPTOR INVERSE AGONIST
Ro15-4513 ANTAGONIZES ETHANOL-INDUCED BEHAVIORS
IN THE RAT

The ability of Ro15-4513 to antagonize the behavioral effects of ethanol
has been studied using several model systems. The effects of Ro15-4513
were initially examined in the Vogel anticonflict paradigm and by its ability to reverse gross motor intoxication. At relatively low doses, ethanol
produces an anticonflict action in several species (Glowa and Barrett,
1976; Koob et al., 1980). In the modified Vogel paradigm (Vogel et al.,
1971), ethanol (1 mg/kg) resulted in a significant increase in punished
responding (Suzdak et al., 1986b). Pretreatment of rats with Ro15-4513
(3 mg/kg) completely blocked the anticonflict actions of ethanol in this
paradigm. In contrast, the increase in punished responding produced by
pentobarbital (4 mg/kg) was not affected by pretreatment with Ro15-4513
(Suzdak et al., 1986b; Suzdak et al., 1988b). Ro15-4513 alone did not
significantly affect punished or nonpunished responding in these experiments. In latter studies, Britton et al. (1988; Koob et al., 1986) found
that Ro15-4513 effectively reversed the anticonflict action of ethanol, but
only at doses that produced intrinsic effects, that is, doses that caused
suppression of both punished and nonpunished responding. This discrepancy may be due to different sensitivities of the behavioral paradigms
employed to study the behavioral effects of ethanol.

Using the behavioral rating scale of Majchrowicz (1975), ethanol
(1.5-2.5 mg/kg) produces a level of intoxication in rats characterized by
general sedation, staggered gait and impaired righting reflexes (Lister
and Durcan, 1989; Majchrowicz, 1975; Suzdak et al., 1986b). Ro15-4513
dose-dependently (0.5-10 mg/kg) blocked ethanol intoxication (Lister and
Durcan, 1989; Marrosu et al., 1989; Suzdak et al., 1986b), and when
administered after ethanol, reversed the intoxication produced by ethanol
(Suzdak et al., 1986b). These effects were antagonized by the benzodiazepine receptor antagonists Ro15-1788 and CGS-8216. The ability of

Ro15-4513 to block ethanol-induced intoxication was not shared by other benzodiazepine inverse agonists, including β-CCE and FG-7142 (Lister and Durcan, 1989; Marrosu et al., 1989; Suzdak et al., 1986b; Suzdak et al., 1988a). Moreover, coadministration of the other inverse agonists, such as FG-7142 or β-CCE, with Ro15-4513 blocked the ability of Ro15-4513 to inhibit ethanol-induced intoxication (Suzdak et al., 1988a). These data suggest that whereas Ro15-4513 must bind to the central benzodiazepine recognition site to produce its effects, the ability of Ro15-4513 to block ethanol's effects may not be mediated solely by virtue of its "inverse agonist" properties. The fact that other benzodiazepine inverse agonists or antagonists do not produce the same effect on ethanol-induced behavior suggests again that these specific effects of Ro15-4513 are mediated by some unique interaction with the GABA receptor complex.

The administration of ethanol at high doses (7.5-15 g/kg) is lethal to rodents. Initially, it was reported that Ro15-4513 protected rats against the lethal effects of ethanol (Fadda et al., 1987). However, a subsequent study failed to confirm these findings (Nutt et al., 1988). The ability of Ro15-4513 to antagonize various other ethanol-induced behaviors has recently been investigated using doses of Ro15-4513 that are devoid of intrinsic behavioral inverse agonist effects. For example, Ro15-4513 has been shown to (a) attenuate the discriminitive stimulus effects of ethanol, but not pentobarbital, in rats (Rees and Balster, 1988); (b) block oral reinforcement in rats (Samson et al., 1987) and (c) reduce ethanol intake in alcohol-preferring rats (McBride et al., 1988). Ro15-4513 reversed the motor incoordination produced by ethanol in the rotorod (Bonetti et al., 1985; Hoffman et al., 1987) and horizontal wire (Polc, 1985) tests. These latter effects were also blocked by the benzodiazepine receptor antagonist Ro15-1788.

In certain behavioral paradigms, Ro15-4513 has been ineffective in blocking ethanol's effects. Low doses of ethanol (1 g/kg) have been shown to increase generalized locomotor activity and wheel-running behavior in rats (Bixler and Lewis, 1987; Johnson et al., 1987). These behaviors are not antagonized by Ro15-4513. Other "antialcohol" actions of Ro15-4513 have been attributed to its inverse agonist properties. For example, Ro15-4513 decreased the number of exploratory headdippings in a holeboard test as well as the number of headdips produced by ethanol (Lister, 1987). However, both effects are shared by other benzodiazepine inverse agonists (Lister, 1987). In addition, Ro15-4513 reportedly will induce seizures in animals that have been withdrawn from ethanol, although it fails to elicit withdrawal itself (Lister and Karanian, 1987). In squirrel monkeys, low doses of Ro15-4513 blocked the decrease in locomotor activity produced by ethanol. However, higher doses of Ro15-4513 (>1 mg/kg) caused severe tremors in these monkeys (Miscek and Weerts, 1987).

Ro15-4513 reverses the anticonvulsant effects of ethanol against both bicuculline and picrotoxin-induced seizures (Lister and Nutt, 1988) at doses that are not proconvulsant (Nutt and Lister, 1987). However, at the same dose Ro15-4513 failed to reverse the anticonvulsant effect of pentobarbital against picrotoxin-induced seizures (Lister and Nutt, 1988). These data also suggest that the ability of Ro15-4513 to antagonize ethanol's effects are not solely related to its inverse agonist activity.

It should be emphasized that Ro15-4513 has intrinsic pharmacologic actions consistent with its classification as a partial inverse agonist at the central benzodiazepine receptor. These actions include anxiogenic and proconvulsant effects. Although Ro15-4513 has been reported to reverse some of the behavioral effects of ethanol at concentrations that are lacking intrinsic pharmacologic effects, its intrinsic inverse agonist properties make it a difficult drug to administer for behavioral studies. Thus, the selectivity of Ro15-4513 seems to depend on both the dose of Ro15-4513 employed and the nature of the behavioral paradigm. Finally, the ability of Ro15-4513 to selectively reverse certain effects of ethanol (intoxication, anxiolytic, reinforcement) suggests that these effects are mediated by the GABA-benzodiazepine receptor complex. Ro15-4513 has proven to be a useful tool for delineation of the role of the GABA receptor complex in the behavioral manifestations of ethanol.

CHRONIC ETHANOL EXPOSURE DECREASES GABA RECEPTOR-MEDIATED CHLORIDE UPTAKE *IN VITRO*

Chronic exposure of rats to ethanol by inhalation produces physical dependence and tolerance (Goldstein and Pal, 1971; Karanian et al., 1986). These effects are associated with a decrease in the sensitivity of the $GABA_A$ receptor coupled Cl^- channel when blood ethanol levels produced by the ethanol exposure were greater than 150 mg/% (Morrow et al., 1988a). The apparent Emax of muscimol-stimulated

^{36}Cl$^-$ uptake was decreased by 26% following chronic ethanol inhalation (Fig. 6A). In a similar manner, pentobarbital-stimulated ^{36}Cl$^-$ uptake was decreased by 25% after chronic ethanol treatment (Figure 6B). "Direct" stimulation of ^{36}Cl$^-$ uptake by ethanol was not altered by this treatment, as demonstrated in the same tissue preparations where the decreases in muscimol and pentobarbital-stimulated ^{36}Cl$^-$ uptake were observed (Fig. 6C). However, the ability of ethanol (20 mM) to potentiate muscimol-stimulated ^{36}Cl$^-$ uptake was completely lost in cerebral cortical synaptoneurosomes (Fig. 6D) and in cerebellar microsacs (Allan and Harris, 1987) after chronic ethanol administration. Thus, it appears that chronic ethanol exposure produces a cellular "desensitization" of the GABA receptor-coupled Cl$^-$ channel similar to the desensitization of GABA-mediated Cl$^-$ flux that has been demonstrated *in vitro* (Schwartz et al., 1989). The decrease in the Emax of both muscimol- and pentobarbital-stimulated ^{36}Cl$^-$ uptake is not easily reconciled with the lack of effects of chronic ethanol exposure on GABA$_A$ receptor density measured using *in vitro* binding methods. The loss of the ability of ethanol to potentiate muscimol-stimulated ^{36}Cl$^-$ uptake suggests that there may be an alteration in the membrane mechanism(s) by which ethanol interacts with the GABA$_A$ receptor complex. Chronic ethanol administration has previously been reported to produce tolerance to the membrane disordering effects of ethanol (Goldstein et al., 1980; Johnson et al., 1980; Rottenberg et al., 1981; Taraschi et al., 1986).

Several days after withdrawal from ethanol, the subsensitivity in both muscimol- and pentobarbital-stimulated ^{36}Cl$^-$ uptake is reversed (Morrow et al., 1988a). At this time, the signs of ethanol withdrawal have also remitted (Karanian et al., 1986). We have suggested, therefore, that subsensitivity of the GABA-barbiturate receptor-coupled Cl$^-$ channel may be involved in the ethanol withdrawal syndrome. This hypothesis is substantiated by a recent report that behavioral responses to intranigral muscimol administration are also reduced after chronic ethanol administration (Gonzalez and Czachura, 1989). This decrease in GABA receptor-gated chloride channel function could also account for the effectiveness of benzodiazepines in the clinical management of the ethanol withdrawal syndrome (Sellers and Kalant, 1976). During ethanol withdrawal, benzodiazepines probably compensate for the reduced effectiveness of GABA on Cl$^-$ flux by enhancing GABA's potency, as we have previously demonstrated *in vitro* (Morrow and Paul, 1988).

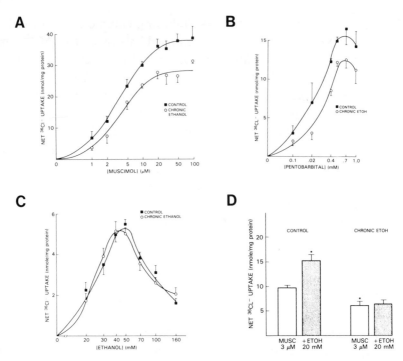

Figure 6. Chronic ethanol administration alters the function of the $GABA_A$ receptor complex. Rats were administered ethanol by inhalation for 14 days. Data represent the mean $\pm$SEM of 4 to 5 independent experiments, each conducted in quadruplicate. **A.** Muscimol stimulation of $^{36}Cl^-$ uptake is reduced following chronic ethanol inhalation. The apparent Emax of muscimol-stimulated $^{36}Cl^-$ uptake is reduced 26% ($p<.01$) with no significant change in the mean EC_{50}. **B.** Pentobarbital-stimulated $^{36}Cl^-$ uptake is decreased after chronic ethanol administration. The apparent Emax was decreased 25% ($p<.05$) and the EC_{50} was increased 39% ($p<.05$) after chronic ethanol exposure. **C.** Direct stimulation of $^{36}Cl^-$ uptake by ethanol is not altered in cerebral cortical synaptoneurosomes after chronic ethanol administration. Ethanol, muscimol and pentobarbital responses were measured simultaneously in the same tissue preparation. **D.** Ethanol enhancement of muscimol-stimulated $^{36}Cl^-$ uptake is abolished after chronic ethanol inhalation. Muscimol and ethanol (where indicated) were added simultaneously and uptake was terminated after 5 sec. There was a significant potentiation of muscimol stimulation by ethanol in control synaptoneurosomes (55%, $p<.001$), but there was no potentiation by ethanol in synaptoneurosomes from ethanol-treated rats. Muscimol stimulation of $^{36}Cl^-$ uptake was decreased after ethanol administration (40%, $p<.001$, n = 6). Adapted from Morrow et al. (1988): Chronic ethanol administration alters γ-aminobutyric acid, pentobarbital and ethanol-mediated $^{36}Cl^-$ uptake in cerebral cortical synaptoneurosomes. *J Pharmacol Exp Ther* 246:158-164.

Table 1. Chronic Pentobarbital Administration Alters Muscimol- and Pentobarbital-Stimulated ^{36}Cl$^-$ Uptake

	Muscimol Stimulation (%)		Pentobarbital Stimulation (%)	
	V_{max}	EC$_{50}$(μM)	V_{max}	EC$_{50}$(μM)
Control	417 $\pm$ 36	4.3 $\pm$ 0.5	328 $\pm$ 30	0.13 $\pm$ 0.03
Pentobarbital-treated	317 $\pm$ 35	5.3 $\pm$ 0.4	220 $\pm$ 20	0.15 $\pm$ 0.04
% Change	-24.5**	$+23.2$	-32.9*	$+15.4$

Muscimol and pentobarbital concentration-response curves were conducted simultaneously using tissue from 4 rats/treatment group. Data are expressed as percent stimulation by muscimol or pentobarbital above basal levels of ^{36}Cl$^-$ uptake. Data shown are the mean $\pm$SEM of 4 independent experiments, each conducted in quadruplicate. The values were compared statistically using the student's t test (two-tailed). *$p<.05$, ** $p<.001$.

Repeated pentobarbital administration to rats produced a similar decrease in the maximal responses in ^{36}Cl$^-$ uptake produced by muscimol and pentobarbital (Table 1). Fig. 7 illustrates the effects of pentobarbital on GABA$_A$ receptor-mediated ^{36}Cl$^-$ uptake in cerebral cortical synaptoneurosomes after 2 weeks of daily administration. The Emax of muscimol-stimulated ^{36}Cl$^-$ uptake is decreased 24.5% with a small increase in the EC$_{50}$ (Fig. 7A). Pentobarbital stimulation of ^{36}Cl$^-$ uptake is reduced 33% in the cerebral cortical synaptoneurosomes after chronic administration of pentobarbital (Fig. 7B).

Tolerance to the sedative and intoxicating effects of ethanol has been postulated to result from a compensatory decrease in GABA-mediated inhibition in the brain (Hunt, 1983). Alterations in endogenous GABA concentrations and turnover rates after chronic ethanol administration are inconsistent (Hunt, 1983), and probably cannot account for the ethanol withdrawal syndrome. Radioligand binding studies with [^{3}H] muscimol (Volicer, 1980; Volicer and Biagioni, 1982), [^{3}H] flunitrazepam (Davis and Ticku, 1981; Rastogi et al. 1986; Volicer and Biagioni, 1982) and [^{35}S] TBPS (Rastogi et al., 1986; Thyagarajan and Ticku, 1985) to quantify the density of GABA$_A$ receptors in the CNS do not support consistent receptor down regulation resulting from chronic ethanol administration. However, there are suggestions that the sensitivity of the GABA and benzodiazepine recognition sites to GABA may be reduced after chronic ethanol exposure (deVries et al. 1987; Ticku and Burch, 1980).

The decrease in the sensitivity of the GABA$_A$ receptor after chronic ethanol and barbiturate administration may be due to altered biosynthesis or processing of receptor subunit proteins that comprise the GABA$_A$ receptor complex itself or to their post-translational modification. Re-

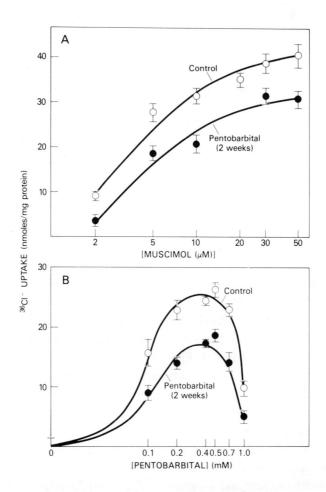

Figure 7. Chronic pentobarbital administration reduces GABA$_A$ receptor function in cerebral cortical synaptoneurosomes. Rats were injected with pentobarbital (30 mg/kg) once daily for 14 days. Control rats received saline injections. Data are from a representative experiment conducted in quadruplicate and repeated twice A: Chronic pentobarbital administration decreases the apparent Emax of muscimol stimulated ^{36}Cl$^-$ uptake by 25% with no significant effect on the EC$_{50}$ (see Table 1). B. The apparent Emax of pentobarbital-stimulated ^{36}Cl$^-$ uptake is decreased by 33% after repeated pentobarbital administration.

duced synthesis of the receptor would be expected to result in decreased binding capacity of the various ligands that bind to the GABA$_A$ receptor complex. The lack of consistent reduction in the density of GABA or benzodiazepine binding sites on the GABA$_A$ receptor complex after chronic ethanol and barbiturate administration may be because radioligand binding studies detect binding sites in all cellular compartments, that is, at various stages of synthesis and degradation. This limitation may result in the masking of a decrease in a "functionally available" pool of receptors localized to the synapse. Alternatively, alterations in the normal population of GABA$_A$ receptors expressed in cerebral cortex may result in structurally different GABA$_A$ isoreceptors that could account for the reduction in GABA$_A$ receptor function. We have hypothesized that an alteration in biosynthesis and/or post-translational modification of the GABA$_A$ receptor may be associated with ethanol-induced receptor subsensitivity.

CHRONIC ETHANOL ADMINISTRATION REDUCES THE LEVELS OF GABA$_A$ RECEPTOR α-SUBUNIT mRNA IN RAT CEREBRAL CORTEX

To test the hypothesis that chronic ethanol administration alters the expression of GABA$_A$ receptors in the CNS, a human GABA$_A$ receptor α-subunit complementary deoxyribonucleic acid (cDNA) was used to synthesize a [^{32}P]-labeled complementary riboprobe for Northern analysis. Hybridization of total ribonucleic acid (RNA) purified from rat cerebral cortex with this cRNA probe results in the detection of several α-subunit transcripts of different sizes (Montpied et al. 1988). Fig. 8 illustrates a representative northern blot of RNA from several regions of the rat brain. In all brain regions at least two messenger RNAs (mRNAs) of 4.4 and 4.8 Kb are detected (Montpied et al., 1989). In the cerebellum and hippocampus two smaller transcripts (2.9 and 3.0 Kb) are also detected, although both are present in lower abundance. The levels of the 4.4- and 4.8-Kb transcripts are comparable within each brain region but are variable among brain regions. The highest levels were observed in the cerebellum, followed by the cerebral cortex, thalamus, and hippocampus, with lower levels in the pons, striatum and medulla (Montpied et al., 1988). Recently, we (Montpied et al., submitted) and others (Wisden et al., 1988) have demonstrated that both the 4.4- and 4.8-Kb mRNAs represent α_1-subunit transcripts of the GABA$_A$ receptor.

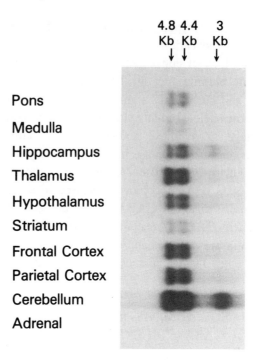

Figure 8. Regional distribution of GABA$_A$ benzodiazepine receptor α-subunit mRNAs in the rat brain. Northern blot analysis was performed on total RNA and hybridization signals were adjusted to be within the linear range. Three different species of mRNA are observed: 4.8 Kb, 4.4 Kb and 3.0 Kb (based on standard DNA markers). Adapted from Montpied et al. (1988): Regional distribution of the GABA$_A$/benzodiazepine receptor (α-subunit) mRNA in rat brain. *J Neurochem* 51:1651-1654.

Chronic ethanol administration, using the inhalation method, results in a reduction in the levels of these α_1-subunit mRNAs in the cerebral cortex of the rat. The level of the 4.8-Kb mRNA species was reduced $47\pm5.0\%$ compared to control animals, while the 4.4 Kb species was reduced $42.5\pm4.7\%$ (Fig. 9). Rehybridization of these northern blots with a β-actin riboprobe revealed no change in the level of β-actin mRNA after chronic ethanol administration. Poly(A)+ RNA levels were also measured to control for a possible "nonspecific" reduction of mRNAs resulting from repeated ethanol administration. Chronic ethanol inhalation also had no effect on the levels of poly(A)+ RNA in the cerebral cortex of ethanol-treated rats compared to control rats.

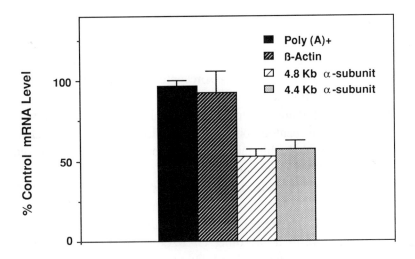

Figure 9. Chronic ethanol inhalation reduces the level of GABA_A receptor α_1-subunit mRNA in the rat cerebral cortex. Total RNA was prepared from individual rats and northern blot analysis was conducted on 2 to 3 blots for each experiment. The 4.8- and 4.4-Kb species of α-subunit mRNA were detected in cerebral cortex from these animals. The same blots were rehybridized with the β-actin riboprobe. Densitometric measurements were made without knowledge of the treatment group. For the measurement of poly(A)+ RNA, total RNA was directly applied under vacuum to separate nitrocellulose membranes and hybridized with the [^{32}P]-labelled deoxythymidine oligonucleotide probe (specific for poly(A)+ RNA). Chronic ethanol administration reduced the level of the 4.8-Kb species of α-subunit mRNA by 47% (p<.01) and reduced the level of the 4.4 Kb species by 43% (p<.01). The levels of β-actin mRNA and poly(A)+ RNA were not altered by chronic ethanol administration. Adapted from Morrow et al. (1990): Chronic ethanol and pentobarbital administration in the rat: effects on GABA_A receptor function and expression in brain. *Alcohol* 7:237-244.

In contrast to ethanol, repeated pentobarbital administration had no effect on the level of GABA_A receptor α_1-subunit mRNA in the rat cerebral cortex. The levels of the 4.8- and 4.4-Kb mRNA species were not altered in rats treated with pentobarbital (see Fig. 5). β-actin mRNA levels were also similar in control and pentobarbital-treated animals.

The reduction in the level of GABA_A receptor α_1-subunit mRNA after chronic ethanol administration suggests that the reduction in the function of the GABA_A receptor complex may be associated with an alteration in transcription of GABA_A receptor subunit genes or an alteration in α_1-subunit mRNA processing/turnover in the cerebral cortex. The functional significance of a specific reduction in α_1-subunit mRNAs is not known at present, but it is conceivable that such an alteration could result in (a) fewer "functionally available" $GABA_A$ receptor proteins, (b) functionally different $GABA_A$ isoreceptors, or (c) a population of desensitized or non-functional receptors.

The lack of alteration in the levels of $GABA_A$ receptor α_1-subunit mRNA after chronic pentobarbital administration does not rule out the possibility that chronic barbiturate administration alters $GABA_A$ receptor transcription or mRNA processing/turnover. We have shown that several other α-subunit mRNA transcripts are expressed in rat cerebral cortex and are detectable by Northern analysis (Montpied et al. 1988). The levels of these mRNAs were not studied in the present set of experiments. Furthermore, there are other $GABA_A$ receptor protein subunits that have been recently identified and whose expression may be modified by pentobarbital administration.

The mechanisms that underlie the effects of repeated ethanol administration on the levels of α-subunit mRNA in the brain are unknown. However, we have recently shown that exposure of cultured chick brain neurons to GABA for several days results in a marked reduction in the cellular level of α_1-subunit mRNA. This effect was concentration-dependent and receptor-mediated (Montpied et al., submitted). Conceivably, ethanol-induced potentiation of GABA receptor-mediated Cl^- conductance could augment the tonic inhibition of receptor gene expression induced by GABA.

Recent studies on the expression of the various subunits of the $GABA_A$ receptor complex have demonstrated that different combinations of $GABA_A$ receptor subunits produce receptors with different gating properties (Blair et al., 1988; Levitan et al., 1988; Pritchett et al., 1989a; Pritchett et al., 1989b). Our studies on the effects of ethanol and pentobarbital on the expression of $GABA_A$ receptor α_1 subunit mRNAs represent only the initial step toward understanding whether any alteration in the structural properties of $GABA_A$ receptors in brain result from repeated ethanol or pentobarbital administration. Clearly, further studies will be required to confirm the hypotheses that repeated ethanol or pentobarbital administration alters the expression of $GABA_A$ receptors in the central nervous system.

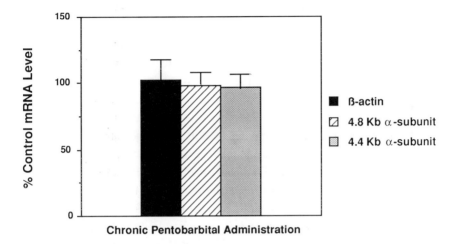

Figure 10. Repeated pentobarbital administration (30-90mg/kg/day for 2 weeks) does not alter the level of GABA$_A$ receptor α_1-subunit mRNA in the rat cerebral cortex. Total RNA was processed and northern blots were analysed as described in Fig. 9. There was no effect of pentobarbital administration on the levels of the 4.8-Kb or the 4.4-Kb species of GABA$_A$ receptor α-subunit mRNA. β-actin mRNA levels were not altered after repeated pentobarbital administration. Adapted from Morrow et al. (1990): Chronic ethanol and pentobarbital administration in the rat: effects on GABA$_A$ receptor function and expression in brain. *Alcohol* 7:237-244.

CONCLUDING REMARKS

Ethanol is one of man's oldest and most commonly used psychoactive drugs. The exact neurochemical mechanisms mediating its myriad pharmacologic actions are still under investigation. Although it is generally accepted that many of the pharmacologic actions of ethanol result from relatively nonspecific interactions with biological membranes, there is increasing evidence that at least some of ethanol's effects may be due to specific actions on defined neurotransmitter systems. For example, it now seems apparent that the relatively "nonspecific" membrane effects of ethanol appear to result in rather specific effects on ligand-gated ion channels, including the GABA receptor-gated Cl$^-$ channel. The actions of ethanol at GABA receptor-gated chloride ion channels are blocked selectively by the imidazobenzodiazepine inverse agonist Ro15-4513. Indeed, these same nonspecific membrane effects of short chain alcohols can result in specific alterations in the conformation of other receptor proteins such as those coupled to adenylate cyclase and comprising other ion channels, including excitatory amino acid receptor-coupled calcium channels. Thus, ethanol has been shown to affect N-Methyl D-Aspartic Acid (NMDA) (Hoffman et al., 1989; Lima-Landman and Albuquerque, 1989; Lovinger et al., 1989) and adenylate cyclase-linked (Mochly-Rosen et al., 1988; Nagy et al., 1988) receptor systems at pharmacologically relevant concentrations. Although the role of these systems in mediating the behavioral effects of ethanol is unclear at this time, the simultaneous activation and/or inhibition of ethanol-sensitive neurochemical systems [e.g. augmentation of inhibitory (GABA-mediated) and inhibition of excitatory (NMDA-mediated) synaptic events] in the CNS probably underly many ethanol-induced behaviors. It is conceivable, therefore, that among the myriad of neurochemical actions of ethanol, several neurotransmitter systems will emerge as being relevant to explain the important pharmacological properties of this drug.

ACKNOWLEDGMENTS

The authors acknowledge Dr. Peter Suzdak (Novo Industries, Bagsvaerd, Denmark) for collaboration with the chloride flux experiments, Dr. John W. Karanian (NIAAA) for collaboration with the ethanol inhalation studies, Dr. Ann Lingford-Hughes for collaboration with the chronic pentobarbital experiments and Drs. Edward I. Ginns and Brian M. Martin (NIMH) for isolation of the cDNA clones used to synthesize the GABA$_A$ receptor α-subunit riboprobe.

REFERENCES

Allan AM, Harris RA (1986): Gamma-aminobutyric acid and alcohol actions: neurochemical studies of long sleep and short sleep mice. *Life Sci* 39:2005-2015

Allan AM, Harris RA (1987): Acute and chronic ethanol treatments alter GABA receptor-operated chloride channels. *Pharmacol Biochem Behav* 27:665-670

Bixler MA, Lewis MJ (1987): The partial inverse benzodiazepine agonist Ro15-4513 potentiates ethanol induced suppression of wheel-running in the rat. *Neurosci Abstr* 13:967

Blair LAC, Levitan ES, Marshall J, Dionne VE, Barnard EA (1988): Single subunits of the GABA$_A$ receptor form ion channels with properties of the native receptor. *Science* 242:577-579

Boisse NN, Okamoto M (1980): Ethanol as a sedative-hypnotic: comparison with barbiturate and non-barbiturate sedative-hypnotics. In: *Alcohol Tolerance and Dependence*. Rigter H, Crabbe JC, eds. Amsterdam: Elsevier, pp 265-292

Bonetti EP, Burkard WP, Gabl M (1985): A partial inverse benzodiazepine agonist Ro15-4513 antagonizes acute ethanol effects in mice and rats. *Br J Pharmacol* 86:463P

Britton KT, Ehlers CL, Koob GF (1988): Is ethanol antagonist Ro15-4513 selective for ethanol? *Science* 239:648-649

Celentano JJ, Gibbs TT, Farb DH (1988): Ethanol potentiates GABA- and glycine-induced chloride currents in chick spinal cord neurons. *Brain Res* 455:377-380

Cott J, Carlsson J, Engel JA, Lindqvist S (1976): Suppression of ethanol-induced motor stimulation by GABA-like drugs. *Arch. Pharmacol* 297:203-209

Davidoff RA (1973): Alcohol and presynaptic inhibition in a isolated spinal cord preparation. *Arch Neurol* 28:60-63

Davis WC, Ticku MK (1981): Ethanol enhances [^{3}H]diazepam binding at the benzodiazepine-GABA receptor ionophore complex. *Mol Pharmacol* 20:287

deVries DJ, Johnston GAR, Ward LC, Wilce PA, Shanley BC (1987): Effects of chronic ethanol inhalation on the enhancement of benzodiazepine binding to mouse brain membranes by GABA. *Neurochem Intl* 10:231-235

Fadda F, Mosca E, Colombo G, Gessa GL (1987): Protection against ethanol mortality in rats by the imidazobenzodiazepine Ro15-4513. *Eur J Pharmacol* 136:265-266

Glowa JR, Barrett JE (1976): Effects of alcohol on punished and unpunished responding. *Pharmacol Biochem Behav* 4:169-174

Goldstein DB (1978): Alcohol withdrawal reactions in mice: effects of drugs that modify neurotransmission. *J Pharmacol Exp Ther* 186:1

Goldstein DB, Chin JH, McComb JA, Parsons LM (1980): Chronic effects of alcohols on mouse biomembranes. *Adv Exp Med Biol* 126:1-5

Goldstein DB, Pal N (1971): Alcohol dependence produced in mice by inhalation of ethanol: grading the withdrawal reaction. *Science* 172:288-290

Gonzalez LP, Czachura JF (1989): Reduced behavioral responses to intranigral muscimol following chronic ethanol. *Physiol Behav* 46:473-477

Greenberg DB, Cooper EC, Gordon A, Diamond I (1984): Ethanol and the GABA-benzodiazepine receptor complex. *J Neurochem* 42:1062-1068

Harrison NL, Majewska MD, Harrington JW, Barker JL (1987): Structure-activity relationships for steroid interaction with the gamma-aminobutyric acid-A receptor complex. *J Pharmacol Exp Ther* 241:346-353

Hoffman PL, Rabe CS, Moses F, Tabakoff B (1989): N-methyl-D-aspartate receptors and ethanol: inhibition of calcium flux and cyclic GMP production. *J Neurochem* 52:1937-1940

Hoffman PL, Tabakoff B, Szabo G, Suzdak PD, Paul SM (1987): Effect of an imidazobenzodiazepine, Ro15-4513, on the incoordination and hypothermia produced by ethanol and pentobarbital. *Life Sci* 41:611-619

Hunt WA (1983): The effect of ethanol on GABAergic transmission. *Neurosci Biobehav Rev* 7:87-95

Johnson DA, Lee NM, Cooke R, Loh H (1980): Adaptation to ethanol-induced fluidization of brain lipid bilayers: cross tolerance and reversibility. *Mol Pharmacol* 17:52-55

Johnson HT, June HL, Lewis MJ (1987): The effects of Ro15-4513 on generalized motor activity. *Neurosci Abstr* 13:967

Karanian JW, Yergey J, Lister R, D'Souza N, Linnoila M, Salem N (1986): Characterization of an automated apparatus for precise control of inhalation chamber ethanol vapor and blood ethanol concentrations. *Alcohol Clin Exp Res* 10:443-447

Koob GF, Braestrup C, Britton KT (1986): The effects of FG 7142 and Ro15-1788 on the release of punished responding produced by chlordiazepoxide and ethanol in the rat. *Psychopharmacology* 90:173-178

Koob GF, Percy L, Britton KT (1988): The effects of Ro15-4513 on the behavioral actions of ethanol in an operant reaction time test and a conflict test. *Pharmacol Biochem Behav* 31:757-760

Koob GF, Strecker RE, Bloom F (1980): Effects of naloxone on the anticonflict properties of alcohol and chlordiazepoxide. *Alcohol Actions Misuse* 1:447-457

Le AD, Khanna JM, Kalant H, Grossi F (1986): Tolerance to and cross-tolerance among ethanol pentobarbital and chlordiazepoxide. *Pharmacol Biochem Behav* 24:93-98

Levitan ES, Schofield PR, Burt DR, Rhee LM, Wisden W, Kohler M, Fujita N, Rodriguez HF, Stephenson FA, Darlison MG, Barnard EA, Seeburg PH (1988): Structural and functional basis for GABA receptor heterogeneity. *Nature* 335:76-79

Liljequist S, Engel JA (1982): Effects of GABAergic agonists and antagonists on various ethanol-induced behavioral changes. *Psychopharmacology* 78:71-75

Liljequist S, Engel, JA (1984): The effects of GABA and benzodiazepine receptor antagonists on the anti-conflict action of diazepam or ethanol. *Pharmacol Biochem Behav* 21:521-526

Lima-Landman MT, Albuquerque EX (1989): Ethanol potentiates and blocks NMDA-activated single-channel currents in hippocampal pyramidal cells. *FEBS Lett* 247:61-67

Lister RG (1987): The benzodiazepine receptor inverse agonists FG 7142 and Ro15-4513 both reverse some of the behavioral effects of ethanol in a hole-board test. *Life Sci* 41:1481-1489

Lister RG (1988): Interactions of ethanol with benzodiazepine receptor ligands in tests of exploration, locomotion and anxiety. *Pharmacol Biochem Behav* 31:761-765

Lister RG, Durcan MJ (1989): Antagonism of the intoxicating effects of ethanol by the potent benzodiazepine receptor ligand Ro19-4603. *Brain Res.* 482: 141-144

Lister RG, Karanian JW (1987): Ro15-4513 induces seizures in DBA/2 mice undergoing ethanol withdrawal. *Alcohol* 4:409-411

Lister RG, Nutt DJ (1988): Interactions of the imidazobenzodiazepine Ro15-4513 with chemical convulsants. *Br J Pharmacol* 93:210-214

Lovinger DM, White G, Weight FF (1989): Ethanol inhibits NMDA-activated ion currents in hippocampal neurons. *Science* 243:1721-1724

Majchrowicz E (1975): Induction of physical dependence upon ethanol and the associated behavioral changes. *Psychopharmacologia* 43:245-254

Mancillas JR, Siggins JR, Bloom FE (1986): Systemic ethanol: enhancement of responses to acetylcholine and somatostatin in hippocampus. *Science* 231:161-163

Marrosu F, Carcangui G, Passino N, Aramo S, Mereu G (1989): Antagonism of ethanol effects by Ro15-4513: an electrophysiological analysis. *Synapse* 3:117-128

McBride WJ, Murphy JM, Lumeng L, Li TK (1988): Effects of Ro15-4513, fluoxetine and desipramine on intake of ethanol water and food in alcohol preferring and non-preferring lines of rats. *Pharmacol Biochem Behav* 30:1045-1050

McCreery MJ, Hunt WA (1978): Physiochemical correlates of alcohol intoxication. *Neuropharmacology* 17:451-461

Mehta G, Ticku MK (1988): Ethanol potentiation of GABAergic transmission in cultured spinal cord neurons involves γ-aminobutyric acid-gated chloride channels. *J Pharmacol Exp Ther* 246:558

Mereu G, Gessa GL (1985): Low doses of ethanol inhibit the firing of neurons in the substantia nigra pars reticulata: a GABAergic effect? *Brain Res* 360:325-330

Miscek KA, Weerts EM (1987): Seizures in drug treated animals. *Science* 235:1127-1128

Mochly-Rosen D, Chang FH, Cheever L, Kim M, Diamond I, Gordon AS (1988): Chronic ethanol causes heterologous desensitization of receptors by reducing alpha s messenger RNA. *Nature* 333:848-850

Montpied P, Ginns EI, Martin BM, Stetler D, O'Carroll A-M, Lolait SJ, Mahan LC, Paul SM (1989): Multiple GABA$_A$ receptor α-subunit mRNAs revealed by developmental and regional expression in rat, chicken and human brain. *FEBS Lett* 258:94-98

Montpied P, Martin BM, Cottingham SL, Stubblefield BK, Ginns EI, Paul SM (1988): Regional distribution of the GABA$_A$/benzodiazepine receptor (α-subunit) mRNA in rat brain. *J Neurochem* 51:1651-1654

Morrow AL, Montpied P, Lingford-Hughes A, Paul SM (1990): Chronic ethanol and pentobarbital administration in the rat: effects on GABA$_A$ receptor function and expression in brain. *Alcohol* 7:237-244

Morrow AL, Paul SM (1988): Benzodiazepine enhancement of γ-aminobutyric acid mediated Cl^- ion flux in rat brain synaptoneurosomes. *J Neurochem* 50:302-306

Morrow, AL, Suzdak, PD, Karanian JR, Paul SM (1988a): Chronic ethanol administration alters γ-aminobutyric acid, pentobarbital and ethanol-mediated $^{36}Cl^-$ uptake in cerebral cortical synaptoneurosomes. *J Pharmacol Exp Ther* 246:158-164

Morrow AL, Suzdak PD, Paul SM (1988b): Benzodiazepine, barbiturate, ethanol and hypnotic steroid hormone modulation of GABA-mediated chloride ion transport in rat brain synaptoneurosomes. In: *Chloride Channels and Their Modulation by Neurotransmitters and Drugs*. Biggio G, Costa E, eds. New York: Raven Press pp 247-261

Nagy LE, Diamond I, Gordon A (1988): Cultured lymphocytes from alcoholic subjects have altered cAMP signal transduction. *Proc Natl Acad Sci USA* 85:6973-6976

Nestores JN (1980): Ethanol specifically potentiates GABA-mediated neurotransmission in the feline cerebral cortex. *Science* 209:708-710

Nutt DJ, Lister RG (1987): The effect of the imidazobenzodiazepine Ro15-4513 on the anti-convulsant effects of diazepam, sodium pentobarbital and ethanol. *Brain Res* 413:193-196

Nutt DJ, Lister RG, Rusche D, Bonetti EP, Reese RE, Rufener R (1988): Ro15-4513 does not protect against the lethal effects of ethanol. *Eur J Pharmacol* 151:127-129

Olsen RW (1982): Drug interactions at the GABA receptor ionophore complex. *Ann Rev Pharmacol Toxicol* 22:245

Palmer MR, van Horne CG, Harlan JT, Moore EA (1988): Antagonism of ethanol effects on cerebellar purkinje neurons by the benzodiazepine inverse agonists Ro15-4513 and FG 7142: electrophysiological studies. *J Pharmacol Exp Ther* 247:1018-1024

Polc P (1985): Interactions of partial inverse agonists Ro15-4513 and FG-7142 with ethanol in rats and cats. *Br J Pharmacol* 86:465P

Pritchett DB, Luddens H, Seeburg PH (1989a): Type I and type II GABA$_A$-benzodiazepine receptors produced in transfected cells. *Science* 245:1389-1392

Pritchett DB, Sontheimer H, Shivers BD, Ymer S, Kettenmann H, Schofield PR, Seeburg PH (1989b): Importance of a novel GABA$_A$ receptor subunit for benzodiazepine pharmacology. *Nature* 338:582-585

Rastogi SK, Thyagarajan R, Clothier J, Ticku MK (1986): Effect of chronic treatment of ethanol on benzodiazepine and picrotoxin sites on the GABA receptor complex in regions of the brain of the rat. *Neuropharmacology* 25:1179-1184

Rees DC, Balster RL (1988): Attenuation of the discriminitive stimulus properties of ethanol and oxazepam, but not pentobarbital, by Ro15-4513 in mice. *J Pharmacol Exp Ther* 244:592-598

Rottenberg H, Waring A, Rubin E (1981): Tolerance and cross-tolerance in chronic alcoholics: reduced membrane binding of ethanol and other drugs. *Science* 213:583-584

Samson HH, Tolliver GA, Pfeffer AU, Sadeghi KG, Mills FG (1987): Oral ethanol reinforcement in the rat: effect of the partial inverse benzodiazepine agonist Ro15-4513. *Pharmacol Biochem Behav* 27:517-519

Schwartz RD, Suzdak PD, Paul SM (1989): γ-aminobutyric acid (GABA) and barbiturate receptor-mediated $^{36}Cl^-$ uptake in rat brain synaptoneurosomes: evidence for rapid desensitization of the GABA receptor-coupled chloride ion channel. *Mol Pharmacol* 30:419-426

Seeman P (1972): The membrane actions of anesthetics and tranquilizers. *Pharmacol Rev* 24:583-655

Sellers EM, Kalant H (1976): Alcohol intoxication and withdrawal. *N Eng J Med* 294:757-760

Skolnick P, Paul SM (1982): Molecular pharmacology of the benzodiazepines. *Intl Rev Neurobiol* 23:103-140

Suzdak PD, Glowa JR, Crawley JN, Schwartz RD, Skolnick P, Paul SM (1986b): A selective imidazobenzodiazepine antagonist of ethanol in the rat. *Science* 234:1243-1247

Suzdak PD, Glowa JR, Crawley JN, Skolnick P, Paul SM (1988b): Is ethanol antagonist Ro15-4513 selective for ethanol? Response to K.T. Britton et al. *Science* 239:649-650

Suzdak PD, Paul SM, Crawley JN (1988a): Effects of Ro15-4513 and other benzodiazepine inverse agonists on alcohol induced intoxication in the rat. *J Pharmacol Exp Ther* 245:880-886

Suzdak PD, Schwartz RD, Skolnick P, Paul SM (1986a): Ethanol stimulates γ-aminobutyric acid receptor-mediated chloride transport in rat brain synaptoneurosomes. *Proc Natl Acad Sci (USA)* 83:4071

Suzdak PD, Schwartz RD, Paul SM (1987): Alcohols stimulate GABA receptor-mediated chloride uptake in brain vesicles: correlation with intoxication potency. *Brain Res* 444:340-344

Taraschi TF, Ellinsson JS, Wu A (1986): Membrane tolerance to ethanol is rapidly lost after withdrawal: a model for studies of membrane adaptation. *Proc Natl Acad Sci (USA)* 83:3669-3673

Thyagarajan R, Ticku MK (1985): The effect of in vitro and in vivo ethanol administration on [^{35}S]t-butylbicyclophosphorothionate binding in C57 mice. *Brain Res Bull* 15:343-345

Ticku MK, Burch T (1980): Alterations in γ-aminobutyric acid receptor sensitivity following acute and chronic ethanol treatments. *J Neurochem* 34:417-423

Ticku MK, Lorimore P, Lehoullier P (1986): Ethanol enhances GABA-induced ^{36}Cl^{-} flux in primary spinal cord cultured neurons. *Brain Res Bull* 17:123-126

Vogel JR, Beer B, Clody DE (1971): A simple and reliable conflict procedure for testing anti-anxiety agents. *Psychopharmacologia* 21:1-7

Volicer L (1980): GABA levels and receptor binding after acute and chronic ethanol administration. *Brain Res Bull* 5:809-813

Volicer L, Biagioni TM (1982): Effect of ethanol administration and withdrawal on benzodiazepine receptor binding in the rat brain. *Neuropharmacology* 21:283-286

Volicer L, Biagioni TM (1982): Effect of ethanol administration and withdrawal on GABA receptor binding in rat cerebral cortex. *Alcohol Actions-Misuse* 3:31-39

Wisden W, Morris BJ, Darlison MG, Hunt SP, Barnard EA (1988): Distinct GABA$_A$ α-subunit mRNAs show differential patterns of expression in bovine brain. *Neuron* 1:937-947

The GABA$_A$ Receptor Complex: Is it a Locus of Action for Inhalation Anesthetics?

Eric J. Moody, Herman J.C. Yeh and Phil Skolnick

The mechanism(s) by which chemically diverse compounds produce general anesthesia (i.e., reversible unconsciousness) remains one of the enigmas of modern pharmacology despite intensive investigation for almost a century. While the structural diversity of general anesthetics (which range from barbiturates, alcohols and steroids to gases) has complicated the search for a common target site, the physical characteristics (high vapor pressure, low solubility in aqueous media and low potency) of commonly used inhalation agents such as halothane renders many pharmacological, neurochemical and electrophysiological approaches problematic.

The independent observations of Meyer (1905) and Overton (1901) that the lipid solubilities of a series of structurally diverse anesthetics were highly correlated with their anesthetic potencies provide compelling evidence that lipids are a target of anesthetic action. Many current theories of anesthetic action are based on lipid components of neural membranes as putative targets. Such lipid based theories incorporate the concept of anesthetics producing a physical change in the neural membrane environment such as an alteration in membrane fluidity, thickness or tension (Haydon et al., 1977) or a critical volume of anesthetic in the membrane (Miller, 1985) resulting in disruption of neural transmission. Many of the measured physical changes in membranes induced by anesthetics are small, and there is no satisfactory explanation of how these physical interactions between the anesthetic and membrane lipids produce anesthesia. The issue of whether lipids represent a viable target for anesthetic action remains a topic of considerable debate (Elliott 1988; Franks and Lieb, 1987; Miller, 1985; Scholfield 1988). However, a cogent demonstration of the difficulties associated with a lipid target has been presented by

Franks and Lieb (1987). Using a simple calculation based on the concentration of halothane (0.3 mM) corresponding to the ED_{50}, these authors estimate a concentration of 25 mM in the lipids of a typical plasma membrane (assuming a partition coefficient of 37 and assuming no significant binding to membrane proteins). Under these conditions, Franks and Lieb estimate the ratio of halothane to lipid molecules would approach 1:80! If this estimate even closely approximates the situation *in vivo*, it would certainly be consistent with the modest changes in membrane characteristics produced by anesthetics, particularly if the lipid bilayer is already in a disordered fluid state, and make lipids an inefficient (and unlikely) target of anesthetic action.

More recent work has provided perhaps equally compelling evidence that membrane proteins are the primary targets of anesthetics. Thus, Franks and Lieb have demonstrated that the potencies of a series of chemically diverse anesthetics to inhibit the activity of a purified (lipid free) firefly luciferase are highly correlated with their anesthetic potencies (Franks and Lieb, 1984, 1986, 1987). This correlation is similar to that obtained when lipid solubilities were correlated with anesthetic potencies over a similar (5 orders of magnitude) concentration range. These findings stimulated studies examining the effect of general anesthetics on transmembrane proteins such as ion channels, since there is a general consensus that they represent the ultimate targets of anesthetic action. This chapter summarizes some recent work from our laboratory demonstrating that general anesthetics, and in particular inhalation agents, can perturb the chloride ionophore associated with the $GABA_A$ receptor complex.

γ-aminobutyric acid (GABA) is the principal inhibitory transmitter in the mammalian central nervous system. It has been estimated that one third of all synapses utilize GABA as a transmitter substance. Application of GABA or GABAmimetics can hyperpolarize sensitive neurones, resulting in a reduced rate of firing. GABA affects this hyperpolarization by regulating ("gating") the opening of a population of ion channels exhibiting a high degree of specificity toward monovalent anions. The oligomeric group of proteins that constitute this GABA-gated anion (chloride) channel possesses recognition sites (receptors) for GABA as well as for many substances that are generically classified as depressants, such as benzodiazepines and barbiturates (see Skolnick and Paul, 1988 for review). The amino acid sequences of several of the constituent proteins of this "supramolecular complex" have recently been elucidated (Levitan et al., 1988; Pritchett et al., 1989; Schofield et al., 1987, 1989). While the stoichiometry and arrangement of these subunits to form a fully functional channel is still under investigation (cf. Pritchett et al., 1989; Schofield et al., 1987), this receptor complex appears to be a member of a superfamily of transmitter-gated ion channel that includes the nicotinic acetylcholine receptor and the glycine receptor (Stevens, 1987).

Electrophysiological and biochemical data accumulated during the past decade strongly indicates that pharmacologically relevant concentrations of anesthetics such as barbiturates and steroids affect GABAergic transmission (reviewed in Keane and Biziere, 1987). Other findings such as the observations that cross tolerance exists between various classes of anesthetics, including inhalation agents, also supports a role for the GABA$_A$ receptor complex in anesthesia. For example, tolerance to ethanol is associated with an increased requirement for general anesthetics in both animals and man (Johnstone et al., 1975; Koblin et al., 1980). In addition, animals tolerant to ethanol exhibit cross tolerance to barbiturate anesthesia (Curran et al., 1988). The cross tolerance between ethanol (which is thought to exert some of its pharmacological effects at the GABA$_A$ receptor complex) and other general anesthetics suggests a common mechanism of action.

A biochemical technique that has been successfully applied to the study of agents that affect the GABA$_A$ receptor complex is the measurement of Cl^- flux in synaptoneurosomes (Hollingsworth et al., 1985). Synaptoneurosomes release (if preloaded) or take up ^{36}chloride ($^{36}Cl^-$) in response to pharmacologically relevant concentrations of substances that perturb the GABA$_A$ receptor complex including barbiturates, GABA and GABAmimetics, anesthetic steroids and alcohols (Cash and Subbarao, 1987; Majeweska et al., 1986; Schwartz et al., 1985, 1986; Suzdak et al., 1986a,b, 1988). Moreover, using this preparation, Schwartz et al. (1985) have demonstrated that the ability of a series of anesthetic barbiturates to stimulate chloride flux from this preparation was highly correlated with anesthetic potency. We examined the effect of inhalation anesthetics such as ether, enflurane and halothane on chloride uptake in synaptoneurosomes (Moody et al., 1988). Inhalation anesthetics directly increase ^{36}chloride influx into synaptoneurosomes in a concentration dependent manner (Fig. 1) at concentrations within the therapeutic range. The increases in $^{36}Cl^-$ uptake elicited by volatile anesthetics are reduced to near baseline by the "cage" convulsant picrotoxin, which has been shown to block GABA-gated chloride channels (Akaike et al., 1985). However, even within this limited framework, inhalation agents differ from non-volatile anesthetics such as barbiturates and steroids in several respects. For example, in our hands they appear to inhibit rather than augment muscimol (a GABAmimetic)-stimulated $^{36}Cl^-$ uptake, and they fail to enhance the binding of radiolabeled benzodiazepines. Moreover, their efficacies (maximum increase in Cl^- uptake) are lower than observed with barbiturates, anesthetic steroids and ethanol (Majewska et al., 1986; Moody et al., 1988; Suzdak et al., 1986a,b). However, using a slightly different cellular preparation (in which neither barbiturates nor alcohols have been reported to directly increase $^{36}Cl^-$ uptake), Huidobro-Toro et al. (1987) have reported that inhalation agents like ether can augment muscimol-stimulated Cl^- uptake.

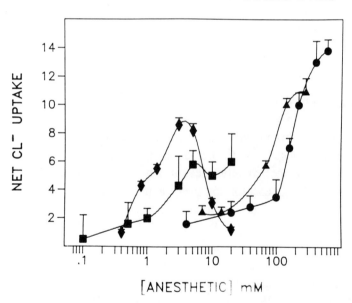

Figure 1. General anesthetics stimulate chloride uptake in rat cortical synapto-neurosomes. Data are from Moody et al. (1988). Net Cl^- uptake is expressed in nmol/mg protein/5 sec and represents the effect of the drug alone. Values represent a quadruplicate determination of a representative experiment. Circles, ether; squares, enflurane; triangles, urethane; diamonds, halothane.

The effects of volatile anesthetics on the binding of [^{35}S]t-butyl-bicyclophosphorothionate (TBPS) to the GABA$_A$ receptor complex in rat cerebral cortical membranes were also examined. This "cage" con-vulsant is structurally related to picrotoxin, and binds with high affinity to sites on or near the chloride ionophore (Havoundjian et al., 1986; Squires et al., 1983) that are functionally coupled to but distinct from receptors for GABA or benzodiazepines (Lewin et al., 1989). Inhalation anesthetics such as methoxyflurane, enflurane, and halothane, as well as other general anesthetics such as pentobarbital and chloralose inhibit [^{35}S]TBPS binding in a concentration dependent manner (Huidobro-Toro et al., 1987; Moody et al., 1988) within their therapeutic ranges. Further-more, a good correlation is obtained between the potencies of these agents to inhibit [^{35}S]TBPS binding and their anesthetic potencies (Fig. 2). Al-though these data indicate that the GABA-gated chloride channel could represent a common locus of action for a diverse series of volatile and nonvolatile anesthetics, these agents do not appear to inhibit [^{35}S]TBPS binding through a common mechanism. Thus, some anesthetics like

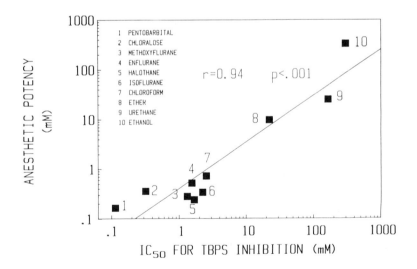

Figure 2. Inhibition of [^{35}S]TBPS binding by general anesthetics: correlation with anesthetic potency. Data is from Moody et al. (1988). [^{35}S]TBPS binding was determined in well washed rat cortical membranes. Note that the values are plotted on log scales.

ether (Moody et al., 1988) and chlormethiazole (Moody and Skolnick, 1989) decrease the apparent affinity of [^{35}S]TBPS while others like pentobarbital (Moody and Skolnick, 1989; Ramanjaneyulu and Ticku, 1984) effect a reduction in the maximum number of binding sites. Anesthetic steroids (Majewska et al., 1986) appear to reduce both the apparent affinity and number of [^{35}S]TBPS binding sites.

In a related series of experiments, we examined the abilities of a series of anesthetic n-alcohols to inhibit [^{35}S]TBPS binding to rat cerebral cortical membranes. These experiments were performed to determine whether a "cut-off" effect could be observed with these n-alcohols. The cut-off effect is the observation that the anesthetic potencies of a series of both alkanes and alkanols (alcohols) (Pringle et al., 1981) increase with chain length, followed by an abrupt loss in anesthetic activity between tri- and tetradecanol (Alifimoff et al., 1989; Pringle et al., 1981), depending on the animal model and experimental procedures employed. The cut-off phenomenon has been invoked (Franks and Lieb, 1986) to support a protein target of anesthesia, since lipid solubility should continue to increase with chain length, although this line of reasoning has been questioned (Alifimoff et al., 1989; Janoff and Miller, 1982; Pringle et al., 1981). We observed (Fig. 3) that the potencies of n-alcohols to inhibit [^{35}S]TBPS binding increased with increasing chain length. When $C > 10$, their potencies decreased and at $C > 12$, these n-alcohols were not sufficiently potent to effect a complete inhibition of [^{35}S]TBPS binding, even at supersaturated concentrations. When the potencies of these n-alcohols to inhibit [^{35}S]TBPS binding were compared with their anesthetic potencies (using loss of righting reflex in tadpoles as an endpoint) (Alifimoff et al., 1989), an excellent correlation ($r = .94$; $p < .001$) was obtained.

These data indicate that the GABA$_A$ receptor complex could mediate the anesthetic actions of n-alcohols. Moreover, these findings are also consistent with the reports that pharmacologically relevant concentrations of ethanol as well as short and branched chain alcohols increase $^{36}Cl^-$ uptake in synaptoneurosomes and potentiate the effects of both muscimol and barbiturates in this regard (Suzdak et al., 1986a, 1988).

The demonstration that inhalation anesthetics enhance chloride uptake at GABA-gated chloride channels and inhibit [^{35}S]TBPS binding

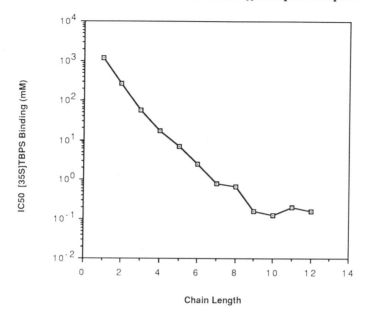

Figure 3. Inhibition of [^{35}S]TBPS binding by n-alcohols exhibits the "cut-off" effect. [^{35}S]TBPS binding was determined in well washed rat cortical membranes as described in Moody et al., 1988. IC_{50} values represent the mean of at least three experiments. The potency of the alcohols to inhibit [^{35}S]TBPS binding increased with chain lengths up to 10 carbons. The potency of longer chain alcohols did not increase potency, and alcohols with C>13 did not completely inhibit [^{35}S]TBPS binding, even at supersaturated concentrations. The potencies of these compounds to inhibit [^{35}S]TBPS binding was significantly correlated with their anesthetic potencies (Alifimoff et al., 1988) (r = .94, p<.001).

indicate some similarity of actions to ethanol and other short chain alcohols (Suzdak et al., 1986a, 1988). These findings, together with the demonstration of a cut-off effect of n-alcohols at the GABA_A receptor complex prompted us to examine the effects of Ro15-4513 on the anesthetic properties of an inhalation agent. Ro15-4513 is a specific, high affinity ligand for benzodiazepine receptors (Sieghart et al., 1987) that has been reported to antagonize some of the biochemical, electrophysiological and pharmacological actions of alcohol (recently reviewed in Harris and Lal, 1988).

In these experiments, groups of 12 mice were placed in a 7-liter chamber filled with oxygen and anesthetized with the inhalational agent methoxyflurane (3.2% in oxygen for 30 minutes at a flow rate of 1 liter/minute). The animals were then removed from the chamber and immediately injected with drug(s) or vehicle. The mice were then placed on their backs in room air, and the time required to regain the righting reflex was determined (Moody and Skolnick, 1988). In this paradigm, Ro15-4513 (4-32 mg/kg) produced a dose-dependent reduction in the time required to regain the righting reflex, with a maximum ~40% reduction in sleep time at 16 mg/kg (Fig. 4). Other investigators have reported similar effects of Ro15-4513 using different experimental conditions. In tadpoles, Keck et al. (1988) demonstrated that Ro15-4513 antagonized the loss of righting reflex induced by alcohols and inhalation agents. Using rats Tessel et al. (1987), showed that Ro15-4513 could partially antagonize methoxyflurane-induced sleep.

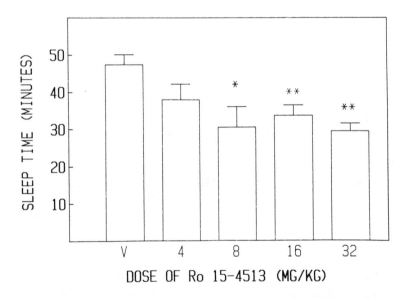

Figure 4. The imidazobenzodiazepine Ro15-4513 antagonizes methoxyflurane anesthesia. Data are from Moody and Skolnick (1988). Groups of mice were anesthetized with 3.2% methoxyflurane for 30 min and then placed in room air, injected with drug and the recovery time for regaining righting reflex was measured. Values represent the mean ±SEM of groups of at least 12 animals. Ro15-4513 produced a significant [ANOVA $p < .0001$] decrease in methoxyflurane sleep time. Symbols * $p < .05$; ** $p < .01$ (Scheffe's test) relative to vehicle treated group.

It is possible that even more robust effects of Ro15-4513 could be obtained by either reducing the depth of anesthesia or administering multiple injections of Ro15-4513. The reductions in methoxyflurane-induced sleep time elicited by Ro15-4513 could be blocked by administration of the benzodiazepine receptor antagonist Ro15-1788 (flumazenil) at a dose (16 mg/kg) that did not affect anesthesia when administered alone (Moody and Skolnick, 1988). These effects strongly indicate that the reduction in methoxyflurane-induced sleep time by Ro15-4513 is mediated at benzodiazepine receptors (Schweri et al., 1982), and lends support to the hypothesis that inhalation anesthetics mediate some of their actions at the GABA$_A$ receptor complex.

Ro15-4513 has properties characteristic of a benzodiazepine receptor "partial inverse agonist" (reviewed in Harris and Lal, 1988). It is this profile [proconvulsant (convulsant under certain conditions in primates) and anxiogenic effects presumably mediated through a reduction in GABA-gated chloride movement] that has resulted in controversy over the "selectivity" of Ro15-4513 in reversing some of the pharmacological and toxicological (e.g., anticonflict and intoxicant) properties of ethanol (Suzdak et al., 1986b), or in the present situation, methoxyflurane. While these issues are clearly beyond the scope of this chapter, they have recently been reviewed in detail (Harris and Lal, 1988) and will also be discussed in other chapters of this book. Nonetheless, if other benzodiazepine receptor inverse agonists can also reverse a drug effect (e.g., methoxyflurane sleep time), the "selectivity" of Ro15-4513 must be questioned. We attempted to reverse methoxyflurane-induced sleep time with both a structurally unrelated benzodiazepine receptor partial inverse agonist (FG 7142) and a full inverse agonist (DMCM). At pharmacologically relevant doses, neither substance affected methoxyflurane sleep time, but both blocked the effect of Ro15-4513 on methoxyflurane-induced sleep time, which strongly supports the concept that this effect occurs at the benzodiazepine receptor. However, it should be noted that whereas Miller et al. (1989) have confirmed that intraperitoneal administration of Ro15-4513 antagonizes the duration of methoxyflurane-induced anesthesia, and that this effect is reversed by Ro15-1788, these investigators were also able to reduce the duration of anesthesia by intravenous administration of the benzodiazepine receptor inverse agonist 3-carboethoxy-β-carboline. These findings are at variance with our observation that neither a partial (FG 7142) nor a full (DMCM) inverse agonist mimicked the actions of Ro

15-4513. It should be noted that different species and routes of administration were employed in the two studies. Moreover, Miller et al. (1989) did not test the latter β-carbolines under their experimental conditions, which makes comparison and interpretation of both data sets problematic. However, if more rigorous testing demonstrates that the effect of Ro15-4513 on methoxyflurane-induced anesthesia cannot be mimicked by benzodiazepine receptor antagonists or inverse agonists, what is the mechanism of action? The ability of Ro15-1788, FG 7142 and DMCM to reverse Ro15-4513's effect on methoxyflurane-induced sleep time indicates that occupation of benzodiazepine receptors is necessary but not sufficient for this action. Ro15-4513 differs from Ro15-1788 by a linear, zwitterionic azido group substituted for a fluorine atom. If the anesthetic action of inhalation agents are mediated via the $GABA_A$ receptor complex, perturbation of lipids or a lipid/protein boundary by the azido group of Ro15-4513 could impart these unusual properties. This hypothesis is particularly attractive since the benzodiazepine receptor may be comprised of a domain formed by at least three distinct subunits (Pritchett et al., 1989). Rigorous testing of this hypothesis will require synthesis of other analogs with similar physicochemical and molecular characteristics.

In summary, the actions of many general anesthetics, including inhalation agents, may be mediated at the $GABA_A$ receptor complex. The effects of inhalation agents at the $GABA_A$ receptor complex mimic, in some respects, the neurochemical actions of other anesthetics such as barbiturates, alcohols, and steroids. Moveover, n-alcohols exhibit a cut-off effect on [^{35}S]TBPS binding at a similar chain length to that observed for anesthesia *in vivo*. Finally, Ro15-4513, which binds to benzodiazepine receptors with high affinity and specificity, reduces sleep time produced by an inhalation anesthetic.

The report (Evers et al., 1987) that pharmacologically relevant concentrations of halothane exhibit saturable binding in rat brain appears to be of potential significance in defining the molecular locus of anesthetic action. Using ^{19}F nuclear magnetic resonance spectroscopy (^{19}F NMR), these investigators reported saturable binding of halothane in the brains of rats exposed to halothane (an apparent saturation at 1.2 mM halothane was achieved with 2.5% inspired anesthetic). Moreover, these investigators reported a unique environment for halothane in brain characterized by a short spin-spin relaxation time (T_2=3.6 ms). In view of the evidence implicating the $GABA_A$ receptor complex in anesthetic action, we performed similar studies in brains and other tissues (red blood cells and liver) of rats exposed to halothane. Using similar methodologies, no evidence for saturable binding was obtained in brain, even at concentrations more than one order of magnitude higher than previously reported to saturate (Evers et al., 1987). Furthermore, the relatively short spin-spin relaxation time in brain, proposed to represent a unique saturable environment for halothane, was also present in other tissues such as red blood cells.

We found that halothane uptake in brain correlated with the concentration of inspired anesthetic. Brain halothane concentrations of 2.4 $\pm$ 0.2 mM were obtained in rats exposed to 4% (v/v) halothane for 60 min. (Fig. 5), in general agreement (brain halothane concentration of $\sim$ 1.6 mM at 2.5% inspired anesthetic and a T_2 of 3.6 msec) with the report of Evers et al. (1987). However, >95% of the halothane was present in the short T_2 environment (3.9 $\pm$ 0.2 msec), which showed no sign of saturability in rats exposed to limiting concentrations of anesthetic (4% inspired for 60 minutes). To further test the extent of halothane uptake in this environment, measurements were also made in brains equilibrated with buffer that had been saturated with halothane. Incubating the brains of anesthetized rats (original halothane concentration, 2.4 mM) with HEPES/Tris buffer equilibrated with halothane (11.5 mM) resulted in anesthetic concentrations of 17 $\pm$ 2.8 mM with >95% of the NMR signal in the short T_2 environment (Fig. 5). We have also extended these measurements to brains from unanesthetized rats equilibrated with various volumes of halothane-saturated buffer solution (Fig. 5, inset). In these experiments ^{19}F NMR spectra revealed a linear relationship between the apparent "brain concentrations" of halothane and the final concentrations of anesthetic in the resulting supernatants (Fig. 5, inset). Under these conditions, brain concentrations of up to 20 mM were achieved, with >95% of the signal in a short T_2 environment. Finally the T_2 relaxation times in red blood cells (RBC) from halothane anesthetized rats were examined. RBC pellets from rats inspiring 4% anesthetic for 60 minutes exhibited a T_2 of 3.0 $\pm$ 0.1 msec (halothane concentration, 2.6 $\pm$ 0.3 mM) comparable to brain, indicating this environment is not unique to brain (Fig. 5, legend). Similar findings were made in other peripheral tissues such as liver (data not shown). These results clearly demonstrate the initial report that halothane exhibits saturable binding in brain (Evers et al., 1987) is due solely to the self-limiting depressant effect of anesthetic.

While this manuscript was in press, Evers et al. (1989) also reported a lack of saturability using techniques like those described here. Nonetheless, these investigators maintain that the short T_2 may still have relevance to the anesthetic action of halothane. *In toto*, our data strongly suggest that although the presence of a highly immobilized environment for halothane in brain (and other tissues) may be of interest, it is unrelated to the anesthetic actions of halothane.

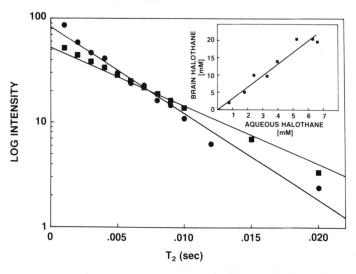

Figure 5. ^{19}F NMR spin-echo T_2 relaxation curves of halothane in brain. Male Sprague-Dawley rats (200-250 g) were anesthetized with 4% halothane for 1 hr. Rats were decapitated and cerebral cortex (from individual animals) was transferred to a gas-tight syringe fitted with an 18-gauge needle. The tissue was injected into 5-mm NMR tubes that had been calibrated to a volume of 0.5 ml. This volume of tissue was used in all subsequent studies. Sealed NMR coaxial inserts (Wilmad Glass Co., No. WGS-5BL) containing 60 μl of known concentrations of CF_3COOH containing a trace of Mn^{2+} in D_2O (for field/frequency lock) were inserted into the 5-mm NMR tubes to serve as an integration and chemical shift reference. In spin-echo T_2 experiments, a concentric capillary containing 60 μl of D_2O was used for field/frequency lock. The halothane concentration in brain was measured based on a 0.5 ml sample volume without any correction. ^{19}F NMR measurements (observed at 282.2 MHz without proton decoupling) were carried out at 22°C using a Varian XL-300 spectrometer equipped with a 5-mm probe. For determination of halothane concentrations in brain, the ^{19}F resonances of halothane and external reference (CF_3COOH) were taken using a 60° pulse and a delay time >5 T_1. The spin-echo experiments were carried out using the Carr-Purcell-Meiboom-Gill pulse sequence. Approximately 12 to 18 echo evolution times ranging from 0.0004 to 0.5sec were used in each experiment

and 64 to 512 transients were collected at each evolution time. In some experiments, mixed trunk blood from anesthetized rats was collected in NMR tubes. After centrifugation, spin-spin relaxation times were determined in 0.5 ml of the RBC pellet as described for cerebral cortex. Symbols: circles, cerebral cortex after inhalation of 4% halothane for 1 hr; squares, the same tissue after equilibration for 1 hr in the NMR tube with 1.5 ml of HEPES/TRIS buffer saturated with halothane (11.5 mM) followed by centrifugation (IEC Centrifuge, Model SBV; 700 rpm for 15 min) and removal of the supernatant. The halothane concentrations of brain tissues (0.5 ml) before and after equilibration with halothane saturated buffer were determined to be 2.5 and 20 mM, respectively. The logarithm of the ^{19}F-halothane signal (intensity in arbitrary units) is plotted as a function of echo evolution time. T_2 values were determined from these plots by fitting to a single exponential function, with >95% of the signal resolved in the short T_2 component. These results indicate that additional halothane can be taken up by the tissue, and this halothane predominantly exists in a short T_2 microenvironment even at brain halothane concentrations (20 mM) one order of magnitude greater than the "saturation" concentration (1.8 mM) reported by Evers et al. (1987).

Inset: Nonsaturable uptake of halothane in brain: Rat cerebral cortices (0.5 ml) were placed in NMR tubes and equilibrated for 1 hr with 1.5 ml of buffer solution containing various halothane concentrations. After centrifugation, the aqueous portion was transferred into another NMR tube. Halothane concentrations were determined (as above) in both the brain and aqueous fractions. Each value represents a single experiment. T_2 relaxation times were determined on representative samples and >95% of the halothane signal in the brain pellet was found to be in an environment with a short T_2 (5.3 ± 0.3 msec). Brain halothane concentrations were highly correlated with the final halothane concentrations in the aqueous fraction ($r = .97$, $p < .001$). Brain halothane concentrations of up to 50 mM could be achieved by repeated washings with saturated halothane solutions. A similar linear relationship was obtained with tissues from anesthetized rats (data not shown).

While the data presented here as well as many other studies (Keane and Biziere, 1987) indicate that anesthetics, including inhalation agents have actions at the GABA$_A$ receptor complex, they do not clearly distinguish between a protein, lipid or protein-lipid boundary as a specific target site. Moreover, given the existence of channel "superfamilies" (Stevens, 1987) with homologies in both sequence and molecular organization, similar phenomena to those described here may be also evinced in other systems (Forman and Miller, 1989). Our laboratory is currently investigating this possibility.

REFERENCES

Alifimoff JK, Firestone LL, Miller KW (1989): Anaesthetic potencies of primary alkanols: implications for the molecular dimensions of the anaesthetic site. *Br J Pharmacol* 96:9-16

Akaike N, Hattori K, Oomura Y, Carpenter D (1985): Bicuculline and picrotoxin block γ-aminobutyric acid gated Cl⁻ conductance by different mechanisms. *Experientia* 41:70-71

Cash DJ, Subbarao K (1987): Desensitization of γ-amino-butyric acid receptor from rat brain: two distinguishable receptors on the same membrane. *Biochemistry* 26:7556-7562

Curran MA, Newman LM, Becker GL (1988): Barbiturate anesthesia and alcohol tolerance in a rat model. *Anesth Analg* 67:868-71

Elliott J (1988): Protein pockets and anaesthesia. *Trends Pharmacol Sci* 9:10-11

Evers AS, Berkowitz BA, d'Avignon DA (1987): Correlation between the anesthetic effect of halothane and saturable binding in brain. *Nature* 328:157-160

Evers AS, Berkowitz BA, d'Avignon DA (1989): Correction: correlation between the anesthetic effect of halothane and saturable binding in brain. *Nature* 341:766

Forman S, Miller K (1989): Molecular sites of anesthetic action in postsynaptic nicotinic membranes. *Trends Pharmacol Sci* 10:449-452

Franks NP, Lieb WR (1984): Do general anaesthetics act by competitive binding to specific receptors? *Nature* 310:599-601

Franks NP, Lieb WR (1986): Partitioning of long-chain alcohols into lipid bilayers: Implications for mechanisms of general anesthesia. *Proc Natl Acad Sci (USA)* 83:5116-5120

Franks NP, Lieb WR (1987): What is the molecular Nature of general anaesthetic target sites? *Trends Pharmacol Sci* 8:169-174

Harris CM, Lal H (1988): Central nervous system effects of the imidazobenzodiazepine Ro15-4513. *Drug Dev Res* 13:187-203

Havoundjian H, Paul SM, Skolnick P (1986): The permeability of γ-aminobutyric acid-gated chloride channels is described by the binding of a "cage" convulsant, t-butylbicyclophosphoro[³⁵S]thionate. *Proc Natl Acad Sci (USA)* 83:9241-9244

Haydon DA, Hendry BM, Levinson SR, Requena J (1977): The molecular mechanisms of anaesthesia. *Nature* 268:356-358

Hollingsworth E, McNeal E, Burton J, Williams R, Daly R, Creveling D, (1985): Biochemical characterization of a filtered synaptoneurosome preparation from guinea pig cerebral cortex: cyclic adenosine 3'5'-monophosphate generating systems, receptors, and enzymes. *J Neurosci* 5:2240-2253

Huidobro-Toro JP, Bleck V, Allan AM, Harris RA (1987): Neurochemical actions of anesthetic drugs on the γ-aminobutyric acid receptor-chloride channel complex. *J Pharmacol Exp Ther* 242:963-969

Janoff AS, Miller KW (1982): A critical assessment of the lipid theories of general anesthetic action. In: *Biological membranes.* Chapman D, ed. London:

Academic Press, pp417-476

Janoff AS, Pringle MJ, Miller KW (1981): Correlation of general anesthetic potency with solubility in membranes. *Biochim Biophys Acta* 649:125-128

Johnstone RE, Kulp RA, Smith TC (1975): Effects of acute and chronic ethanol administration on isoflurane requirement in mice. *Anesth Analg* 58:277-282

Keane PE, Biziere K (1987): The effects of general anaesthetics on gabaergic synaptic transmission. *Life Sci* 41:1437-1448

Keck K, Firestone L, Nemoto E, Winter P (1988): Ro15-4513, a benzodiazepine (BDZ) inverse agonist, antagonizes the potencies of general anesthetics in rana pipens tadpoles. *FASEB Journal 2: Abstract #6320*

Koblin DD, Deady JE, Dong DE (1980): Mice tolerant to nitrous oxide are also tolerant to alcohol. *J Pharmacol Exp Ther* 213:309-316

Levitan ES, Schofield P, Burt D, Rhee L, Wisden W, Kohler M, Fujita N, Rodriguez H, Stephenson A, Darlison M, Barnard EA, Seeburg P (1988): Structural and functional basis for GABA$_A$ receptor heterogeneity. *Nature* 335:76-79

Lewin AH, de Costa BR, Rice KC, Skolnick P (1989): Meta- and para- isothio-cyanato-t-butylbicycloorthobenzoate: irreversible ligands of the gamma-aminobutyric acid-regulated chloride ionophore. *Mol Pharmacol* 35:189-194

Majewska M, Harrison N, Schwartz R, Barker J, Paul S (1986): Steroid hormone metabolites are barbiturate-like modulators of the GABA receptor. *Science* 232:1004-1007

Meyer HH: The theory of narcosis. *Harvey Lect* 1905-6. 11-17

Miller D, Yourick D, Tessel R (1989): Antagonism of methoxyflurane-induced anesthesia in rats by benzodiazepine inverse agonists. *Eur J Pharmacol* 173:1-10

Miller KW (1985): The nature of the site of general anesthesia. *Intl Rev Neurobiol* 27:1-61

Moody EJ, Skolnick P (1988): The imidazobenzodiazepine Ro15-4513 antagonizes methoxyflurane anesthesia. *Life Sci* 43:1269-1276

Moody EJ, Skolnick P (1989): Chormethiazole: neurochemical actions at the γ-aminobutyric acid receptor complex. *Eur J Pharmacol* 164:153-158

Moody EJ, Suzdak PD, Paul SM, Skolnick P (1988): Modulation of the benzodiazepine/gamma-aminobutyric aacid chloride channel complex by inhalation anesthetics. *J Neurochem* 51:1386-1393

Overton E (1901): Studien uber die narkose zugleich ein beintrag zur allgemeinen pharmakologie. Jena : Verlag Gustav Fischer

Pringle MJ, Brown KB, Miller KW (1981): Can the lipid theories of anesthesia account for the cutoff in anesthetic potency in homologous series of alcohols? *Mol Pharmacol* 19:49-55

Pritchett DB, Sontheimer H, Shivers BD, Ymer S, Kettenmann H, Schofield PR, Seeburg PH (1989): Importance of a novel GABA$_A$ receptor subunit for benzodiazepine pharmacology. *Nature* 338:582-585

Ramanjaneyulu R, Ticku M (1984): Binding characteristics and interactions of depressant drugs with [^{35}S]t-butylbicyclophosphorothionate, a ligand that binds to the picrotoxinin site. *J Neurochem* 42:221-229

Schofield PR, Darlison MG, Fujita N, Burt DR, Stephenson FA, Rodriguez H, Rhee LM, Ramachandran J, Reale V, Glencorse TA, Seeburg PH, Barnard EA (1987): Sequence and functional expression of the GABA$_A$ receptor shows a ligand-gated receptor superfamily. *Nature* 328:221-227

Schofield PR, Pritchett DB, Sontheimer H, Kettenmann H, Seeburg PH (1989): Sequence and expression of human GABA$_A$ receptor α_1 and β_1 subunits. *FEBS Letts* 244:361-364

Scholfield, CN (1988): Molecular mechanism of general anaesthetic action? *Trends Pharmacol Sci* 9:11-12

Schwartz R, Jackson J, Weigart D, Skolnick P, Paul S (1985): Characterization of barbiturate-stimulated chloride efflux from rat brain synaptoneurosomes. *J Neurosci* 5:2963-2970

Schwartz R, Skolnick P, Seale T, Paul S (1986): Demonstration of GABA/barbiturate-receptor-mediated chloride transport in rat brain synaptoneurosomes: a functional assay of GABA receptor-effector coupling. In: *GABAergic Transmission and Anxiety.* Biggio G, Costa E, eds. New York: Raven Press, pp 33-49

Schweri M, Cain M, Cook J, Paul S, Skolnick P (1982): Blockade of 3-carbomethoxy-β-carboline induced seizures by diazepam and the benzodiazepine antagonists, Ro15-1788 and CGS 8216. *Pharmacol Biochem Behav* 17:457-460

Sieghart W, Eichinger A, Richards JG, Mohler H (1987): Photoaffinity labeling of benzodiazepine receptor proteins with the partial inverse agonist [^{3}H] Ro 15-4513: biochemical and autoradiographic study. *J Neurochem* 48:46-52

Skolnick P, Paul S (1988): The benzodiazepine/GABA receptor chloride channel complex. *ISI Atlas Pharmacol* 2:19-22

Squires RF, Casida JE, Richardson M, Saederup E (1983): [^{35}S]t-Butylbicyclophosphorothionate binds with high affinity to brain specific sites coupled to γ-aminobutyric acid-A and ion recognition sites. *Mol Pharmacol* 23:326-336

Stevens C (1987): Channel families in the brain. *Nature* 328:198-199

Suzdak PD, Glowa JR, Crawley JN, Schwartz RD, Skolnick P, Paul SM (1986b): A selective imidazobenzodiazepine antagonist of ethanol in the rat. *Science* 234:1243-1247

Suzdak P, Schwartz R, Skolnick P, Paul S (1986a): Ethanol stimulates γ-aminobutyric acid-mediated chloride transport in rat brain synaptoneurosomes. *Proc Nat Acad Sci (USA)* 83:4071-4075

Suzdak P, Schwartz R, Skolnick P, Paul S (1988): Alcohols stimulate γ-aminobutyric acid receptor mediated chloride uptake in brain vesicles: correlation with intoxication potency. *Brain Res* 444:340-345

Tessel RE, Miller DW, Yourick DL (1987): Evidence for the involvement of GABA-chloride channels in a behavioral effect of methoxyflurane. *Pharmacologist 29: Abstract #357* (p 172)

Ethanol and the NMDA Receptor:
Insights into Ethanol Pharmacology

Boris Tabakoff, Carolyn S. Rabe, Kathleen A. Grant,
Peter Valverius, Michael Hudspith and Paula L. Hoffman

The relationship between lipid solubility and the pharmacological actions of ethanol and other alcohols was demonstrated many years ago (Meyer and Gottlieb, 1926). Since then it has been shown that alcohols can partition into cell membranes and perturb the structure of the bulk membrane lipids (Chin and Goldstein, 1977), and that the intoxicating potency of alcohols is positively correlated with their lipid-perturbing capacity (Lyon et al., 1981). These results led to the hypothesis that the pharmacological actions of ethanol stem from its nonspecific effects on membrane lipid "fluidity" and subsequently a perturbation of the activities of membrane-bound proteins (e.g., receptors, enzymes). However, relatively high concentrations of ethanol are necessary to produce significant increases in membrane lipid fluidity (Chin and Goldstein, 1977; Lyon et al., 1981), and inspection of the literature reveals that the function of few membrane-bound proteins is significantly affected by concentrations of ethanol that are relevant *in vivo*. There are some exceptions to this observation, including the effects of low concentrations of ethanol on the stimulatory guanine nucleotide binding protein, G_s (Saito et al., 1985; Valverius et al., 1987), and the GABA receptor-coupled chloride channel (Allan and Harris, 1987; Suzdak et al., 1986), which is the major inhibitory neurotransmitter system in the brain. The activity of each of these membrane-bound proteins or protein complexes can be influenced (enhanced) by physiologically relevant concentrations of ethanol. Sensitive systems like these have been postulated to represent "receptive areas" for ethanol in the cell membrane, at which this drug may exert its pharmacological effects (Tabakoff and Hoffman, 1987). Possible sites of action of ethanol in these "receptive areas" include the lipid-protein interface or hydrophobic portions of the proteins themselves. It is apparent that the identification of such "receptive areas" is necessary for an understanding of the spectrum of actions of ethanol in the central nervous system (CNS).

The major excitatory neurotransmitter in the brain is the amino acid glutamate. An inhibitory effect of ethanol on the function of this transmitter would be complementary to the reported potentiation by ethanol of the response to GABA, and might be expected to contribute to the depressant effects of ethanol. The effects of glutamate are mediated by at least three subtypes of receptor, designated on the basis of ligand binding and electrophysiological studies as kainate, quisqualate and N-methyl-D-aspartate (NMDA) receptors (Cull-Candy and Usowicz, 1987; Foster and Fagg, 1984; Mayer and Westbrook, 1987). All of these receptor subtypes are coupled to cation channels, and the quisqualate and NMDA receptors may also be coupled to the phosphatidylinositol second messenger system. There is both biochemical and electrophysiological evidence that NMDA receptors may be coupled to channels that are functionally distinct from those coupled to kainate and quisqualate receptors (MacDermott et al., 1986; Nowak et al., 1984). For example, NMDA receptor-gated channels, when open, are permeable to monovalent cations and Ca^{++}, and the actions of NMDA are blocked selectively and non-competitively by phencyclidine (PCP) and Mg^{++} in a voltage-dependent manner (suggesting sites of action of PCP and Mg^{++} within the channel). Furthermore, glycine enhances the actions of NMDA, but not kainate or quisqualate (Anis et al., 1983; Johnson and Ascher, 1987), and has been suggested to be necessary in order for NMDA to exert its effects (Kleckner and Dingledine, 1988). The actions of agonists at the NMDA receptor are also regulated by Zn^{++} ions, which inhibit responses (Peters et al., 1987), and by polyamines such as spermine, which enhance the affinity of the NMDA receptor-channel complex for compounds that bind within the channel, possibly by an interaction at the glycine binding site (Ransom and Stec, 1988; Sacaan and Johnson, 1989). The properties of the NMDA receptor-channel complex have been studied in some detail because of its implicated role in neuronal plasticity (long-term synaptic potentiation) (Harris et al., 1984), hypoxic damage (Simon et al., 1984), epileptiform seizure activity (Dingledine et al., 1986) and neuronal development (Pearce et al., 1987). Thus, *a priori*, a role of the NMDA receptor could be suggested in the cognitive deficits produced by ethanol intake, as well as in the teratogenic effects of ethanol and in the seizures that accompany ethanol withdrawal.

In our laboratories, the effects of ethanol on biochemical responses to NMDA and other glutamate receptor agonists were initially examined in primary cultures of cerebellar granule cells (Hoffman et al., 1989). In these cells, kainate and NMDA stimulate calcium uptake in a dose-dependent manner. The action of NMDA can be blocked, as expected, by addition of Mg^{++} to the assay. The response to NMDA can also be selectively blocked by the receptor antagonist D-2-amino-5-phosphono-valeric acid (2-APV). We found that the effect of NMDA (used at its EC_{50} concentration) on calcium uptake in these cells was also potently inhibited by ethanol, with significant inhibition observed at 10 mM ethanol, and an IC_{50} of approximately 40 mM. Similarly, ethanol (25-100 mM) has been found to inhibit the NMDA-induced increase in intracellular calcium levels, measured by fura-2 fluorometry, in dissociated cells from whole brain of neonatal rats (Dildy and Leslie, 1989). In cerebellar granule cells, the response to kainate was much less effectively blocked by ethanol than the NMDA response, with an IC_{50} for ethanol of approximately 120 mM (Hoffman et al., 1989). In contrast to the selective inhibitory effect of ethanol in this system, pentobarbital was more effective at inhibiting kainate- than NMDA-evoked increases in calcium uptake in cerebellar granule cells, whereas benzodiazepines (e.g., flurazepam, diazepam) had no effect on the response to NMDA (Tabakoff et al., in press).

In addition to these biochemical findings, electrophysiological studies using whole cell patch-clamp preparations of dissociated embryonic hippocampal neurons in culture have demonstrated that ethanol selectively inhibits NMDA-induced ion currents (Lovinger et al., 1989). In one study (Lovinger et al., 1989), low concentrations of ethanol (threshold, 5 mM) inhibited the response to NMDA, while in another the effect of ethanol was reported to be biphasic, with lower ethanol concentrations (approximately 2-9 mM) enhancing the NMDA response, and higher concentrations (approximately 90-170 mM) producing inhibition (Lima-Landman and Albuquerque, 1989). Responses to kainate and quisqualate were less sensitive to inhibition by ethanol than the response to NMDA (Lovinger et al., 1989). NMDA-activated ion currents in fetal hippocampal cells were also inhibited by other short-chain alcohols, and the inhibitory potencies of these alcohols (approximate IC_{50}s: methanol, 117 mM; 1-butanol, 1.1 mM; isopentanol, 0.32mM) were linearly related to their hydrophobicity and to their potency for producing intoxication (Lovinger et al., 1989). These data suggested a hydrophobic site of action for ethanol and the other alcohols.

More recently, electrophysiological studies have been expanded to include studies in neurons and brain slices from adult animals. Ethanol was found to be a potent inhibitor (IC_{50}, 10 mM) of NMDA-induced ion currents measured by whole cell patch-clamp techniques in isolated neurons from the dorsal root ganglion (White et al., 1990). In addition, in slices from adult rat hippocampus, 50 mM ethanol significantly inhibited NMDA receptor-mediated population excitatory postsynaptic potentials (EPSPs), while having little effect on the responses mediated by non-NMDA glutamate receptors (Lovinger et al., 1990b). It has also been reported that electrophysiological responses to NMDA are reduced in hippocampal slices of adult rats that were prenatally exposed to ethanol (Morrisett et al., 1989).

NMDA and kainate, as well as glutamate, stimulate cyclic guanosine monophosphate (GMP) production in cerebellar granule cells (Hoffman et al., 1989; Novelli et al., 1987), and this stimulation is Ca^{++}-dependent (Hoffman et al., 1989; Novelli et al., 1987). Thus, this cell culture preparation provided the opportunity to evaluate the effect of ethanol on a functional consequence of NMDA-induced calcium uptake. Our results showed that ethanol had little or no effect on basal cyclic GMP levels, but was a potent inhibitor of the response to NMDA (Hoffman et al., 1989). In contrast, even 100 mM ethanol did not significantly inhibit the cyclic GMP response to kainate (Hoffman et al., 1989). The similarity in the effect of ethanol on NMDA-induced increases in Ca^{++} uptake and cyclic GMP production suggested that ethanol may inhibit NMDA-stimulated production of cyclic GMP by its action at the NMDA receptor-gated channel, that is, blocking NMDA-mediated calcium uptake. Another consequence of NMDA-activated calcium influx is the release of neurotransmitters. Studies in slices and synaptosomal preparations of rat cerebral cortex and hippocampus have indicated that NMDA stimulates the release of norepinephrine (NE), but not serotonin, acetylcholine, glutamate or GABA (Göthert and Fink, 1989). In striatal slices, NMDA stimulates acetylcholine and dopamine release (Göthert and Fink, 1989; Woodward and Gonzales, 1990). The effect of NMDA on NE release in the cortex was inhibited by low concentrations of ethanol (IC_{50} approximately 40 mM). In this system, ethanol did not inhibit depolarization-

or calcium-induced neurotransmitter release, and the results are compatible with the hypothesis that a primary site of action of ethanol in the cortex is the NMDA receptor-gated ion channel. Ethanol also inhibited NMDA-activated acetylcholine release in striatal slices, but with about one-fourth the potency observed for NE release in cortex. On the other hand, ethanol was a potent inhibitor of endogenous dopamine release in striatal slices, with a significant effect observed at 10 mM ethanol (Woodward and Gonzales, 1990). The differences in the potency of ethanol could reflect the characteristics of the different cell types and the NMDA receptors involved. Tetrodotoxin blocked NMDA stimulation of cortical NE release and striatal dopamine release, suggesting that NMDA receptors are not localized on presynaptic noradrenergic or dopaminergic terminals in these brain areas (Göthert and Fink, 1989; Woodward and Gonzales, 1990). NMDA was hypothesized to affect cortical NE release via activation of an excitatory interneuron. However, NMDA receptors may be localized directly on cholinergic neurons in the striatum (Göthert and Fink, 1989). In addition, cortical and striatal NMDA receptors have been reported to differ with respect to agonist and antagonist binding, as well as responsiveness to glycine (Monaghan et al., 1988).

The diverse data described above support the hypothesis that the function of the NMDA receptor-gated ion channel is very sensitive to ethanol, and several studies have been performed to investigate the site of action of ethanol within the receptor-channel complex. As mentioned above, PCP is another drug that inhibits the action of NMDA, by acting at a site within the NMDA receptor-gated ion channel (Anis et al., 1983). It seemed possible that inhibition by ethanol and PCP might involve a similar site(s) or mechanism(s) of action. However, when the effects of ethanol and PCP on NMDA-stimulated cyclic GMP production in cerebellar granule cells were examined in combination, these effects appeared to be additive (Hoffman et al., 1989). In contrast, ethanol reduced the ability of glycine to enhance NMDA-stimulated cyclic GMP production (Hoffman et al., 1989). Conversely, when NMDA-stimulated calcium flux was measured in cerebellar granule cells, high concentrations of glycine reversed the inhibition produced by ethanol (Rabe and Tabakoff, 1989; Rabe and Tabakoff, in press). It has also been reported that ethanol (25 mM)-induced inhibition of NMDA-stimulated dopamine release in slices of rat striatal tissue can be reversed by addition of glycine (Woodward and Gonzales, 1990). As noted above, glycine has been suggested to be *required* for the action of NMDA (i.e., glycine was suggested to be a "coagonist" at the NMDA receptor (Kleckner and Dingledine, 1988)), and these data suggest that ethanol may particularly affect the interaction of glycine with the NMDA receptor-channel complex. Results of electrophysiological studies in hippocampal neurons were similar to the biochemical findings in that NMDA receptor-gated ion channel blockers (Zn^{++}, Mg^{++} or ketamine) did not alter ethanol-induced inhibition. However, in this system, the response to ethanol was also unaffected by glycine (Lovinger et al., 1990a). This difference may reflect the fact that only low concentrations of glycine (<1 μM) were used in the electrophysiological studies. In fact, more recently it has been found that higher concentrations of glycine (10 μM) *can reduce* ethanol-induced inhibition of NMDA responses in mouse hippocampal neurons (White et al., 1990). Further investigation of the effect of ethanol on the NMDA-glycine interaction is warranted.

It has been demonstrated that benzodiazepines can alter cerebellar cyclic GMP levels (Boireau et al., 1988), and ethanol has been reported to increase neuronal membrane chloride ion flux by an action at the benzodiazepine-GABA receptor-channel complex (Allan and Harris, 1987; Suzdak et al., 1986). However, picrotoxin, a chloride channel blocker, did not antagonize the effects of ethanol either on NMDA-stimulated calcium uptake or cyclic GMP accumulation in cerebellar granule cells (Hoffman et al., 1989). In addition, in slices of adult rat hippocampus, the $GABA_A$ antagonist bicuculline did not alter ethanol-induced inhibition of NMDA-mediated population EPSPs (Lovinger et al., 1990b). Therefore it may be postulated that ethanol's inhibition of the NMDA-mediated responses occurs independently of any action of ethanol at the GABA receptor-gated chloride ion channel. On the other hand, increased intracellular calcium has been reported to reduce the activity of GABA receptor-coupled chloride channels (Inoue et al., 1986). Thus, it may be speculated that the previously-observed potentiating effects of ethanol on chloride flux could be secondary to an inhibition of receptor-gated calcium channel activity.

In addition to the selective sensitivity to ethanol of the NMDA receptor-gated ion channel (as opposed to the kainate receptor-coupled channel), it is important to note that the concentrations of ethanol that alter the responses to NMDA are those that are found in the brains of humans who have consumed moderate amounts of alcohol. Thus, inhibition of NMDA receptor-coupled responses can be expected to occur *in vivo* after ethanol ingestion and may contribute to the pharmacological (intoxicating, sedative and/or cognitive) effects of ethanol. In order to assess the possibility that certain of ethanol's behavioral effects are mediated by its actions at the NMDA receptor, studies of the discriminative stimulus properties of ethanol have been performed. These studies are designed to investigate whether interoceptive cues produced by ethanol are recognized by animals as being similar to cues produced by other drugs that act at the NMDA receptor-gated ion channel. White Carneau pigeons or CD-1 mice were trained to discriminate between ethanol and water by standard drug discrimination techniques (Grant et al., 1990; Schuster and Balster, 1977). That is, the animals were given ethanol or vehicle and were placed in a chamber equipped with two keys. The animals were given a food (pigeons) or milk (mice) reinforcement after 30 or 20 responses, respectively, on the correct key (i.e., the key associated with ethanol or that associated with vehicle, depending on the pretreatment). During training, only responding on the appropriate key resulted in reinforcement; responding on the incorrect key had no consequences. For testing, the conditions were changed so that responding on either key produced reinforcement. Under these conditions animals were given various drugs that act as antagonists at the NMDA receptor-gated channel (PCP, ketamine or MK-801, a compound that binds to the PCP site), and responding on the ethanol- and vehicle-associated keys was monitored. Both pigeons and mice given PCP or ketamine responded more than 80% on the ethanol-associated key. Similarly, MK-801 administration to pigeons resulted in more than 90% responding on the ethanol-appropriate key (Grant et al., 1990). In anthropomorphic terms, the results of these studies suggest that the animals perceive the effects of PCP and other noncompetitive antagonists of NMDA function as being similar to those of ethanol.

While the acute effect of ethanol at the NMDA receptor is inhibitory, it is possible that chronic ethanol ingestion could result in an adaptive change that would lead to increased NMDA-mediated responses. Since the NMDA receptor is involved in epileptiform seizure activity (Dingledine et al., 1986), "up-regulation" of this receptor could contribute to ethanol withdrawal seizures. To evaluate this possibility, C57BL/6NCR mice were made physically dependent on ethanol by feeding them ethanol in a liquid diet for 7 days (Ritzmann and Tabakoff, 1976). The ethanol-containing diet was then replaced with control diet, and withdrawal symptomatology (including tremors, spasms, handling-induced and spontaneous seizures) was monitored (Grant et al., 1990). Some mice were injected with the NMDA antagonist MK-801 three times during the initial 24 hours of withdrawal, while others received vehicle. MK-801 reduced withdrawal seizure severity in a dose-dependent manner. In contrast, when mice were injected with NMDA itself, ethanol withdrawal seizure severity increased, and a higher proportion of lethal seizures occurred in the NMDA-treated mice than in vehicle-injected animals (NMDA at the dose used did not produce seizures in control mice) (Grant et al., 1990). These results are consistent with the hypothesis that changes in NMDA receptor-gated ion channel function occur during chronic ethanol ingestion, and that these changes may contribute to the symptoms of ethanol withdrawal (i.e., seizures). Similar results have been reported with respect to voltage-gated calcium channels in brain, in that dihydropyridine calcium channel antagonists reduced ethanol withdrawal seizures (Little et al., 1986). Thus, increased sensitivity of several types of calcium channels in the brain may be involved in the overt manifestations of the ethanol withdrawal syndrome. The up-regulation of the NMDA receptor complex can also be observed by ligand binding studies. [^{3}H]MK-801 binding (Foster and Wong, 1987), measured in the presence of glutamate and glycine, was significantly increased in hippocampal membranes of ethanol-fed mice at the time of withdrawal (Grant et al., 1990). The number of binding sites was still increased at 8 hours after withdrawal, and had returned to the control value by 24 hours after withdrawal when overt withdrawal signs had dissipated (Gulya et al., submitted). The hippocampus, among other brain areas, has previously been shown to be involved in ethanol withdrawal seizure activity (Walker and Zornetzer, 1974). An increase in hippocampal NMDA receptor number would be expected to result in increased sensitivity to endogenous glutamate and contribute to the CNS hyperexcitability that is characteristic of ethanol withdrawal. The increase in receptor number may be envisioned as a form of receptor supersensitivity that may develop as an adaptation to the continued inhibition of channel activity produced by ethanol.

To further investigate the role of NMDA receptors in ethanol withdrawal, MK-801 binding was measured in brains of mice selectively bred to be prone or resistant to ethanol withdrawal seizures (Valverius et al., 1990). Such selected lines of mice are ideally genetically invariant for the genes that contribute to the selected trait, while all other gene frequencies remain variable. Thus, if environmental conditions are constant, a biochemical difference between the lines is assumed to play a role in producing the difference in the selected trait (Kosobud and Crabbe, 1986). There was a higher number of hippocampal MK-801 binding sites in untreated withdrawal seizure-prone (WSP) mice than in the withdrawal seizure-resistant (WSR) mice. In contrast, there was no difference in the number of cerebral cortical NMDA receptor-channel complexes between the selected lines. After WSP and WSR mice were fed ethanol in a liquid diet for 6 days, and were physically dependent on ethanol, the number of hippocampal MK-801 binding sites increased in mice of both lines. This increase, however, resulted in the ethanol-fed WSP mice having an even higher number of binding sites than the ethanol-fed WSR mice. In fact, the number of hippocampal binding sites in the ethanol-fed WSR mice did not exceed the number of sites in *untreated* WSP mice. There was no change in number of cerebral cortical MK-801 binding sites after chronic ethanol ingestion (Valverius et al., 1990). These data are consistent with a role for the hippocampal NMDA receptor-gated ion channel complex in mediating ethanol withdrawal seizures, as well as other signs of ethanol withdrawal that differ in WSP and WSR mice (Kosobud and Crabbe, 1986).

It should be noted that chronic ethanol exposure has also been reported to result in an increase in voltage-gated calcium channels, both in cultured cells (Messing et al., 1986) and in the brain (Dolin et al., 1987). The precise contributions of changes in each of these types of calcium channel to ethanol withdrawal symptomatology needs further elucidation. However, the function of the NMDA receptor-gated channel is clearly more sensitive to the acute inhibitory effect of ethanol than that of voltage-gated Ca^{++} channels (Hoffman et al., 1989; Leslie et al., 1983).

These findings regarding the biochemical, electrophysiological and behavioral interactions of ethanol and the NMDA receptor provide evidence that the NMDA receptor-gated ion channel in brain may be a specific site of action of ethanol. As mentioned, the selective and potent inhibition by ethanol of the actions of glutamate at the NMDA receptor may well be involved in the cognitive deficits produced by even moderate ethanol intake (Lister et al., 1987). Furthermore, increased sensitivity to glutamate at the NMDA receptor following chronic ethanol ingestion appears to contribute to ethanol withdrawal seizure activity and could also be involved in chronic ethanol-induced neurotoxicity. The findings to date are consistent with a key role of the NMDA receptor complex in certain of the pharmacological effects of ethanol, and suggest a unique and specific mechanism of action of ethanol in the brain. Further studies of this mechanism, including a search for the biochemical or molecular basis of the selective and potent responses to ethanol, and the specificity of these responses in comparison to responses to other drugs should greatly enhance the understanding of the CNS effects of ethanol, and may eventually yield therapies to counter certain of ethanol's deleterious actions.

ACKNOWLEDGMENTS

This work was supported in part by the Banbury Foundation. We are grateful to Drs. D.M. Lovinger, G. White and F.F. Weight for providing us with preprints of their work, and to Ms. Robin DuBeau for secretarial assistance.

REFERENCES

Allan AM, Harris RA (1987): Acute and chronic ethanol treatments alter GABA receptor-operated chloride channels. *Pharmacol Biochem Behav* 27:665-670

Anis NA, Berry SC, Burton NR, Lodge D (1983): The dissociative anesthetics, ketamine and phencyclidine selectively reduce excitation of central mammalian neurones by N-methyl-D-aspartate. *Br J Pharmacol* 79:565-575

Boireau A, Martel M, Farges G, Dubdat P, Laduron PM, Blanchard JC (1988): *In vivo* determination of the profile of benzodiazepine ligands by comparing the inhibition of 3H-RO15-1788 binding to the modulation of cGMP levels in mouse cerebellum. *Biochem Pharmacol* 37:3765-3769

Chin JH, Goldstein DB (1977): Drug tolerance in biomembranes: a spin label study of the effects of ethanol. *Science* 196:684-685

Cull-Candy SG, Usowicz MM (1987): Multiple-conductance channels activated by excitatory amino acids in cerebellar neurons. *Nature* 325:525-528

Dildy JE, Leslie SW (1989): Ethanol inhibits NMDA-induced increases in free intracellular Ca^{2+} in dissociated brain cells. *Brain Res* 499:383-387

Dingledine R, Hynes MA, King GL (1986): Involvement of N-methyl-D-aspartate receptors in epileptiform bursting in the rat hippocampal slice. *J Physiol* 380:175-189

Dolin S, Little H, Hudspith M, Pagonis C, Littleton J (1987): Increased dihydro-pyridine-sensitive calcium channels in rat brain may underlie ethanol physical dependence. *Neuropharmacology* 26:275-279

Foster AC, Fagg GE (1984): Acidic amino acid binding sites in mammalian neuronal membranes: their characteristics and relationship to synaptic receptors. *Brain Res Rev* 7:103-164

Foster AC, Wong EHF (1987): The novel anticonvulsant MK-801 binds to the activated state of the N-methyl-D-aspartate receptor in rat brain. *Br J Pharmacol* 91: 403-409

Göthert M, Fink K (1989): Inhibition of N-methyl-D-aspartate (NMDA)- and L-glutamate-induced noradrenaline and acetylcholine release in the rat brain by ethanol. *Arch Pharmacol* 340: 516-521

Grant KA, Valverius P, Hudspith M, Tabakoff B (1990): Ethanol withdrawal seizures and the NMDA receptor complex. *Eur J Pharmacol* 176:289-296

Grant KA, Knisely JS, Tabakoff B, Barrett JE, Balster RL (submitted): Ethanol-like discriminative stimulus effects of noncompetitive N-methyl-D-aspartate antagonists. *Behav Pharmacol*

Gulya K, Grant KA, Valverius P, Hoffman PL, Tabakoff B (submitted): Brain regional specificity and time course of changes in the NMDA receptor-ionophore complex during ethanol withdrawal. *Brain Res*

Harris EW, Ganong AH, Cotman CW (1984): Long-term potentiation in the hippocampus involves activation of N-methyl-D-aspartate receptors. *Brain Res* 323: 132-137

Hoffman PL, Moses F, Tabakoff B (1989): Selective inhibition by ethanol of glutamate-stimulated cyclic GMP production in primary cultures of cerebellar granule cells. *Neuropharmacology* 28:1239-1243

Hoffman PL, Rabe CS, Moses F, Tabakoff B (1989): NMDA receptors and ethanol: inhibition of calcium flux and cyclic GMP production. *J Neurochem* 52:1937-1940

Inoue M, Oomura Y, Yakushiji T, Akaike N (1986): Intracellular calcium ions decrease the affinity of the GABA receptors. *Nature* 324:156-158

Kleckner NW, Dingledine R (1988): Requirement for glycine in activation of NMDA receptors expressed in Xenopus oocytes. *Science* 241:835-837

Kosobud A, Crabbe JC (1986): Ethanol withdrawal in mice bred to be genetically prone or resistant to ethanol withdrawal seizure. *J Pharmacol Exp Ther* 238:170-177

Leslie SW, Barr E, Chandler J, Farrar RP (1983): Inhibition of fast- and slow-phase depolarization-dependent synaptosomal calcium uptake by ethanol. *J Pharmacol Exp Ther* 225:571-575

Lima-Landman MTR, Albuquerque EX (1989): Ethanol potentiates and blocks NMDA-activated single-channel currents in rat hippocampal pyramidal cells. *FEBS Lett* 247:61-67

Lister RG, Eckardt M, Weingartner H (1987): Ethanol intoxication and memory. Recent developments and new directions. In: *Recent Developments in Alcoholism. Vol 5.* Galanter M, ed. New York: Plenum Press, pp 111-125

Little HJ, Dolin SJ, Halsey MJ (1986): Calcium channel antagonists decrease the ethanol withdrawal syndrome. *Life Sci* 39:2059-2065

Lovinger DM, White G, Weight FF (1989): Ethanol inhibits NMDA-activated ion current in hippocampal neurons. *Science* 243:1721-1724

Lovinger DM, White G, Weight FF (1990a): Ethanol (EtOH) inhibition of NMDA-activated ion current is not voltage-dependent and EtOH does not interact with other binding sites on the NMDA receptor/ionophore complex. *FASEB J* 4:A678

Lovinger DM, White G, Weight FF (1990b): NMDA receptor-mediated synaptic excitation selectively inhibited by ethanol in hippocampal slice from adult rat. *J Neurosci* 10:1372-1379

Lyon RC, McComb JA, Schreurs J, Goldstein DB (1981): A relationship between alcohol intoxication and the disordering of brain membranes by a series of short-chain alcohols. *J Pharmacol Exp Ther* 218:669-675

MacDermott AB, Mayer ML, Westbrook GL, Smith SJ, Barker JL (1986): NMDA-receptor activation increases cytoplasmic calcium concentration in cultured spinal cord neurones. *Nature* 321:519-522

Mayer ML, Westbrook GL (1987): The physiology of excitatory amino acids in the vertebrate nervous system. *Prog Neurobiol* 28:197-276

Messing RO, Carpenter CL, Diamond I, and Greenberg DA (1986): Ethanol regulates calcium channels in clonal neural cells. *Proc Natl Acad Sci (USA)* 83:6213-6215

Meyer HH, Gottlieb R (1926): Theory of narcosis. In: *Experimental Pharmacology as a Basis for Therapeutics*, (2nd ed) (Henderson VE, trans) Philadelphia: Lippincott, pp 116-129

Monaghan DT, Olverman HJ, Nguyen L, Watkins JC, Cotman CW (1988): Two classes of N-methyl-D-aspartate recognition sites: differential distribution and differential regulation by glycine. *Proc Natl Acad Sci (USA)* 85:9836-9840

Morrisett RA, Martin D, Wilson WA, Savage DD, Swartzwelder S (1989): Prenatal exposure to ethanol decreases the sensitivity of the adult rat hippocampus to N-methyl-D-aspartate. *Alcohol* 6:415-420

Novelli A, Nicoletti F, Wroblewski JT, Alho H, Costa E, Guidotti A (1987): Excitatory amino acid receptors coupled with guanylate cyclase in primary cultures of cerebellar granule cells. *J Neurosci* 7:40-47

Nowak L, Bregestovski P, Ascher P, Herbet A, Prochiantz A (1984): Magnesium gates glutamate-activated channels in mouse central neurones. *Nature* 307:462-465

Pearce IA, Cambray-Deakin MA, Burgoyne RD (1987): Glutamate acting on NMDA receptors stimulates neurite outgrowth from cerebellar granule cells. *FEBS Lett* 223:143-147

Peters S, Koh J, Choi DW (1987): Zinc selectively blocks the action of N-methyl-D-aspartate on cortical neurons. *Science* 236:589-593

Rabe CS, Tabakoff B (1989): Glycine antagonizes ethanol-mediated inhibition of NMDA-stimulated calcium uptake into primary cultures of cerebellar neurons. *Soc Neurosci Abstr* 15:202

Rabe CS, Tabakoff B (in press): Glycine site directed agonists reverse ethanol's actions at the NMDA receptor. *Mol Pharmacol*

Ransom RW, Stec NL (1988): Cooperative modulation of [^{3}H]-MK-801 binding to the N-methyl-D-aspartate receptor-ion channel complex by L-glutamate, glycine and polyamines. *J Neurochem* 51:830-836

Ritzmann RF, Tabakoff B (1976): Body temperature in mice: a quantitative measure of alcohol tolerance and physical dependence. *J Pharmacol Exp Ther* 199:158-170

Sacaan AI, Johnson KM (1989): Spermine enhances binding to the glycine site associated with the N-methyl-D-aspartate receptor complex. *Mol Pharmacol* 36:836-839

Saito T, Lee JM, Tabakoff B (1985): Ethanol's effects on cortical adenylate cyclase activity. *J Neurochem* 44:1037-1044

Schuster CR, Balster RL (1977): The discriminative stimulus properties of drugs. In: *Advances in Behavioral Pharmacology*. Thompson T, Dews PB, eds. New York: Academic Press, pp 85-138

Simon RP, Swan JH, Griffiths T, Meldrum BS (1984): Blockade of N-methyl-D-aspartate receptors may protect against ischemic damage in brain. *Science* 226:850-852

Suzdak PD, Schwartz RD, Skolnick P, Paul SM (1986): Ethanol stimulates gamma-aminobutyric acid receptor-mediated chloride transport in rat brain synaptoneurosomes. *Proc Natl Acad Sci (USA)* 83:4071-4075

Tabakoff B, Hoffman PL (1987): Biochemical pharmacology of alcohol. In: *Psychopharmacology: The Third Generation of Progress*. Meltzer HY, ed. New York: Raven Press, pp 1521-1526

Tabakoff B, Rabe CS, Hoffman PL (in press): Selective effects of sedative/hypnotic drugs on excitatory amino acid receptors in brain. *Ann. NY Acad Sci*

Valverius P, Crabbe JC, Hoffman PL, Tabakoff B (1990): NMDA receptors in mice bred to be prone or resistant to ethanol withdrawal seizures. *Eur J Pharmacol* 184:185-189

Valverius P, Hoffman PL, Tabakoff B (1987): Effect of ethanol on mouse cerebral cortical beta-adrenergic receptors. *Mol Pharmacol* 32: 217-222

Walker DW, Zornetzer SF (1974): Alcohol withdrawal in mice: electroencephalographic and behavioral correlates. *Electroenceph Clin Neurophysiol* 36:233-
244

White G, Lovinger DM, Weight FF (1990): Ethanol inhibits NMDA-activated
current but does not affect GABA-activated current in an isolated adult mammalian neuron. *Brain Res* 507:332-336

White G, Lovinger DM, Peoples RW, Weight FF (1990): Analysis of ethanol
(EtOH) interaction with glycine potentiation of NMDA-activated in current.
Soc Neurosci Abstr 16:1041

Woodward JJ, Gonzales RA (1990): Ethanol inhibition of N-methyl-D-aspartate-
stimulated endogenous dopamine release from rat striatal slices: reversal by
glycine. *J Neurochem* 54:712-715

Molecular and Genetic Approaches to Understanding Alcohol-Seeking Behavior

Ting-Kai Li, David W. Crabb and Lawrence Lumeng

In alcoholism research, two fundamental and related questions are: "why do people drink?" and "why do some people drink too much despite having experienced negative consequences?" Drinking normally occurs in a social setting. Environmental factors and how individuals react to them can therefore have powerful influences on drinking behavior. On the other hand, the neuropsychopharmacological actions of ethanol and how different individuals react to these effects can be important biological determinants. Ethanol's action is biphasic, that is, it can be reinforcing or rewarding at low concentrations, but aversive at high concentrations (Pohorecky, 1977). Perception by the individual of the reinforcing actions of ethanol might be expected to maintain alcohol-seeking behavior, whereas aversive effects would be expected to extinguish it. The disorder alcoholism can be defined in experimentally approachable terms as a state of abnormally intense alcohol-seeking behavior that over time leads to the alcohol dependence syndrome (Edwards and Gross, 1976). Identification of both the environmental and the biological variables that promote and maintain high alcohol-seeking or alcohol self-administration behavior is key to our understanding of this disorder.

Little is known about specific biological factors that promote problem drinking and alcoholism in humans, but there is now convincing evidence for identifiable genetic risk in a large segment of the alcoholic population (Cloninger, 1986; Cloninger et al., 1981). Thus, there is biological predisposition for "drinking too much" in some individuals; what this inherited propensity (or propensities) might be is currently a subject of intense research interest. In looking at various biological responses to ethanol that can serve as feedback loops to influence alcohol ingestion in humans and experimental animals, it is noteworthy that a number of them, as well as drinking behavior itself, have shown large degrees of between-individual variability that is partly genetically determined. These include in humans: alcohol pharmacokinetics and metabolism, the sensitivity of the brain to ethanol as revealed by electroencephalographic measurements, and systemic reactivity to ethanol metabolism (e.g., the alcohol-flush reaction). In experimental animals, genetic influence has been documented for alcohol preference, alcohol metabolic rate, neuronal sensitivity to the acute effects of ethanol, the capacity to develop tolerance, and severity of withdrawal reactions (Li, 1985; McClearn and Erwin, 1982).

It has been postulated that inherited differences in sensitivity to the rewarding and aversive effects of ethanol in part underlie the genetic predisposition to excessive ethanol consumption. Recent studies in humans and experimental animals have provided strong support for this viewpoint. The human studies have examined the molecular genetic basis of the alcohol-flush reaction and have related this phenotype and the genes that determine it to drinking behavior. The animal studies have employed genetic methodology to produce experimental animals exhibiting high and low alcohol-seeking behaviors. These animals are now being used to identify the neuronal, endocrine, and neurotransmitter systems that subserve abnormal alcohol-seeking behavior.

HUMAN STUDIES

Alcohol Metabolism and the Alcohol-flush Reaction

Ethanol is eliminated from the body mostly by oxidative metabolism in the liver, first to acetaldehyde and then to acetate. Acetate, in turn, is oxidized by peripheral tissues to carbon dioxide and water. The enzymes that are principally responsible for the hepatic metabolism of ethanol and acetaldehyde are alcohol dehydrogenase (ADH) and aldehyde dehydrogenase (ALDH), respectively. There are multiple forms of both these enzymes in humans and the molecular and kinetic properties of the isozymes of ADH and ALDH have been studied in considerable detail (Bosron et al., 1988). Genetic polymorphism involving a number of the ADH and ALDH isozymes has been detected. The variant forms of ADH exhibit different kinetic properties that are likely to contribute to individual differences in alcohol elimination rates. As reviewed in this section, the variant form of ALDH has been shown to produce a pronounced sensitivity in response to alcohol metabolism that influences drinking behavior.

Approximately 50% of Japanese and Chinese have the so-called "null" variant of the mitochondrial form of ALDH (ALDH2) (Goedde et al., 1979; Harada et al., 1980; Teng, 1981). This isozyme is normally the principal enzyme form that oxidizes acetaldehyde to acetate in liver, because it possesses the highest affinity for acetaldehyde, in comparison with the other ALDH isozymes that are situated in the cytosol. Individuals who have the "null" variant or ALDH2-deficient phenotype are less able to oxidize acetaldehyde. Consequently, their blood levels of acetaldehyde after ingestion of ethanol are 10 or more times higher than in individuals with the normal ALDH2 phenotype (Mizoi et al., 1979). Individuals who have the ALDH2-deficient phenotype also exhibit the alcohol-flush reaction after drinking (Harada et al., 1981). This dysphoric reaction is commonly characterized by facial flushing, vasodilation, tachycardia and headaches. When the reaction is severe, nausea, vomiting, edema, and hypotension can occur. The reaction is similar to the reaction seen in alcoholic patients receiving Antabuse (disulfiram), a potent inhibitor of ALDH, if they ingest or are exposed to ethanol.

The Molecular Genetic Basis of ALDH2 Deficiency

The ALDH2 phenotypes (active and deficient) can be determined by starch gel electrophoresis or by isoelectric focusing of liver tissue extracts or hair root extracts, and staining for aldehyde oxidizing activity (Harada et al., 1980). Population studies have shown that, in addition to Asians, a high prevalence of the ALDH2-deficient phenotype is found in South American Indians. Prevalence of the deficient phenotype is very low or zero in North American Indians, European Germans, white Americans, and African Americans (Bosron et al., 1988).

ALDH is a tetrameric protein composed of four identical subunits. In ALDH2-deficient subjects, an immunoreactive band that migrates cathodally to the active ALDH2 isozyme has been identified (Impraim et al., 1982; Johnson et al., 1987). Amino acid sequencing has shown that the protein subunit from the active and inactive isozymes differ in only 1 of 500 amino acid residues. The glutamic acid at position 487 in the subunit of the normal active isozyme is replaced by lysine in the inactive variant form (Hempel et al., 1984; Yoshida et al., 1984). The structural gene for ALDH2 has been cloned and large parts of it (all 13 exons and intron–exon boundaries) have been sequenced (Hsu et al., 1988). The single amino acid alteration resulting in loss of activity of ALDH2 arises from a point mutation, a G to A nucleotide base change in exon 12 of the gene (Hsu et al., 1987).

Knowledge of the nucleotide sequence surrounding the mutation site has enabled the synthesis of allele-specific oligonucleotide probes and the direct genotyping of subjects with use of leukocyte deoxyribonucleic acid (DNA). This has been accomplished both with and without amplification of the relevant DNA segments (exon 12) by means of the polymerase chain reaction (PCR) (Crabb et al., 1989; Hsu et al., 1987). Until these studies were performed, it was assumed that individuals with the deficient phenotype are homozygous for the $ALDH_2$ variant allele ($ALDH_2^2/ALDH_2^2$), and those with the normal phenotype are homozygous for the normal allele ($ALDH_2^1/ALDH_2^1$) or are heterozygous ($ALDH_2^1/ALDH_2^2$). Those who are heterozygous would be expected to exhibit lowered ALDH2 activity, but not to be deficient. The genotyping studies yielded surprising and interesting results. As shown in Table I, 20 Japanese liver specimens were both phenotyped by means of starch gel electrophoresis and genotyped by use of allele-specific oligonucleotide probes after DNA amplification. It was found that, contrary to expectation, most of the ALDH2-deficient specimens were heterozygous ($ALDH_2^1/ALDH_2^2$). Thus, the presence of a single $ALDH_2^2$ allele results in the ALDH2-deficient phenotype; that is, this phenotype is inherited as an autosomal dominant trait. Based on these data, it can be calculated that the gene frequency of $ALDH_2^2$ is about 0.25 in the Japanese population and not 0.65 as predicted by the old autosomal recessive gene model (Crabb et al., 1989).

The mechanism by which the $ALDH_2^2$ gene product, that is, the inactive ALDH2 subunit, produces the ALDH2-deficient phenotype in heterozygous individuals is not understood. The ALDH2 enzyme is a homotetrameric protein, and the random association of active and inactive subunits, equally expressed, should generate about 6% normal tetramers. If all tetramers containing one or more mutant subunits were inactive, there would be only 6% activity in individuals who are heterozygous. This amount of activity would likely be below the detection limit of activity staining of the gels. Whether the tetramers containing one or more of the variant subunits are indeed inactive and whether such heterotetramers are inherently unstable are unknown and merit further study.

Table 1.   Correlation of ALDH2 Phenotype and Genotype.

Liver Specimen	Phenotype	Genotype
433	active	1,1
807	active	1,1
810	active	1,1
819	active	1,1
821	active	1,1
824	active	1,1
825	active	1,1
826	active	1,1
827	active	1,1
829	active	1,1
480	deficient	1,2
483	· deficient	1,2
529	deficient	1,2
530	deficient	1,2
806	deficient	1,2
808	deficient	1,2
809	deficient	1,2
818	deficient	2,2
820	deficient	1,2
828	deficient	1,2

Twenty autopsy liver specimens were homogenized and the activities of the ALDH isozymes in homogenate supernatants were visualized by staining with propionaldehyde as substrate after electrophoresis on starch gels (Johnson et al., 1987). The DNA from these livers was extracted and exon 12 of the $ALDH_2$ gene was amplified by use of the polymerase chain reaction. The genotyping was performed by hybridization with allele-specific oligonucleotides for $ALDH_2^1$ and $ALDH_2^2$ (Crabb et al., 1989). Genotype 1,1 is $ALDH_2^1/ALDH_2^1$; genotype 1,2 is $ALDH_2^1/ALDH_2^2$; genotype 2,2 is $ALDH_2^2/ALDH_2^2$.

The ALDH2 Phenotype and Alcohol-Drinking Behavior

Studies from Japan and recent studies from our laboratory indicate that the ALDH2 gene has a major influence on drinking behavior and the development of alcoholism. It has been shown that the ALDH2 phenotype is uncommon in Japanese alcoholic individuals and in Japanese individuals with alcoholic liver disease. Only fewer than 5% of alcoholic persons with or without liver disease were ALDH2-deficient when phenotyped by hair-root analysis, as compared with the 44% ALDH2 deficiency in the Japanese general population (Harada et al., 1983).

The influence of the ALDH2 phenotype on drinking behavior has recently been studied in many Japanese subjects who are social drinkers, as well as in alcoholic persons (Shigemori et al., 1988). The prevalence of this deficiency as determined by hair-root analysis of the enzyme is about 50% in non-alcoholics, but it is only 9% in alcoholics. Further, in non-alcoholic individuals, drinking frequency and amount was significantly lower in the ALDH2-deficient subjects. This inverse relationship was less pronounced in women than in men. The reason for this gender difference is unclear, but it may be that Japanese women as a group tended to drink less than the men. Among alcoholic individuals, initial drinking, habitual drinking, and first hospitalization occurred later in life in those who are ALDH2-deficient. The data indicate that the ALDH2-deficient phenotype is protective against heavy drinking and alcoholism.

A recent study from our laboratory examined the genotypes for the ALDH2 enzyme in Atayal Taiwanese aborigines and Han Chinese living in Taiwan (Thomasson et al., 1989). As expected from the incidence of the alcohol-flush reaction in Chinese and Japanese, the $ALDH_2^2$ allele was found in about 50% of the Chinese in Taiwan. However, the variant allele was seen in only 15% of the aborigines. The two groups also differed in rate of alcoholism, which is high among the aborigines and low in the Chinese. Part of this difference may arise from environmental factors, but a striking difference in $ALDH_2^2$ allele prevalence was seen in the alcoholic and nonalcoholic Chinese. The large majority (85%) of the Chinese alcoholics exhibited the homozygous $ALDH_2^1/ALDH_2^1$ genotype, in contrast to the 50% in the nonalcoholic Chinese population. No significant difference in the distribution of $ALDH_2$ alleles was seen in the alcoholic and nonalcoholic aborigines. These findings are consistent with the Japanese study summarized above. The results show that the $ALDH_2^2$ allele is protective against heavy drinking, whereas the $ALDH_2^1$ allele is permissive of heavy drinking and alcoholism. The $ALDH_2^2$ allele appears to be prevalent only among Asian populations. This mutation has not been detected in populations of European descent, although other kinds of ALDH mutations in these populations are currently being sought.

ANIMAL STUDIES

Genetic Animal Models for the Study of Alcoholism

Understanding of the neurobiology of alcoholism can be gained from studying animals that exhibit abnormally intense alcohol-seeking behavior in comparison with other animals. Through the years a number of investigators have attempted to develop suitable animal models of alcoholism for experimental study. However, most species of laboratory animals do not show a drinking preference for unflavored aqueous solutions containing moderate to high concentrations of ethanol, and a number of approaches to increasing oral consumption of ethanol have been explored (Deitrich and Melchior, 1985; Pohorecky, 1981). The most successful of these has been genetic. McClearn and Rodgers (1959) first showed that inbred strains of mice differed widely in their preference for a 10% ethanol solution versus water, an indication of a genetic influence on that trait. Capitalizing on this potential, rat lines that differ in alcohol preference have been developed through selective breeding. Selective breeding is the process by which subjects exhibiting the most extreme levels of a chosen phenotype (e.g., high and low voluntary consumption) are mated in successive generations. Over time, the selected lines would have a high or low frequency of the genes influencing that trait, while the frequency of the genes not affecting that trait should remain randomly distributed. These pharmacogenetically different animal lines provide useful tools for investigating mechanisms, since associated traits are likely to share common mechanisms through common gene action.

Currently, there are three pairs (high and low) of established rat lines that differ in alcohol preference, developed through selective breeding from different foundation stocks (Eriksson and Rusi, 1981; Li et al., 1979; Mardones and Segozia-Riquelene, 1983). One of these pairs, the high preference P and the low preference NP line, was developed in our laboratory (Li et al., 1987). The P rats have been shown to meet the major requirements proposed for an animal model of alcoholism (Lester and Freed, 1973), and comparison of the P and NP lines has identified associated traits, opening up avenues for exploration of the neurobiological basis of alcohol-seeking behavior.

More recently, we initiated a new selective breeding experiment for high and low alcohol drinking preference, using as a heterogeneous foundation stock the N/Nih rat (Hansen and Spuhler, 1984), which was developed from the cross of eight inbred strains. The new duplicate lines are the HAD-1 and HAD-2 (high alcohol-drinking) and the LAD-1 and LAD-2 (low alcohol-drinking) lines. The purpose of this new selection study is to address the issue of generality of the phenotypic associations of high alcohol-seeking behavior discovered in the P and NP lines and to establish the HAD line as another useful animal model for alcoholism research. Studies to date indicate that the HAD rats are similar to the P rats in many ways, behaviorally (in response to ethanol) and neurochemically.

The P/NP and the HAD/LAD Rat Lines as Animal Models for the Study of Alcohol-seeking Behavior and Alcoholism

Studies in the last 12 years have shown that the P rats satisfy all the major criteria for an animal model of alcoholism (Cicero, 1979; Lester and Freed 1973). Specifically, the P rats:

1. voluntarily drink ethanol solutions (10–30% in water, v/v) in quantities that elevate blood alcohol concentrations (BACs) into pharmacologically meaningful ranges (Li et al., 1979, Lumeng and Li, 1986, Murphy et al., 1986)
2. develop tolerance and physical dependence with chronic drinking (Gatto et al., 1987a; Waller et al., 1982)
3. work through operant responding to obtain ethanol in concentrations as high as 30%, (Fig. 1) but not because of the caloric value, taste, or smell of the ethanol solutions (Murphy et al., 1989; Penn et al., 1978; Waller et al., 1984).

More importantly, comparison of the P rats with the selectively bred, alcohol-nonpreferring NP line of rats has revealed differences that suggested new avenues for exploration of the neurobiological basis of alcohol-seeking behavior. When compared with the NP rat,

1. Ethanol-naive P rats exhibit lower levels of serotonin (5-HT) and dopamine (DA) in certain brain regions (Murphy et al., 1982), most notably the nucleus accumbens (NA) (Murphy et al., 1987). Higher densities of 5-HT receptors in some of these regions (cerebral cortex and hippocampus) have been found in the P rats as compared with NP rats (Wong et al., 1988). Preliminary immunocytochemical studies suggest that the P rats may have fewer 5-HT fibers in the affected regions as compared with NP rats (unpublished observations).

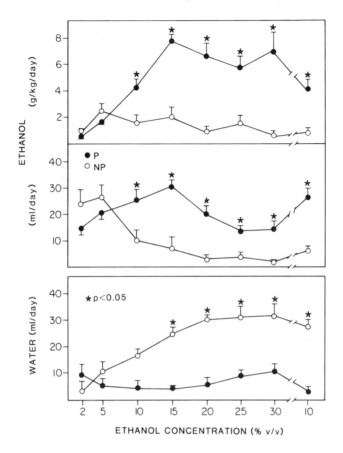

Figure 1.   Daily consumption by P and NP rats responding to a two-bar operant task for water and different concentrations of ethanol. Each point represents an average over 3 days. * p <0.05 by ANOVA and Newman-Keuls post-hoc test for the P compared with the NP group. Reproduced with permission of Pergamon Press from Murphy et al. (1989): Operant responding for oral ethanol in the alcohol-preferring P and alcohol non-preferring NP lines of rats. *Alcohol* 6:127-131.

The administration of 5-HT uptake inhibitors attenuates the alcohol-seeking behavior of the P rats (McBride et al., 1988).

2. The P rats are behaviorally stimulated by low doses of ethanol and are less affected by sedative-hypnotic doses of ethanol (Waller et al., 1986).

3. The P rats develop tolerance more quickly within a single session

of exposure to a sedative-hypnotic dose of ethanol (acute tolerance), and this tolerance persists (as tested by a second dose of ethanol) for a much longer period of time (Gatto et al., 1987b; Waller et al., 1983).

The difference between lines in response to ethanol suggested to us the general hypothesis that an enhanced responsiveness to the low-dose, reinforcing effects of ethanol, together with the rapid development and persistence of tolerance to high-dose, aversive effects of ethanol promotes high alcohol-seeking behavior. Recent comparison studies in HAD and LAD rats have shown that, as with the P rats, selection for ethanol drinking preference (10% ethanol vs. H_2O) produced lines (HAD) that exhibit operant responding for ethanol as reward in concentrations as high as 30%. As with NP rats, LAD rats responded very little for ethanol when alcohol concentration exceeded 5% (Levy et al., 1988). Furthermore, as was found in the P and NP rats, HAD animals exhibit longer persistence of tolerance after a single sedative-hypnotic dose of ethanol than do the LAD animals (Froehlich et al., 1987). Therefore, the salient features of the hypothesis formulated from the studies of the P and NP rats appear generalizable.

More recently, the contents of dopamine (DA), serotonin (5-HT), and their primary acid metabolites were assayed in 10 brain regions of HAD and LAD lines of rats (Gongwer et al., 1989). Compared with the LAD line, the contents of 5-HT and/or 5-hydroxyindoleacetic acid were lower in several brain regions (cerebral cortex, striatum, nucleus accumbens, septal nuclei, hippocampus and hypothalamus) of the HAD line. The levels of DA, 3,4-dihydroxyphenylacetic acid, and homovanillic acid were also lower in the nucleus accumbens and anterior striatum of the HAD rats. These data generally agree with the findings in P and NP rats and implicate the involvement of 5-HT and DA pathways in mediating alcohol-drinking behavior. Another neurotransmitter system that may have an important role in ethanol preference is gamma-aminobutyric acid (GABA). Immunocytochemical and morphometric studies have revealed more GABAergic terminals in the nucleus accumbens of the P rats than in that of the NP rats (Hwang et al., 1988). How the GABAergic system interfaces with the 5-HT and DA systems in the brain-reward pathways is not well-understood.

MOLECULAR AND GENETIC STUDIES IN ANIMAL MODELS: PRESENT AND FUTURE

Our ultimate goal in studying the selectively bred alcohol-preferring and nonpreferring rats is to identify the genes responsible for the neurobiological abnormalities that lead to excessive alcohol-seeking behavior. Alcohol drinking is a quantitative trait and is most likely influenced by multiple genes. However, there are indications that only a few genes are involved in exerting a major influence on alcohol preference. In the development of both the P and NP lines and the HAD and LAD lines, differences in the average drinking scores of the high and low lines began to emerge in the early generations, suggesting that a few genes may be controlling a major portion of the variation in alcohol drinking in these lines. From a triple-test cross analysis of ethanol preference, Drewek and Broadhurst (1981, 1983) concluded that an additive-dominance model proved adequate in the rat, and a strong directional dominance for low alcohol preference was found. Studies in the B × D recombinant inbred (C57BL/6J × DBA/2J) mice have revealed a potential single gene effect for ethanol acceptance or preference (Crabbe et al., 1983). A panel of recombinant inbred (RI) strains exhibited a bimodal distribution for ethanol acceptance (shown to be genetically equivalent to ethanol preference), implying that a single gene exerts a major control on this trait. A genetic correlation between high ethanol acceptance and the basic (electrophoretic) form of the brain protein LTW-4 was found in studies of inbred mouse strains and in the B × D RI strains. The finding suggests that a locus-determining ethanol intake is near the gene for the LTW-4 protein on chromosome 1 of the mouse (Goldman et al., 1987).

Recently, we tested the P and NP rats for 17 different biochemical markers and found that the NP line was homozygous at all 17 loci. The P rats were identical to the NP rats at 14 loci and exhibited heterozygosity at 3 loci. Thus, the P rats still have some genetic heterogeneity, whereas the NP rats appear now to be highly inbred. Interestingly, whereas the NP rats exhibited the *ll* phenotype at the RT1-A locus of the major histocompatibility complex (MHC), the P rats were predominantly *uu*, with about 20% having the *ul* heterozygous phenotype. The mean drinking score of the *uu* animals was significantly higher than that of the *ul* animals, suggesting a genetic association of ethanol preference with the RT1-A locus of the rat (Fig. 2). We have also recently discovered a polymorphism involving the mitochondrial aldehyde dehydrogenase isozyme that appears to have an association with alcohol preference. These findings indicate that it is now timely to initiate more extensive biochemical/genetic marker studies to examine not only gene product markers but also DNA markers.

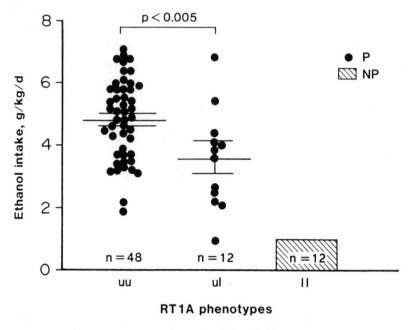

Figure 2. Relationship between RT1-A phenotypes and alcohol-drinking behavior in the P and NP rats. Sixty P rats and 12 NP rats were tested for voluntary ethanol intake (10% (v/v) ethanol, water, and food *ad lib*) and their RT1-A phenotypes were determined by hemagglutination assay (Charles River Professional Services, Wilmington, MA).

Unfortunately, compared with humans and mice, there is relatively little information about the gene map of the rat. Fewer than 100 rat genes have been mapped (Cramer, 1988). A restriction fragment length polymorphism (RFLP) linkage map for the rat genome is nonexistent. The rat MHC locus on chromosome 14 (linkage group IX) is actually the best characterized region of the rat genome. The RT1 is flanked by the polymorphic glyoxalase and neuraminidase genes, and several mouse and human MHC complementary DNA (cDNA) probes have detected polymorphism within the RT1 region. These marker enzymes and cDNA probes can be used to further characterize a potential genetic relationship to alcohol preference.

When a complete linkage map of RFLPs is established, it should be possible to resolve quantitative traits into mendelian factors and discern the number of quantitative trait loci (QTLs) and assign them to the appropriate chromosomal locations (Paterson et al., 1988). Rat genetics is currently far from this stage, but a reasonable beginning might be to explore the relationship of ethanol preference to a number of "candidate" genes for which cDNA probes are available. Since the P and NP rats differ in 5-HT, DA, and GABA neuronal systems, it appears reasonable to examine the genes and messenger ribonucleic acids (mRNAs) of the receptors and enzymes of synthesis and metabolism associated with these neurotransmitter systems. This can be done on a qualitative level, that is, RFLP analysis of genomic DNA, and on a quantitative level, through *in situ* and solution hybridization methodology, of the relevant mRNAs.

Other approaches to identifying potential genetic markers of ethanol preference are to screen for differences between P and NP lines in brain proteins, as has been done in the inbred and the B × D RI mouse strains (Goldman et al., 1987). The use of subtractive hybridization probing techniques can also be used to identify unique (to P or NP) mRNAs in brain cDNA libraries (Milner et al., 1987; Travis and Sutcliffe, 1988). A future technique that can provide genetic markers for ethanol preference may come from the use of polymorphisms involving the variable numbers of tandem repeat (VNTR) sequences (White and Lalouel, 1988). These loci are highly polymorphic in man. A development that shows promise for screening VNTR polymorphisms is the 2D-gel chromatography method recently reported by Uitterlinden et al. (1989).

SUMMARY

Alcohol drinking is influenced in different ways by different neuropharmacological responses to ethanol. The use of selective breeding methodology to produce animal lines with high and low alcohol preference has demonstrated convincingly that there is genetic influence on alcohol-seeking behavior. Studies that compare preferring and nonpreferring animals have shown that not only are the rewarding properties of ethanol important for high consumption, but tolerance developed to the aversive effects of ethanol may also be a major factor. Aversive reactions produce decreased consumption, as exemplified by the alcohol-flush reaction in humans and by conditioned taste aversion studies in the P and NP rats (Froehlich et al., 1988).

An association of various neurotransmitter systems with high alcohol-seeking behavior has been identified in rats. How these systems interface in producing alcohol-seeking behavior is currently under active investigation. Finally, characterization of the differences between the preferring and nonpreferring animals by means of molecular biology techniques can now be undertaken, with the ultimate goal of identifying the genes that are responsible for alcohol-seeking behavior.

REFERENCES

Bosron WF, Lumeng L, Li T-K (1988): Genetic polymorphism of enzymes of alcohol metabolism and susceptibility to liver disease. *Mol Aspects Med* 10:147-158

Cicero TJ (1979): A critique of animal analogues of alcoholism. In: *Biochemistry and Pharmacology of Ethanol, Vol. 2.* Majchrowicz E, Noble EP, eds. New York: Plenum Press

Cloninger CR (1986): Genetics of alcoholism. *Alcoholism: Clin Exp Res* 9:479-482

Cloninger CR, Bohman M, Sigvardsson S (1981): Inheritance of alcohol abuse: cross-fostering analysis of adopted men. *Arch Gen Psychiatry* 38:861-868

Crabb DW, Edenberg HJ, Bosron WJ, Li T-K (1989): Genotypes for aldehyde dehydrogenase deficiency and alcohol sensitivity: the inactive $ALDH_2^2$ allele is dominant. *J Clin Invest* 83:314-316

Crabbe JC, Kosobud A, Young ER, Janowsky JS (1983): Polygenic and single-gene determination of responses to ethanol in BXD/Ty recombinant inbred mouse strains. *Neurobehav Toxicol Teratol* 5:181-187

Cramer DV (1988): Biochemical loci of the rat (Rattus Norvegicus). *Rat News Lett* 20:15-19

Deitrich RA, Melchior CL (1985): A critical assessment of animal models for testing new drugs for altering ethanol intake. In: *Research Advances in New PsychoPharmacological Treatments for Alcoholism.* Naranjo CA, Sellers EM, eds. Amsterdam: Excerpta Medica

Drewek KJ, Broadhurst PL (1981): A simplified triple-test cross analysis of alcohol preference in the rat. *Behav Genet* 11:517-531

Drewek KJ, Broadhurst PL (1983): The genetics of alcohol preference in the female rat confirmed by a full triple-test cross. *Behav Genet* 13:107-116

Edwards G, Gross MM (1976): Alcohol dependence: provisional description of a syndrome. *Br Med J* 1:1058-1061

Eriksson K, Rusi M (1981): Finnish selection studies on alcohol-related behaviors: general outline. In : *NIAAA Research Monograph-6. Development of Animal Models as Pharmacogenetic Tools.* McClearn GE, Deitrich RA, Erwin VG, eds. Washington, DC: U.S. Government Printing Office

Froehlich JC, Harts J, Lumeng L, Li T-K (1988): Differences in response to the aversive properties of ethanol in rats selectively bred for oral ethanol preference. *Pharmacol Biochem Behav* 31:215-222

Froehlich JC, Hostetter J, Lumeng L, Li T-K (1987): Association between alcohol preference and acute tolerance. *Alcoholism: Clin Exp Res* 11:199 (Abstract)

Gatto GJ, Murphy JM, Waller MB, McBride WJ, Lumeng L, Li T-K (1987a): Chronic ethanol tolerance through free-choice drinking in the P line of alcohol-preferring rats. *Pharmacol Biochem Behav* 28:111-115

Gatto GJ, Murphy JM, Waller MB, McBride WJ, Lumeng L, Li T-K (1987b): Persistence of tolerance to a single dose of ethanol in the selectively bred alcohol-preferring P rats. *Pharmacol Biochem Behav* 28:105-110

Goedde HW, Harada S, Agarwal DP (1979): Racial differences in alcohol sensitivity: a new hypothesis. *Hum Genet* 51:331-334

Goldman D, Lister RG, Crabbe JC (1987): Mapping of a putative genetic locus determining ethanol intake in the mouse. *Brain Res* 420:220-226

Gongwer MA, Lumeng L, Murphy JM, McBride WJ, Li T-K (1989): Regional brain contents of serotonin, dopamine and their metabolites in the selectively bred high- and low-alcohol-drinking lines of rats. *Alcohol* 6:317-320

Hansen C, Spuhler K (1984): Development of the National Institutes of Health genetically heterogeneous rat stock. *Alcoholism: Clin Exp Res* 8:477-479

Harada S, Agarwal DP, Goedde HW (1980): Electrophoretic and biochemical studies of human aldehyde dehydrogenase isozymes in various tissues. *Life Sci* 26:1773-1780

Harada S, Agarwal DP, Goedde HW (1981): Aldehyde dehydrogenase deficiency as cause of facial flushing reaction to alcohol in Japanese. *Lancet* ii:982

Harada S, Agarwal DP, Goedde HW, Ishikawa B (1983): Aldehyde dehydrogenase isoenzyme variation and alcoholism in Japan. *Pharmacol Biochem Behav* 18(Suppl 1):151-153

Hempel J, Kaiser R, Jornvall H (1984): Human liver mitochondrial aldehyde dehydrogenase: a C-terminal segment positions and defines the structure corresponding to the one reported to differ in the Oriental enzyme variant. *FEBS Letters* 173:367-372

Hsu LC, Bendel RE, Yoshida A (1987): Direct detection of usual and atypical alleles on the human aldehyde dehydrogenase-2 (ALDH2) locus. *Am J Hum Genet* 41:996-1001

Hsu LC, Bendel RE, Yoshida A (1988): Genomic structure of the human mitochondrial aldehyde dehydrogenase gene. *Genomics* 2:57-65

Hwang BH, Lumeng L, Wu J-Y, Li T-K (1988): GABAergic neurons in nucleus accumbens: a possible role in alcohol preference. *Alcoholism: Clin Exp Res* 12:306 (Abstract)

Impraim C, Wang G, Yoshida A (1982): Structural mutation in a major human aldehyde dehydrogenase gene results in loss of enzyme activity. *Am J Hum Genet* 34:837-841

Johnson CT, Bosron UF, Harden CA, Li T-K (1987) Purification of human liver aldehyde dehydrogenase by high performance liquid chromatography and identification of isoenzymes by immunoblotting. *Alcoholism: Clin Exp Res* 11:60-65

Lester D, Freed EX (1973): Criteria for an animal model of alcoholism. *Pharmacol Biochem Behav* 1:103-107

Levy AD, McBride WJ, Murphy J, Lumeng L, Li T-K (1988): Genetically selected lines of high- and low-alcohol-drinking rats: operant studies. *Abs Soc Neurosci* 14:41

Li T-K (1985): Genetic variability in response to ethanol in humans and experimental animals. In : *Proceedings: NIAAA-WHO Collaborating Center Designation Meeting and Alcohol Research Seminar*. Towle LH, ed. Washington, DC: U.S. Government Printing Office

Li T-K, Lumeng L, McBride WJ, Murphy JM (1987): Rodent lines selected for factors affecting alcohol consumption. *Alcohol and Alcoholism* (Suppl) 1:91-96

Li T-K, Lumeng L, McBride WJ, Waller MB, Hawkins DT (1979): Progress toward a voluntary oral-consumption model of alcoholism. *Drug and Alcohol Depend* 4:45-60

Lumeng L, Li T-K (1986): The development of metabolic tolerance in the alcohol-preferring P rats: comparison of forced and free-choice drinking of ethanol. *Pharmacol Biochem Behav* 25:1013-1020

Mardones J, Segozia-Riquelene N (1983): Thirty-two years of selection of rats by ethanol preference: UChA and UChB strains. *Neurobehav Toxicol Teratol* 5:171-178

McBride WJ, Murphy JM, Lumeng L, Li T-K (1988): Effects of Ro15-4513, fluoxetine and desipramine on the intake of ethanol, water and food by the alcohol-preferring (P) and -nonpreferring (NP) lines of rats. *Pharmacol Biochem Behav* 30:1045-1050

McClearn GE, Erwin VG (1982): Mechanisms of genetic influence on alcohol-related behaviors. In : *Alcohol and Health Monograph I. Alcohol Consumption and Related Problems*. Washington, DC: U.S. Government Printing Office

McClearn GE, Rodgers DA (1959): Differences in alcohol preference among inbred strains of mice. *J Stud Alcohol* 20:691-695

Milner RJ, Bloom FE, Sutcliffe JG (1987): Brain-specific genes: strategies and issues. In: *Current Topics in Developmental Biology* 12:117-150

Mizoi Y, Ijiri I, Tatsuno Y, Kijima T, Fujiwara S, Adachi J (1979): Relationship between facial flushing and blood acetaldehyde levels after alcohol intake. *Pharmacol Biochem Behav* 10:303-311

Murphy JM, Gatto GJ, McBride WJ, Lumeng L, Li T-K (1989): Operant responding for oral ethanol in the alcohol-preferring P and alcohol-nonpreferring NP lines of rats. *Alcohol* 6:127-131

Murphy JM, Gatto GJ, Waller MB, McBride WJ, Lumeng L, Li T-K (1986): Effects of scheduled access on ethanol intake by the alcohol-deferring P line of rats. *Alcohol* 3:331-336

Murphy JM, McBride WJ, Lumeng L, Li T-K (1982): Regional brain levels of monoamines in alcohol-preferring and nonpreferring lines of rats. *Pharmacol Biochem Behav* 16:145-149

Murphy JM, McBride WJ, Lumeng L, Li T-K (1987): Contents of monoamines in forebrain regions of alcohol-preferring (P) and nonpreferring (NP) lines of rats. *Pharmacol Biochem Behav* 26:389-392

Paterson AH, Lander ES, Hewitt JD, Peterson S, Lincoln SE, Tanksley SD (1988): Resolution of quantitative traits into mendelian factors by using a complete linkage map of restriction fragment length polymorphisms. *Nature* 335:721-726

Penn PE, McBride WJ, Lumeng L, Gaff TM, Li T-K (1978): Neurochemical and operant behavioral studies of a strain of alcohol-preferring rats. *Pharmacol Biochem Behav* 8:475-481

Pohorecky LA (1977): Biphasic action of ethanol. *Biobehav Rev* 1:231-240

Pohorecky LA (1981): Animal analog of alcohol dependence. *Fed Proc* 40:2056-2064

Shigemori K, Higuchi S, Muramatsu T, Saito M, Sasao M, Takagi T, Kono H, Harada S (1988): Effects of the ALDH phenotype on drinking behavior. *Alcohol and Alcoholism* 23:A60

Teng Y-S (1981): Human liver aldehyde dehydrogenase in Chinese and Asiatic Indians: gene deletion and its possible implications in alcohol metabolism. *Biochem Genet* 19:107-114

Thomasson HR, Mai XL, Crabb DW, Li T-K, Hwu HG, Chen CC, Yeh E-K, Wang S-P, Lin Y-T, Lu R-B, Yin S-J (1989): Aldehyde dehydrogenase deficiency: relationship of aldehyde dehydrogenase-2 genotype with risk for alcoholism in Taiwanese. *Clin Res* 37:898A

Travis GH, Sutcliffe JG (1988): Phenol emulsion-enhanced DNA-driven subtractive cDNA cloning: isolation of low-abundance monkey cortex-specific mRNAs. *Proc Natl Acad Sci USA* 85:1696-1700

Uitterlinden AG, Slagboom PE, Knook DL, Vijg J (1989): Two dimensional DNA fingerprinting of human individuals. *Proc Natl Acad Sci USA* 86:2742-2746

White R, Lalouel J-M (1988): Sets of linked genetic markers for human chromosomes. *Ann Rev Genet* 22:259-279

Waller MB, McBride WJ, Gatto GJ, Lumeng L, Li T-K (1984): Intragastric self-infusion of ethanol by the P and NP (alcohol-preferring and nonpreferring) lines of rats. *Science* 225:78-80

Waller MB, McBride WJ, Lumeng L, Li T-K (1982): Induction of dependence on ethanol by free-choice drinking in alcohol-preferring rats. *Pharmacol Biochem Behav* 16:501-507

Waller MB, McBride WJ, Lumeng L, Li T-K (1983): Initial sensitivity and acute tolerance to ethanol in the P and NP lines of rats. *Pharmacol Biochem Behav* 19:683-686

Waller MB, Murphy JM, McBride WJ, Lumeng L, Li T-K (1986): Effect of low dose ethanol on spontaneous motor activity in alcohol-preferring and nonpreferring lines of rats. *Pharmacol Biochem Behav* 24:617-625

Wong DT, Lumeng L, Threlkeld PG, Reid LR, Li T-K (1988): Serotonergic and adrenergic receptors of alcohol-preferring and -nonpreferring rats. *J Neurol Trans* 71:207-218

Yoshida A, Huang I-Y, Ikawa M (1984): Molecular abnormality of an inactive aldehyde dehydrogenase variant commonly found in Orientals. *Proc Natl Acad Sci (USA)* 81:258-261

The Neuropharmacology of Ethanol Self-Administration

F. Weiss and G. F. Koob

The abuse liability of ethanol is thought to derive primarily from its anxiolytic and euphoric effects. Together, these properties are believed to underlie the acute reinforcing actions of ethanol that, in turn, sustain continued abuse and thereby ultimately may lead to the development of dependence. An increasing body of evidence suggests that the rewarding and intoxicating effects of ethanol are mediated by its actions on one or more specific neurotransmitter systems in the brain (Faber and Klee, 1977; Kulonen, 1983; Liljequist and Engel, 1979; Myers, 1978b; Tabakoff, 1977). However, although there is tentative evidence linking certain transmitters—notably the catecholamines, opioids, gamma-amino butyric acid and serotonin—or their receptors to aspects of the intoxicating actions of ethanol, no exclusive role for any transmitter in ethanol reward or dependence has yet been established.

ANIMAL MODELS OF ETHANOL SELF-ADMINISTRATION

Self-administration procedures have been an effective tool to study the neuropharmacology of drug-seeking behavior and reward, particularly in the case of opiate and psychostimulant drugs (Bozarth, 1982; Goeders and Smith, 1983; Koob et al., 1987; Lyness et al., 1979; Wise, 1984). Indeed, on the basis of this work biological theories of drug reinforcement have emerged that center around the assumption that drugs of abuse act on specific neuronal systems that directly or indirectly activate central "reward substrates" that mediate motivated behavior and reinforcement (Bozarth, 1982; Fibiger, 1978; Koob and Goeders, 1988; Wise, 1980, 1984; Wise and Bozarth, 1982).

Relative to the advances made over the past two decades in eluci-
dating critical circuitries for psychostimulant and opiate reward, com-
paratively little is known about the neuropharmacological substrates for
ethanol reward. There are essentially two problems that have hampered
progress toward an understanding of ethanol reward. First, it has been
difficult to establish ethanol as a reinforcer when presented orally. The
failure to obtain spontaneous, voluntary oral ethanol self-administration
in rats is generally attributed to rats' taste aversion to ethanol concentrations greater than 6% (w/v), as well as the long interval between alcohol
ingestion and the onset of its pharmacological (interoceptive) effects (for
review see Meisch, 1982, 1984; Samson, 1987). Second, factors other
than, or in addition to, its central effects may modify self-administration
of ethanol. For example, contextual or environmental variables as well
as ethanol interactions with brain systems involved in drinking behavior
per se such as the angiotensin-renin system may play an important role
in the self-administration of ethanol (Stewart et al., 1988).

In order to develop voluntary ethanol drinking at pharmacologically
meaningful levels, animal studies of alcohol intake have typically relied
on special procedures to initiate ethanol self-administration. In this section, a brief overview of these procedures will be presented. It is not
the purpose of this chapter to exhaust the literature on animal models
of alcoholism (for comprehensive reviews see Lester and Freed, 1973;
Meisch, 1982, 1984; Mello, 1973, 1976; Samson, 1987), but to examine
ethanol self-administration procedures with regard to their implications
for the study of the neuropharmacology of ethanol reward.

Several procedures have been successfully used to initiate oral ethanol intake. The most common of these include alcohol acclimation and
taste adulteration, schedule-induced polydipsia and prandial models. *Alcohol acclimation* typically involves some form of "habituation" procedure to the aversive taste effects of ethanol. Animals are either exposed
to gradually increasing alcohol concentrations (Veale, 1973) or, alternatively, water or ethanol are switched daily as the sole source of fluid over
a period of time. After several forced drinking and deprivation cycles,
ethanol intake increases (Sinclair and Senter, 1967; Wayner and Greenberg, 1972; Wayner et al., 1972; Wise, 1973). Another procedure that
has been successfully used to obtain voluntary oral ethanol intake, the
taste adulteration model, requires the addition of other substances (e.g.,
sweeteners) to the drinking solution to overcome or mask the aversive

taste of ethanol (Amit and Stern, 1971; Eriksson, 1969; Falk et al., 1973; Pekkanen and Rusi, 1979; Samson, 1986). *Prandial* models make use of the postprandial drinking associated with feeding in rats. Food-deprived animals are given access to increasing concentrations of ethanol along with their daily food ration during short daily sessions (Meisch, 1977, 1984; Meisch and Henningfield, 1977; Stewart and Grupp, 1984; Stewart and Perlanski, 1988). Once stable ethanol intake is observed, animals will continue to drink ethanol in the absence of food. Prandial drinking models have essentially evolved from the *schedule-induced polydipsia* technique, which takes advantage of the adjunctive drinking behavior associated with food reinforced responding on some schedules of reinforcement (Falk, 1961; Falk et al., 1972; Meisch and Thompson, 1971). While prandial models have been developed to initiate operant responding for ethanol, they have also been successfully adapted to initiate two-bottle home cage drinking (Linseman, 1987; Stewart and Grupp, 1984; Stewart and Perlanski, 1988).

Two issues are central to the study of ethanol reward. First, it is important to demonstrate that ethanol intake in a given model is maintained by pharmacological motivation rather than factors related to nutritional appetite, thirst, and so forth (Dole, 1986; Lester and Freed, 1973; Mello, 1973). Second, in order to demonstrate that ethanol functions as a reinforcer, ethanol should change and maintain behavior in addition to maintaining ethanol drinking. Indeed, as pointed out by Samson (1987), the major concern of procedures designed to initiate voluntary ethanol intake is to overcome the aversive taste properties of ethanol. If successful, these procedures establish behaviors that are maintained by the reinforcing properties of ethanol.

When evaluated in terms of these criteria, only mixed success has been achieved with most procedures (Meisch, 1977; Samson, 1987, for review). Alcohol intake in acclimated animals typically declines toward pre-exposure levels within a few weeks, although more sustained ethanol drinking has been observed under certain conditions (Wise, 1973; Weiss and Koob, unpublished results). After prandial initiation procedures, ethanol intake decreases substantially upon cessation of food restrictions to the extent that measurable blood alcohol concentrations are no longer reliably obtained (Linseman, 1986; Meisch and Thompson, 1973; Roehrs and Samson, 1982; Samson, 1987).

Despite these largely negative results, several recent reports have shown encouraging results and offer the promise of providing reliable procedures for the initiation and maintenance of alcohol intake. Using taste adulteration procedures (sucrose substitution), Samson and colleagues have shown that reliable, sustained operant responding for 10% ethanol can be obtained in free-feeding and drinking rats even after complete removal of sweetener, provided that the sweetener is slowly withdrawn (Grant and Samson, 1985; Samson, 1986). Comparable levels of ethanol intake have also recently been demonstrated by Linseman (1987) in a two-bottle water ethanol choice situation after modified prandial and acclimation procedures.

However, the vast majority of neuropharmacological investigations of ethanol reward have employed variations of the two-bottle water alcohol choice paradigm originally introduced by Richter and Campbell (1940). In this procedure rats are given continuous 24-hour home-cage access to both water and one or more ethanol solution(s) of varying concentrations. Ethanol preference over water (i.e., choice behavior) serves as a measure of ethanol reinforcement. Rats prefer ethanol at concentrations up to 6% in this model, although the total amount of ethanol consumed over 24 hours is typically far below rats' metabolic capacity (e.g., Meisch, 1977; Wallgren and Barry, 1970). Therefore, the validity of the two-bottle choice model as a measure of ethanol reward has been questioned since ethanol intake is usually not sufficient to demonstrate that it is ingested for its pharmacological effects (Cicero, 1979; Kalant, 1983; Lester and Freed, 1973). To overcome these limitations and to enhance both ethanol and water intake, restricted-access regimens have frequently been employed in which access to both water and ethanol, while concurrently available, is limited to only several hours per day. These procedures that have been devised to increase ethanol intake frequently introduce confounds of their own. As pointed out above, much effort has therefore been expended to develop procedures for the initiation of voluntary ethanol drinking in nondeprived rats. The progress that has been made with the development of such models (see below) should allow a systematic exploration of the neurobiological basis for low-dose ethanol reinforcement in nondependent, nonmotivationally constrained animals.

DEVELOPMENT OF A RELIABLE OPERANT MODEL
OF ETHANOL SELF-ADMINISTRATION

To establish a reliable drinking paradigm suited for the study of the neuro-pharmacological substrate of ethanol reward, Samson and colleagues have developed a sweet solution substitution procedure in which sustained alcohol preference and maintenance of lever-pressing were observed even after complete withdrawal of sweetener (Grant and Samson, 1985; Samson, 1986). Subsequent modification of these procedures where food and water-sated rats, operantly trained to self-administer alcohol, were allowed to obtain water or ethanol reinforcement by responding at one of two levers has yielded an operant choice paradigm that incorporates several important measures relevant to the investigation of ethanol reward. These include maintenance of responding for ethanol as a measure of ethanol reinforcement, an index of preference for ethanol over water independent of changes in the absolute amounts of ethanol consumed, and a control for nonspecific drug effects on ingestive behavior reflected in changes in total fluid intake. In addition to demonstrating maintenance of behavior, this procedure offers the advantage of operant measures of ethanol reward that may allow dissociation of the pharmacological motivation to respond from consummatory behavior.

With this procedure, reliable and reproducible oral ethanol self-administration in genetically heterogenous Wistar and alcohol-preferring (P) rats without food or water deprivation has been established (Weiss et al., 1990). Briefly, rats were trained to lever-press for 0.1 ml reinforcements of an ethanol– (5% v/v) sucrose (5% w/v) solution at either of two levers on a fixed ratio 5 schedule of reinforcement (FR 5). After development of stable FR5, responding rats were exposed to six successive sessions in which the drinking solution was alternated daily from ethanol-sucrose to ethanol (5% v/v) only. After this 6-day alternation procedure, ethanol concentrations in the drinking solution were gradually raised from 0 to 10% (v/v) in the absence of saccharine (Fig. 1). Ethanol intake (10% v/v) stabilized after approximately 45 days of single-solution training. The rats were then introduced to a two-lever, free-choice task in which presses at one lever produced ethanol (0.1 ml; 10% v/v), while responses at the other lever resulted in delivery of water (0.1 ml) into one of two drinking cups. All free-choice responding was conducted on a schedule of continuous reinforcement (CRF). After 17 days of free-choice training, the rats ingested virtually identical volumes of 10% ethanol as

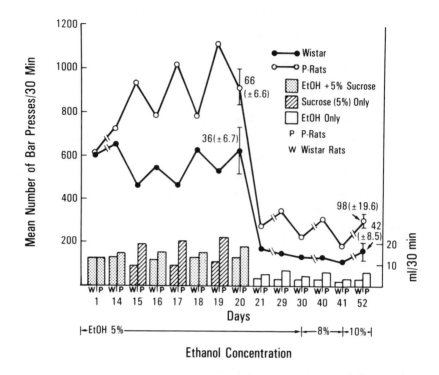

Figure 1.   Mean (±SEM) number of lever presses and mean ethanol intake (ml) during the single-solution training phase. Numbers above frequency polygons indicate mean (±SEM) BALs taken on days 20 and 52. Both alcohol-preferring (P) and genetically heterogenous Wistar rats developed stable levels of responding for 10% (v/v) ethanol by day 52 of single-solution self-administration training. Reprinted with permission of Springer-Verlag, New York, from Weiss et al. (1990): Free-choice responding for ethanol vs. water in alcohol-preferring (P) and unselected Wistar rats differentially altered by naloxone, bromocriptine and methysergide. *Psychopharmacology* 101:178-186.

compared to the end of single-solution training (Fig. 2). While there was no change in total ethanol intake, both strains of rats showed a moderate to marked preference for ethanol over water at the end of free-choice training and attained pharmacologically relevant mean blood alcohol levels (BALs) ranging from 25 to 230 mg% in P-rats and from 27 to 75 mg% in heterogenous Wistar rats (Fig. 3). Ethanol intake was highly correlated with BALs in both strains of rats, although Wistar rats showed considerable dispersion at the upper end of the distribution. Ethanol consumption in both P and Wistar rats exceeded ethanol elimination rates, which have been reported to range from 0.35 g/kg/hour in Wistar to approximately 0.38g/kg/hour in female P rats with comparable history of ethanol drinking (Lumeng et al., 1982; Lumeng and Li, 1986; see also Ferko and Bobyock, 1979).

Although there was no evidence of gross behavioral signs of intoxication in either strain of rats, BALs in the observed range appear to be relevant to the reinforcing actions of ethanol. For example, ethanol at doses that produce BALs in this range have discriminative stimulus properties (i.e., are meaningful to animals) (York, 1978). Similarly, low doses of ethanol (0.25 g/kg) increase dopamine release in the nucleus accumbens and stimulate spontaneous locomotor activity in rats, a finding that has been interpreted as an expression of the positively reinforcing effects of ethanol (Imperato and DiChiara, 1986; Lewis, this volume; Waller et al., 1986). Finally, the BALs and amounts of ingested ethanol by rats of both groups correspond well to those observed in other work with several strains of genetically heterogenous and alcohol-preferring rats (Grant and Samson, 1985; Li et al., 1986; Linseman, 1987; Samson, 1986).

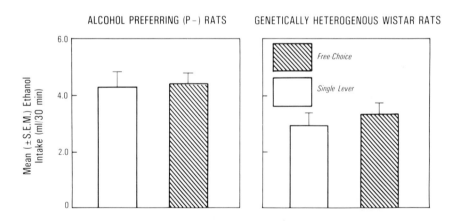

Figure 2. Ethanol (10% v/v) intake in P- and genetically-heterogenous Wistar rats after completion of single-solution and free-choice self-administration training. Data represent the mean (±SEM) ethanol intake across the two final days of single-lever or free-choice training. Ethanol intake remained remarkably stable across training procedures.

These results demonstrate that reliable operant responding for oral ethanol self-administration can be developed in rats without the need for food or water restrictions and confirm that procedures developed by Samson and colleagues provide a reliable model for the induction of ethanol-maintained behavior. Although P-rats consumed greater absolute quantities of ethanol than genetically heterogenous Wistar rats, a marked mean preference for ethanol over water was evident in both groups. More importantly, rats of both strains responded for ethanol reinforcement at rates sufficient to produce pharmacologically relevant BALs.

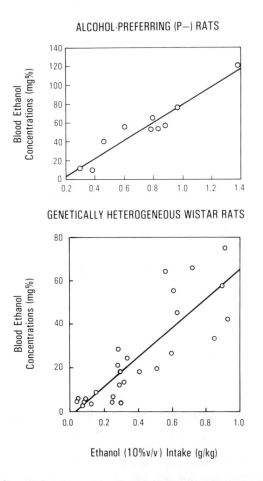

Figure 3. Correlation between ethanol intake (mg/kg) and blood alcohol concentration (BAL) in P-rats (r = .95; p<.0001) and unselected Wistars (r = .85; p<.01).

THE NEUROPHARMACOLOGY OF
ETHANOL-MAINTAINED REINFORCEMENT

Opioids

A possible involvement of endogenous opioid systems in the rewarding and intoxicating effects of ethanol has been suggested by several observations. A link between opiate- and ethanol-seeking behavior has originally been postulated by findings that acetaldehyde, an intermediary metabolite of ethanol, can undergo a condensation reaction with monoamines to form tetrahydroisoquinolines (TIQs) (i.e., compounds structurally related to morphine precursors) (Davis and Walsh, 1970) which can stimulate opiate receptors (Fertel, et al., 1980). More recently, it has been suggested that ethanol may interact indirectly by increasing the levels of endogenous opioid peptides or directly by modifying opiate receptor binding with brain opioid systems to produce its reinforcing effects (Blum et al., 1980; Charness et al., 1984; Froehlich et al., 1987; Naber et al., 1981; Pfeffer et al., 1981; Schulz et al., 1980; Tabakoff and Hoffman, 1983).

The TIQ hypothesis has received some tentative support by reports demonstrating *in vivo* synthesis of aldehyde condensation products contingent upon ethanol administration (Collins and Kahn, 1982; Critcher et al., 1982; Sandler et al., 1982). Specific TIQ interactions with endogenous opioid systems were further suggested by findings that opiate receptor antagonists, including naloxone and naltrexone, inhibit TIQ-induced alcohol self-administration in rats (Critcher et al., 1982; Myers and Critcher, 1982; Pulvirenti and Kastin, 1988). Moreover, specific neuroanatomical substrates exist that modify TIQ-induced alcohol self-administration in rats (Myers and Privette, 1989). Perhaps the most persuasive evidence for a role of TIQs in alcohol-seeking behavior is their ability to elicit drinking of abnormally high quantities of ethanol (see Myers, 1989, for review). TIQs, in particular tetrahydropapaveroline, have also been reported to produce sustained, intense preference for ethanol after discontinuation of TIQ administration, including signs of dependence and withdrawal, although some of these findings have not been unequivocally replicated (Duncan and Dietrich, 1980). But the TIQ hypothesis remains controversial since *in vivo* TIQ formation after ethanol administration can be attributed to dietary factors rather than to direct effects of ethanol exposure (Collins, 1988; Collins and Cheng, 1988).

A role for endogenous opiates in ethanol-seeking behavior has also been implicated by ethanol's ability to modify beta-endorphin and met-enkephalin levels as well as *in vitro* opiate receptor binding (see Gianoulakis, 1989, for review). Acute ethanol increases blood β-endorphin levels in humans and rats, where it also elevates hypothalamic beta-endorphin and met-enkephalin levels. In contrast, after chronic exposure to ethanol, beta-endorphin and met-enkephalin levels are reduced in the hypothalamus (Naber et al., 1981; Patel and Pohorecky, 1989; Schultz et al., 1980; Seizinger et al., 1983). Similarly, the content of β-endorphin in the CSF of human alcoholics was substantially depressed 3 to 10 days after detoxification (Genazzani et al., 1982). Although these results suggest a role for endogenous opioids in the intoxicating effects of ethanol, their precise function in ethanol preference and reward remains unclear. For example, met-enkephalin levels in the hypothalamus and corpus striatum of rats selectively bred for ethanol preference (P-rats) are higher than the corresponding levels of nonpreferring rats (Froehlich et al., 1987), but differ in the opposite direction in ethanol-avoiding and ethanol-preferring C57BL mice (Blum et al., 1982).

A testable prediction common to all accounts of opioid mediation of ethanol reward is that opiate antagonists should selectively block the pharmacological effects of ethanol or inhibit its self-administration. Consistent with the hypothesis that endogenous opioids or their receptors are involved in ethanol reward are the findings that naloxone and naltrexone inhibit TIQ-induced alcohol self-administration in rats as well as ethanol intake in acclimated rats and monkeys (Altshuler et al., 1980; Marfaing-Jallat et al., 1983; Myers and Critcher, 1982; Pulvirenti and Kastin, 1988; Reid and Hunter, 1984; Sandi et al., 1988; Volpicelli et al., 1986). However, the frequent observation that, in contrast to their effects on morphine self-administration, only relatively large opiate antagonist doses reduce ethanol intake, raises some doubt that direct opiate receptor activation by ethanol, its metabolites or TIQs is involved in the mediation of ethanol's reinforcing actions (Beaman et al., 1984; Reid and Hunter, 1984; Samson and Doyle, 1985). Moreover, a recent report in which naloxone failed to produce extinction-like behavior (while suppressing operant responding for ethanol) has questioned the specificity of opiate antagonist actions to ethanol reward (Samson and Doyle, 1985).

Indeed, there is considerable evidence to suggest that endogenous opioids exert inhibitory effects on consummatory behavior in general. For example, systemically administered naloxone and other opiate antagonists suppress food and water intake over a wide dose range (Brown and Holtzman, 1979; Frenk and Rogers, 1979; Holtzman, 1979; Hynes et al., 1981). Inhibitory effects of naloxone on ingestive behavior occur in non-deprived as well as deprived animals and extend to stimuli which are normally potent reinforcers (e.g., sucrose and sweetened milk) (Cooper, 1980; Ostrowski et al., 1980; Stapleton et al., 1979).

To further investigate the role of opioid receptors in ethanol reward, nonmotivationally constrained rats orally self-administering ethanol were given systemic injections of low naloxone doses. At the selected dose range, naloxone effectively alters opiate reinforcement but may have less pronounced effects on ingestive behavior (Ettenberg et al., 1982; Hynes et al., 1981). Naloxone effects were examined in two strains of rats differing in ethanol preference [i.e., genetically heterogenous Wistar and alcohol-preferring (P) rats]. Using the free-choice operant procedures outlined above, naloxone (0.125, 0.25, 0.5 mg/kg) induced changes in ethanol preference and intake were assessed during 30-minute, free-choice (ethanol vs. water), self-administration sessions. After development of stable free-choice responding, rats were first tested in a saline pretest, followed by naloxone tests (three doses), and a saline post test. At least 4 days of baseline ethanol self-administration elapsed between test days in order to re-establish baseline responding.

Rats of both strains responded to naloxone pretreatment with dose-dependent reductions in responding and consequently decreases in the total amount of fluid intake (Fig. 4). The reduction in total fluid intake was the result of decreased responding for ethanol as well as water. Ethanol preference was not altered in either strain of rats since the water-ethanol ratios remained constant across naloxone doses (Fig. 5). In P-rats, naloxone effects on both ethanol and water intake were dose-dependent. In contrast, although naloxone produced dose-dependent (but statistically nonreliable) decreases in water consumption of unselected Wistar rats, identical reductions in ethanol intake were observed at all naloxone doses in these animals.

Interpretation of the motivational effects produced by pharmacological treatments designed to identify drug or ethanol interactions with specific neurotransmitter systems hinges on the concurrent assessment of responding for a second reinforcer. When evaluated in terms of the animals' preference to respond for one of two reinforcers, naloxone pretreatment did not alter ethanol preference, although naloxone reduced the absolute amount of ethanol intake. The general and nonselective decreases in responding for both water and ethanol do not seem to support a selective role for opiate receptors in the reinforcing actions of ethanol, but

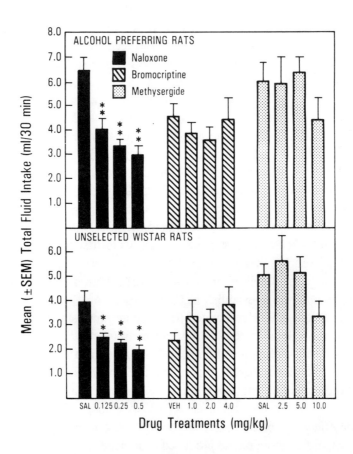

Figure 4. Mean (±SEM) total (ethanol + water) fluid consumption after systemic administration of naloxone (NAL), bromocriptine (BRO), or methysergide (MET) in alcohol-preferring and unselected Wistar rats. (** p<.01, significantly different from SAL−1). Reprinted with permission of Springer-Verlag, New York, from Weiss et al. (1990): Free-choice responding for ethanol vs. water in alcohol-preferring (P) and unselected Wistar rats differentially altered by naloxone, bromocriptine and methysergide. *Psychopharmacology* 101:178-186.

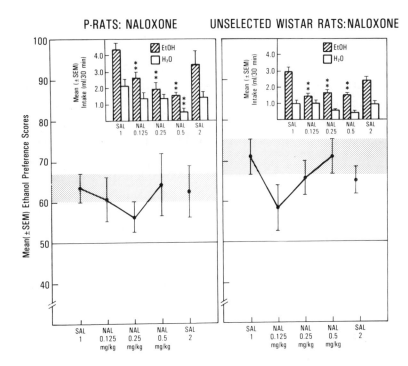

Figure 5. Effects of naloxone (NAL; 0.125, 0.25 and 0.5 mg/kg; SC) and saline (SAL) on free-choice responding for ethanol (EtOH) vs. water in alcohol-preferring (N=10) and genetically heterogenous Wistar (N=12) rats. Data are expressed as mean (±SEM) preference scores [(ethanol/total) * 100] and as the mean (±SEM) total ethanol and water intake (insets) over 30 min. In P-rats, NAL produced marked, dose-dependent reductions in ethanol and water intake but did not alter ethanol preference in either strain of rats. EtOH and water intake returned to pretest (SAL−1) levels at the end of the experiment (SAL −2). (** p<.01; significantly different from SAL−1). Reprinted with permission of Springer-Verlag, New York, from Weiss et al. (1990): Free-choice responding for ethanol vs. water in alcohol-preferring (P) and unselected Wistar rats differentially altered by naloxone, bromocriptine and methysergide. *Psychopharmacology* 101:178-186.

appear more consistent with the well-documented inhibitory effects on consummatory behaviors of this opiate antagonist (Brown and Holtzman 1979; Hynes et al., 1981).

These results are in disagreement with several earlier findings where naloxone selectively reduced ethanol intake in high (HAD) and low

(LAD) alcohol-drinking rats and in genetically heterogenous rats, findings that are consistent with a decrease in ethanol reward (Critcher et al., 1982; Froehlich et al., 1987; Myers and Critcher, 1982; Pulvirenti et al., 1988). There are a number of differences in procedures between these studies in the work described above that may have contributed to these discrepancies. First, selective reductions in voluntary ethanol intake have typically been observed in conjunction with two-bottle, home-cage drinking paradigms. The behavior maintained by ethanol reinforcement in this situation is "drinking choice." The tests used above involve an additional operant: lever-pressing. It is possible that lever-pressing as opposed to drinking recruits different motivational processes. As pointed out by Samson (1987), the demonstration that animals consume ethanol in one situation does not imply that ethanol will generalize to a different situation. Indeed, preliminary data (Weiss and Koob, unpublished observations) suggest that alcohol-acclimated rats ingesting significant amounts of ethanol in a 24-hour, two-bottle choice paradigm (Wise, 1973) failed to acquire or maintain reliable responding when required to lever-press for ethanol reinforcement.

Second, ethanol drinking in most of the two-bottle choice studies that reported selective naloxone effects on ethanol consumption was facilitated by restrictions in fluid access (Critcher et al., 1982; Froehlich et al., 1987; Myers and Critcher, 1982; Pulvirenti et al., 1988). Thus, it is possible that the "selective" suppression of ethanol intake in such "forced drinking" paradigms may occur as the result of water deprivation. In this situation, nonspecific suppressive effects of naloxone on both water and ethanol could be masked since rats have to meet their daily water requirements during the (limited) time of concurrent ethanol availability. Third, the nonselective suppression of total fluid intake in both strains of our nondeprived animals were evident already at considerably lower doses than those used in earlier work (e.g., Froehlich et al., 1987; Pulvirenti et al., 1988). It is possible that different results (i.e., selective effects on ethanol reward) might be obtained with higher naloxone doses. This appears unlikely, however, since high opiate antagonist doses are typically associated with reductions in intake of both alcohol and water as well as a variety of other reinforcers (Beaman et al., 1984; Holtzman, 1979; Reid and Hunter, 1984; Sanger and McCarthy, 1982).

Another important consideration with regard to the specificity of opiate antagonist treatments to ethanol reward are their acute versus chronic actions. Although acute naloxone administration failed to alter ethanol preference in our self-administration paradigm, it remains possible that sustained or chronic opiate receptor blockade is more relevant to endogenous opiate mechanisms presumed to play a role in ethanol reinforcement. Strong and selective inhibitory effects on ethanol intake have been demonstrated in different species after repeated and chronic opiate antagonist administration (Altshuler et al., 1980; Myers and Critcher, 1982). However, under these conditions too, the specificity of opiate antagonists on ethanol reward has not been conclusively established. For example, periodic administration of naloxone reduced ethanol, but not water intake (which was, in fact, increased) over a 24-hour period in food and water-sated rats (Myers and Critcher, 1982). The increase in water intake observed in this work was paralleled by a significant decrease in food intake. Therefore, nonspecific or general aversive naloxone effects may still be apparent. Since the demand for water is less flexible than that for food, it may be argued that water consumption is reinstated over the course of 24 hours despite a naloxone-induced "malaise" and may overshoot as a result of dehydration. Hence, an increase in water intake can be observed. Therefore, general suppressant effects of naloxone cannot be ruled out completely in this situation. In view of the wide procedural differences among studies that have investigated the role of endogenous opiates in ethanol self-administration, it seems important to carefully reconsider the actions of opiate antagonists on ethanol preference under different circumstances and reinforcement contingencies.

Dopamine

Considerable evidence suggests that the rewarding effects of a wide variety of stimuli are dopamine-dependent (e.g., Fibiger, 1978; Wise, 1978). In particular, recent findings have implicated the mesolimbic dopamine system in intracranial self-stimulation and in the self-administration of drugs of abuse (Lyness et al., 1979; Robbins et al., 1983; Roberts et al., 1980, 1982). In fact, it was recently shown that many substances of abuse stimulate mesolimbic dopamine (DA) release (DiChiara and Imperato, 1988). Although there is convincing evidence for a dopaminergic involvement in psychomotor stimulant reward, it is not clear whether this also applies to ethanol as some have proposed (see Wise, 1980, vs. Amit and Brown, 1982). In support of a possibly important role of dopamine in the intoxicating actions of ethanol are the results of numerous biochemical and functional studies. Ethanol, particularly at low and intermediate doses, stimulates dopamine synthesis, metabolism and turnover (Bustos and Roth, 1976; Dar and Wooles, 1984; Fadda et al., 1980; Khatib et al., 1988), produces stimulatory effects on dopamine release from striatal slices *in vitro* (Carmichael and Israel, 1975; Holman and Snape, 1985b) and, after chronic administration, changes the binding characteristics of DA receptors in the striatum and nucleus accumbens (Korpi et al., 1987; Liljeqvist, 1978; Lucchi et al., 1983). Although these biochemical data provide ample evidence for ethanol-dopamine interactions at the cellular level, the precise role of this transmitter in ethanol reward remains unclear.

The results of behavioral work with selective neurotoxin lesions of brain catecholamine systems have suggested a dopaminergic involvement in the behavioral effects of ethanol intoxication, but failed to establish a direct role of dopamine in ethanol self-administration or reward (Brown and Amit, 1977; Kiianmaa et al., 1979; Myers and Melchior, 1975). In fact, evidence from work with selective or combined dopamine and noradrenaline lesions suggested that brain norepinephrine may play a more important role than dopamine in regulating ethanol intake (Amit et al., 1977; Brown and Amit, 1977; Kiianmaa et al., 1975; see also Amit and Brown, 1982). Similarly, in pharmacological work the dopamine antagonist pimozide reduced ethanol-reinforced operant responding, but ethanol intake was unaffected by pimozide treatments when continuously available in the home cage (Brown et al., 1982; Pfeffer and Samson, 1985b).

The strongest, albeit indirect, evidence in favor of a dopaminergic involvement in ethanol reward comes from several independent observations on the locomotor stimulatory effects of ethanol. Low doses of ethanol were shown to stimulate spontaneous locomotor activity in two lines of rats genetically selected for ethanol preference [Maudsley reactive and alcohol-preferring (P) rats], but not in rats outbred for nonpreference (NP-rats) (Waller et al., 1986). Low dose, ethanol-stimulated locomotor effects have also recently been investigated in conjunction with intracranial microdialysis measurements of dopamine release (DiChiara and Imperato, 1988; Imperato and DiChiara, 1986). Systemic administration of ethanol produced marked increases in extracellular dopamine, particularly in the nucleus accumbens where neurotransmitter release was closely time-locked to behavioral stimulation. Moreover, ethanol-induced

DA release, as estimated from DA metabolite levels, was subsequently shown to be greater in alcohol-preferring (P) than nonpreferring (NP) rats (Fadda et al., 1989; Khatib et al., 1988). These findings are of particular significance in view of the evidence that both the rewarding and locomotor-stimulatory effects of psychostimulant drugs depend on increased dopamine activity in the region of the nucleus accumbens (Koob et al., 1987). Thus, it is possible that the alcohol-induced activity increases reflect the reinforcing properties of ethanol and that the reinforcing properties of ethanol derive, in part, from its ability to stimulate mesolimbic dopamine neurotransmission. In support of this account, Samson and colleagues have recently shown that the dopamine receptor antagonists, haloperidol and pimozide, reduce operant responding for ethanol as well as voluntary ethanol drinking in a water ethanol choice situation when session length is limited to 15 to 30 minutes (Pfeffer and Samson, 1985b, 1986, 1988).

Studies using dopamine receptor antagonists to determine whether such treatments decrease ethanol reward can be confounded by nonspecific motor effects (e.g., Ettenberg et al., 1981). An alternative approach, therefore, is to examine the effects of dopamine agonists on ethanol preference or intake. Using cocaine self-administration as a model, the ergot derivative bromocriptine, a long-acting dopamine receptor agonist, produced a dose-dependent decrease in responding for cocaine (Hubner and Koob, 1990). One hypothesis to explain this effect is that bromocriptine blunts the reinforcing actions of cocaine by substituting for the dopamine enhancing action of this drug. This would be analogous to the effects of methadone on opiate self-administration. Considering the hypothesis that low doses of ethanol may produce their reinforcing effects by activating central dopamine neurotransmission, it was of some interest to determine whether dopamine agonists also decrease ethanol self-administration.

Bromocriptine (1.0, 2.0, 4.0 mg/kg), administered according to the same experimental protocol as naloxone, did not alter total fluid intake in either rat strain (Fig. 4). Bromocriptine produced, however, pronounced and dose-dependent shifts in preference from ethanol toward water, particularly in alcohol-preferring rats (Fig. 6). In this strain of rats marked, dose-dependent reductions in ethanol intake paralleled by increases in water consumption were observed. Whereas the magnitude of corresponding changes in ethanol and water intake in unselected Wistar rats were smaller and not consistently dose-dependent, bromocriptine produced a similar reversal of ethanol preference in this group of rats.

In contrast to naloxone, bromocriptine reversed ethanol preference and inhibited ethanol intake without altering the rats' motivation to respond for liquid reinforcement. The selective suppression of ethanol

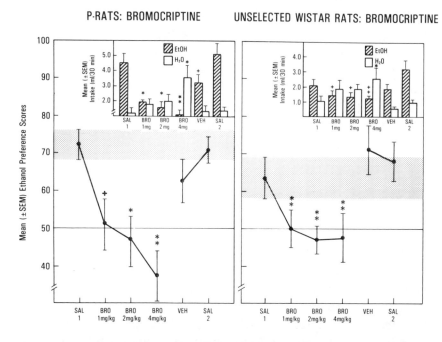

Figure 6. Effects of bromocriptine (BRO; 1, 2 and 4 mg/kg; IP), saline (SAL) and vehicle solution (VEH; propylene glycol) on free-choice responding for ethanol (EtOH) vs. water in alcohol-preferring (N = 10) and heterogenous Wistar (N = 11) rats. Data are represented as mean (±SEM) EtOH preference scores and as the mean (±SEM) total ethanol or water intake in ml (Insets) over 30 min. Bromocriptine clearly reversed ethanol preference in both strains of rats. The drug produced marked, and in P-rats dose-dependent, decreases in ethanol intake while increasing water consumption. Ethanol preference and total volumes of EtOH and water consumed returned to Pretest (SAL−1) when assessed 4 days after the last bromocriptine treatment. (+ p<.05, different from SAL−1; ++ p<.01, different from SAL−1; * p<.05 different from VEH and SAL−1; ** p<.01, different from VEH and SAL−1). Reprinted with permission of Springer-Verlag, New York, from Weiss et al. (1990): Free-choice responding for ethanol vs. water in alcohol-preferring (P) and unselected Wistar rats differentially altered by naloxone, bromocriptine and methysergide. *Psychopharmacology* 101:178-186.

intake suggests that bromocriptine may modify the reinforcing properties of ethanol. In a replication of this work with SDZ 5-152, a novel
mixed D1/D2 dopamine agonist, similar results on ethanol preference
and intake were observed (Rassnick et al., 1989). Together, these findings seem to provide further support for the hypothesis that dopamine
may play an important role in ethanol reinforcement. Such claims,
however, require that several potential confounds be ruled out. First,
in choice situations or situations of concurrent availability of two reinforcers, dopamine agonist treatments can produce some form of "response competition," resulting in a perseveration of responding for one
reinforcer (Lyon and Robbins, 1975). Perseveration of responding at the
water-reinforced lever seems unlikely as an alternative explanation of
these results, since rats consume most of the ethanol at the beginning of
self-administration sessions. Consequently, perseveration at the ethanol-
and not water-associated lever would be expected to occur with a higher
probability. Second, the bromocriptine-induced decrease in ethanol intake
does not appear to be specific to the lever-press response since similar
suppressive effects on both lever-pressing and home-cage drinking have
been noted in related work after pretreatment with the indirect dopamine
agonist, d-amphetamine (Pfeffer and Samson, 1985a,b, 1986).

A final problem for the interpretation of these results with regard
to a dopaminergic reward hypothesis is whether the observed decrease
in responding is a consequence of a decrease in the reinforcement value
of ethanol. The simple interpretation of reductions in responding as
a reflection of a decrease in the rewarding value of a stimulus and,
conversely, an increase in responding as a manifestation of facilitation
of reinforcement is confounded in self-administration studies by several
observations. For example, in the case of amphetamine and cocaine,
partial pharmacological blockade of dopamine receptors produces an *increase* in self-administration rats (DeWit and Wise, 1977; Ettenberg et
al., 1982; Yokel and Wise, 1975). In contrast, decreases in responding
are typically observed in dopamine-denervated rats or after high-dose
dopamine antagonist treatments (Kelly et al., 1975; Roberts et al., 1980;
Yokel and Wise, 1976). Both effects have been interpreted as a decrease
in the reinforcing value of psychostimulant drugs. In the former case,
such increases presumably occur to compensate for the reduced effectiveness of these drugs. The destruction of dopamine terminals, or effective
blockade of DA receptors in the latter case, presumably produces extinc-

tion to the effects of these indirect dopamine agonists. The decrease in responding for ethanol and cocaine (Hubner and Koob, 1990) observed with bromocriptine, a dopamine receptor agonist, are difficult to explain in terms of a reward deficit because the latter is typically associated with high-dose neuroleptic or dopamine denervation treatments. Perhaps the most adequate explanation of the decreases in ethanol intake produced by bromocriptine (and other dopamine agonists) is that these drugs may substitute for the rewarding effects of ethanol via their action at dopamine receptors and/or activation of a "reward-sensitive" subset of dopamine receptors. As a result, the heightened "hedonic state" produced by DA receptor activation may eliminate rats' motivation to respond for ethanol (i.e., make further ethanol consumption redundant; cf. Pfeffer and Samson, 1988).

Results similar to those obtained with bromocriptine have been reported earlier with apomorphine in genetically heterogenous rats (Pfeffer and Samson, 1988). Apomorphine produced a pronounced decrease in responding (single-lever) for ethanol, but this effect was clearly dose-dependent and stronger than that observed with bromocriptine in unselected Wistar rats. A possible explanation for the different potencies and dose-response effects of bromocriptine and apomorphine in these tests may lie in bromocriptine's mechanism of action, which is thought to be different from that of apomorphine. In contrast to the potent direct dopamine receptor agonist apomorphine, bromocriptine seems to require the presence of dopamine or other dopamine agonists in addition to its own actions at dopamine receptors in order to produce observable behavioral effects (Ushijima et al., 1988). In fact, considering the evidence that ethanol enhances dopamine release from mesolimbic terminals (Imperato and DiChiara, 1986) and stimulates dopamine-dependent locomotor activity in alcohol-preferring but not nonpreferring rats (Waller et al., 1986), it is interesting to speculate that the differences with regard to bromocriptine effects between Wistar and P-rats observed above may be a function of the lesser degree of dopamine stimulation by ethanol in the genetically heterogenous Wistar group, and consequently a reduced ability of bromocriptine to express its synergistic effects at postsynaptic dopamine receptors.

In summary, both dopamine antagonist and dopamine agonist drugs decrease ethanol self-administration. Although superficially this appears paradoxical, such results may reflect two different mechanisms of action. Simply speaking, dopamine antagonists may interfere with the low-dose reinforcing effects of ethanol by antagonizing ethanol-stimulated dopamine activity at postsynaptic receptors. Dopamine agonists, on the other hand, may interfere with alcohol reinforcement by substituting for the dopamine-enhancing effects of ethanol. The issue is further complicated, however, by the fact that very low doses of dopamine receptor agonists and antagonists are associated with "paradoxical" effects that produce behaviors opposite to those observed with normal or high doses of these compounds (e.g., Ahlenius and Engel, 1971; DiChiara et al., 1979; Schaefer and Michael, 1984). Explanation of the reductions in ethanol reinforcement observed after low doses of dopamine agonist and antagonist drugs may have to be modified accordingly (Pfeffer and Samson, 1988). Further studies characterizing the specificity of these pharmacological treatments to ethanol reward will be needed to test these hypotheses.

Serotonin

With regard to ethanol interactions with brain neurotransmitters, serotonin is perhaps the most extensively studied transmitter substance. A serotonergic involvement in ethanol preference has long been suggested by the findings that pharmacological manipulation of serotonergic function affects ethanol consumption and modifies the development of tolerance. Thus, treatments designed to increase the synaptic availability of serotonin (5-HT) such as precursor loading (5-hydroxytryptophane), administration of the 5-HT reuptake blockers zimelidine, fluoxetine and chlorimipramine, or central injection of 5-HT itself reduces voluntary ethanol intake and accelerates the development of tolerance (Amit et al., 1984; Daoust et al., 1985; Geller, 1973; Khanna et al., 1979; Lawrin et al., 1986; Myers and Martin, 1973; Rockman et al., 1979, 1982; Zabik et al., 1985). The results of pharmacological alterations in 5-HT function on ethanol self-administration, however, are more difficult to interpret in the case of treatments that reduce brain 5-HT. For example, as might be predicted on the basis of the evidence above, 5-HT depletion by the neurotoxin 5,6-dihydroxytryptamine (DHT) has been reported to increase ethanol intake and to retard tolerance to ethanol (Ho et al., 1974; Khanna et al., 1980; Le et al., 1981), but the effects of DHT lesions on ethanol intake have not been successfully replicated (Kiianmaa, 1976). Moreover, p-chlorophenylalanine (PCPA), p-chloramphetamine and fenfluramine, which are known to decrease central 5-HT levels, inhibit rather than increase voluntary ethanol drinking (Frey et al., 1970; Myers and Veale, 1968; Opitz, 1969; Veale and Myers, 1970). Although the reductions in ethanol consumption produced by PCPA have been attributed by some to nonspecific aversive interoceptive effects and malaise (Nachman et al., 1970; Parker and Radow, 1976; Stein et al., 1977), the effects of pharmacological interference with brain 5-HT remain inconclusive, particularly in view of the inconsistent results of the DHT lesion work (Ho et al., 1974; Kiianmaa, 1976).

Like the behavioral work, biochemical and functional studies of acute or chronic ethanol effects on serotonergic function have remained largely inconclusive. Ethanol can modify midbrain and forebrain turnover and concentrations of 5-HT, but large differences between studies are seen (e.g., Gothoni and Ahtee, 1980; Hunt and Majchrowicz, 1974; Morinan, 1987; Pohorecky et al., 1978; Badawy and Evans, 1983). Increases in 5-hydroxyindoleacetic acid (5-HIAA), the major 5-HT metabolite, are more consistently observed (Hunt and Majchrowicz, 1974, 1983; Pohorecky et al., 1978; Tabakoff and Boggan, 1974), but these have been attributed to inhibition of 5-HIAA transport out of the brain (Tabakoff et al., 1975). Similarly, *in vivo* voltammetry and microdialysis estimations of striatal 5-HT release after systemic injections of ethanol have yielded inconsistent results (Holman and Snape, 1985a; Signs et al., 1987).

Perhaps the strongest support for a serotonergic involvement in ethanol-seeking behavior derives from the differences in regional 5-HT and 5-HT metabolite levels between two lines of alcohol-preferring (P and HAD)-rats and their nonpreferring (NP and LAD) counterparts (Gongwer et al., 1989; Murphy et al., 1982, 1987). The levels of 5-HT and 5-HIAA in the P and HAD lines of rats have been shown to be 10 to 30% lower than for NP and LAD rats in the cerebral cortex, hippocampus, corpus striatum, thalamus and hypothalamus. Reduced brain 5-HT levels have also recently been observed in several alcohol-preferring, inbred strains of mice (Yoshimoto and Komura, 1987; Yoshimoto et al., 1985). These findings suggest that alcohol preference may be associated with decreased 5-HT biosynthesis, functional activity and/or density of forebrain 5-HT pathways. In support of this view, Li and colleagues have shown that the 5-HT reuptake inhibitor, fluoxetine, decreases intragastric and oral ethanol self-administration in P-rats (McBride et al., 1988; Murphy et al., 1988).

The contribution of serotonin to ethanol preference and reward was examined in preliminary work with a free-choice operant task, again using the same experimental protocol as with naloxone and bromocriptine. Ethanol preference and self-administration patterns were examined in alcohol-preferring and heterogenous Wistar rats after acute blockade of 5-HT transmission by the 5-HT antagonist, methysergide.

No major changes in ethanol preference and water or ethanol intake were observed after methysergide at any dose (Figs. 7; see Fig. 4). The drug produced mild increases in ethanol intake and preference in genetically heterogenous Wistar rats at the lowest dose (2.5 mg) as well as some decrement in ethanol and total fluid intake at the highest dose (10 mg/kg) in both strains of rats (Fig. 7). However, these effects were not statistically reliable. Thus, this particular 5-HT antagonist at these doses failed to produce consistent and reliable changes in ethanol preference.

This treatment was of particular importance in view of the evidence suggesting that impaired central 5-HT function may be a neurochemical correlate of alcohol preference in P-rats (Murphy et al., 1982). If impaired functional activity of central 5-HT transmission is a critical factor in the ethanol preference of P-rats, one might expect that pharmacological blockade by 5-HT transmission would induce some degree of ethanol preference in genetically heterogenous Wistars, and possibly further enhance voluntary ethanol intake in P-rats. One may argue that the lack of activity of methysergide in alcohol-preferring (P) rats may be analogous to a "floor effect" resulting from the putative, deficient central 5-HT activity in these animals. However, a biochemical hypothesis that links brain 5-HT dysfunction with alcohol preference nonetheless predicts increased ethanol preference in genetically heterogenous rats after pharmacological blockade of 5-HT neurotransmission. Although not statistically reliable, there was indeed some increase in ethanol intake in genetically heterogeneous Wistars at the lowest dose of methysergide. Even lower doses of methysergide, or perhaps other more selective serotonin antagonists, need to be explored. In addition, since P-rats did not show a tendency to increase ethanol intake, baseline levels of responding may be critical for observing increases in ethanol intake and/or preference. A question of interest, therefore, is whether pharmacological blockade of 5-HT neurotransmission will facilitate the *initiation* of voluntary ethanol intake, although such treatments may not further enhance ethanol preference, once established, in previously alcohol-acclimated animals.

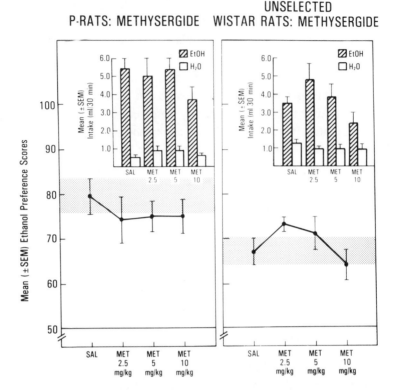

Figure 7. Effects of methysergide (MET; 2.5, 5.0 and 20.0 mg/kg; SC) and saline (SAL) on free-choice responding for ethanol (EtOH; 10% v/v) vs. water in alcohol-preferring (N = 9) and unselected Wistar (N = 9) rats. Data are shown as mean (±SEM) ethanol preference scores and as the mean (±SEM) total ethanol and water intake (insets) over 30 min. Methysergide produced no significant changes in preference or ethanol and water intake in P-rats. A weak but statistically non-reliable increase in ethanol intake and preference was observed in heterogenous Wistar group at the 2.5 mg/kg MET dose.

The mean (±SEM) number of FR 5 responses over the 2 final days (43 and 44) of this phase of the training procedure were 216 (± 27.5) for P-rats and 148.5 (± 28.0) for unselected Wistar rats. At 0.1 ml per reinforcement, these response rates correspond to a mean total ethanol intake of 4.23±0.55 (P-rats) and 2.97±.56 (heterogenous Wistars) over 30 min. Reprinted with permission of Springer-Verlag, New York, from Weiss et al. (1990): Free-choice responding for ethanol versus water in alcohol-preferring (P) and unselected Wistar rats differentially altered by naloxone, bromocriptine and methysergide. *Psychopharmacology* 101:178-186.

As noted above, several studies have shown that *enhancement* of serotonergic activity by 5-HT reuptake inhibitors *reduced* voluntary ethanol consumption in both genetically heterogenous and P-rats (Amit et al., 1984; McBride et al., 1988; Murphy et al., 1988). The discrepancy between these and the results with methysergide is unclear but may be related to several factors. 5-HT reuptake inhibitors can reduce food intake and their inhibitory action on ethanol preference may be secondary to their anorectic effect (Amit et al., 1984; Gill and Amit, 1987). Therefore, 5-HT receptors may not be specifically involved in ethanol preference—a possibility that might account for the inactivity of methysergide. On the other hand, strong evidence in favor of a selective decrease in oral and, in particular, intragastric ethanol intake of alcohol-preferring (P) rats has been reported with the 5-HT reuptake inhibitor, fluoxetine (McBride et al., 1988; Murphy et al., 1988).

An alternative explanation for the methysergide results may derive from the reports that alcohol-preferring (P) and high alcohol drinking (HAD) rats have reduced concentrations of transmitters in addition to 5-HT (Gongwer et al., 1989; Froehlich et al., 1987; Murphy et al., 1982, 1987). These findings suggest that the neurochemical basis of ethanol preference may not be limited or specific, or a single neurotransmitter system. Therefore, the possibility cannot be ruled out that acute blockade of a single transmitter substrate (e.g., by methysergide) is not sufficient to induce or increase voluntary ethanol intake.

Another possible interpretation of the methysergide results is related to the literature on ethanol interactions with the renin-angiotensin system. It has been suggested that activation of the renin-angiotensin system or direct administration of angiotensin II potently reduces ethanol intake (Grupp et al., 1989; Stewart et al., 1988, for review). Moreover, it has been shown that brain 5-HT has a potent stimulatory action on this system (Van de Kar et al., 1981; Zimmerman and Ganong, 1980). It is therefore possible that the reduction in ethanol intake observed with serotonin reuptake inhibitors is not mediated by a primary effect on 5-HT neurotransmission, but through a change in the renin angiotensin system. Strong support for this account comes from the recent finding that angiotensin II synthesis inhibition antagonizes the fluoxetine-induced reductions in ethanol intake, but does not alter ethanol consumption by itself (Grupp et al., 1988). Consequently, the decreases in ethanol preference produced by fluoxetine may be specific to this drug's interactions with the renin-angiotensin system. On the other hand, while decreases in renin-angiotensin activity are associated with increased ethanol preference (Stewart et al., 1988, for review), serotonin receptor blockade by methysergide may not produce a (sufficient) decrease in renin-angiotensin activity so as to enhance alcohol intake. The failure of methysergide to significantly increase ethanol intake is therefore not necessarily in disagreement with some role of central 5-HT in ethanol preference. These results appear, however, more consistent with the view that the enhancement of ethanol intake observed with 5-HT reuptake blockers may be mediated indirectly, via an activation of the renin-angiotensin system, rather than by a direct action at central 5-HT receptors that presumably control ethanol intake and preference.

SUMMARY

Behavioral and neuropharmacological research has implicated a role for several central neurotransmitters in low-dose ethanol reinforcement. However, the role of individual transmitter systems in ethanol reward, abuse and dependence remains to be established. Progress toward the identification of neurobiological substrates of ethanol reward has been hampered, in part, by the unavailability of reliable models of oral ethanol self-administration. New models have been developed in which oral alcohol intake appears to be maintained more clearly by the pharmacological motivation to respond for ethanol rather than by variables related to nutritional appetite or thirst. These models offer the promise of allowing a systematic exploration of the physiological systems involved in the mediation of low-dose ethanol reinforcement. Preliminary work with these procedures designed to assess the role of opioid, catecholaminergic and serotonergic neurotransmitter substrates in ethanol reward suggests that dopamine may be an important neurotransmitter in ethanol reward. Dopamine agonists, including apomorphine, bromocriptine and amphetamine, all reduce ethanol preference and intake, possibly by substituting for activation in dopamine neurotransmission observed with low doses of ethanol. While there is evidence that ethanol may interact directly—by increasing endogenous opioid levels or altering opiate receptor binding—or indirectly—with brain opioid systems to produce its reinforcing effects—ethanol blockade of opiate receptors by naloxone-inhibited ethanol intake in a nonselective fashion. The naloxone effects appear more consistent with a role of opioids in the regulation of consummatory behavior rather than an exclusive role in the mediation of ethanol reward. Blockade of 5-HT transmission by methysergide failed to alter ethanol intake in P-rats and had only mild effects in unselected Wistar rats. Nonetheless, there may be an important serotonergic contribution to ethanol preference, although it remains unclear whether manipulations of 5-HT transmission affects ethanol self-administration directly or via an action on the renin-angiotensin system. Although these investigations examined the role of three transmitters individually, it is possible that neurotransmitter systems interact to produce or maintain ethanol reward. The existence of such interactions has been demonstrated for dopamine and opiates in intracranial self-stimulation reward (for review, see Schaefer, 1988). Future research characterizing the actions of individual transmitters as well as interactions and modulatory effects will be needed to more clearly delineate the neurobiology of ethanol reward.

REFERENCES

Ahlenius S, Engel J (1971): Effects of small doses of haloperidol on timing behavior. *J Pharm Pharmacol* 32:301-302

Altshuler HL, Phillips PE, Feinhandler DA (1980): Alterations of ethanol self-administration by naltrexone. *Life Sci* 26:679-688

Amit S, Sutherland EA, Bill K, Ogren SO (1984): Zimelidine: a review of its effects on ethanol consumption. *Neurosci Biobehav Rev* 8:35-54

Amit Z, Brown ZW (1982): Actions of drugs of abuse on brain reward systems: a reconsideration with specific attention to alcohol. *Pharmacol Biochem Behav* 17:233-238

Amit Z, Levitan DE, Brown ZW, Sutherland EA (1977): Catecholaminergic involvement in alcohol's rewarding properties: Implications for a treatment model for alcoholics. In: *Advances in Experimental Medicine and Biology: Biological Aspects of Ethanol IIIa, vol. 85A.* Gross MM, ed. New York: Plenum Press

Amit Z, Stern MH (1971): A further investigation of alcohol preference in the laboratory rat induced by hypothalamic stimulation. *Psychopharmacologia* 21:317-327

Badawy AA-B, Evans M (1983): Opposite effects of chronic administration and subsequent withdrawal of drugs of dependence on the metabolism and disposition of endogenous and exogenous tryptophane in the rat. *Alcohol* 18:369-382

Beaman CM, Hunter GA, Dunn LL, Reid LD (1984): Opioids, benzodiazepines and intake of ethanol. *Alcohol* 1:39-42

Blum K, Briggs AH, DeLallo L, Elston SFA, Ochoa R (1982): Whole brain methionine enkephalinase of ethanol avoiding and ethanol-preferring C57Bl mice. *Experientia* 38:1469-1470

Blum K, Briggs AH, Elston SFA, Hirst M, Hamilton MG, Verebey KA (1980): A common denominator theory of alcohol and opiate dependence: review of similarities and differences. In: *Alcohol Tolerance and Dependence*, Crabbe J, Rigter R, eds. New York: Elsevier/North Holland Biomedical Press

Bozarth MA (1982): Opiate reward mechanisms mapped by intracranial self-administration. In: *Neurobiology of Opiate Reward*, Smith JE, Lane JD, eds. New York: Raven Press

Brown DR, Holtzman SG (1979): Suppression of deprivation-induced food and water intake in rats and mice by naloxone. *Pharmacol Biochem Behav* 11:567-573

Brown ZW, Amit Z (1977): The effects of selective catecholamine depletions by 6-hydroxydopamine on ethanol preference in rats. *Neurosci Lett* 5:333-336

Brown ZW, Gill K, Abitbol M, Amit Z (1982): Lack of effects of dopamine receptor blockade on voluntary ethanol consumption in rats. *Behav Neural Biol* 36(3):291-294

Bustos G, Roth RH (1976): Effect of acute ethanol treatment on transmitter synthesis and metabolism in central dopaminergic neurons. *J Pharm Pharmacol* 28:580-582

Carmichael FJ, Israel Y (1975): Effects of ethanol on neurotransmitter release by rat cortical slices. *J Pharmacol Exp Ther* 193:824-834

Charness ME, Gordon AD, Diamond I (1984): Ethanol modulation of opiate receptors in cultured neuronal cells. *Science* 222:1246-1248

Cicero TJ (1979): A critique of animal analogues of alcoholism. In: *Biochemistry and Pharmacology of Ethanol, vol. 2*. Majchrowicz E, Noble EP, eds. New York: Plenum Press

Collins MA (1988): Acetaldehyde and its condensation products as markers in alcoholism. In: *Recent Developments in Alcoholism, vol. 6*, Galanter M, ed. New York: Plenum Press

Collins MA, Cheng BY (1988): Oxidative decarboxylation of salsinol-1-carboxylic acid to 1,2-dehydrosalsinol: evidence for exclusive catalysis by particulate fractions in rat kidney. *Arch Biochem Biophys* 263:86-95

Collins MA, Kahn AJ (1982): Attraction to ethanol solutions in mice: induction by a tetrahydroisoquinoline of L-DOPA. *Subs Alc Actions Misuse* 3:299-302

Cooper SJ (1980): Naloxone: effects on food and water consumption in the non-deprived and deprived rat. *Psychopharmacology* 71(1):1-6

Critcher EC, Lin CI, Patel J, Myers RD (1982): Attenuation of alcohol drinking in tetrahydroisoquinoline-treated rats by morphine and naltrexone. *Pharmacol Biochem Behav* 18:225-229

Daoust M, Chretien P, Moore N, Saligaut C, Lhuintre JP, Boismare F (1985): Isolation and striatal (^{3}H) serotonin uptake: role in the voluntary intake of ethanol by rats. *Pharmacol Biochem Behav* 22:205-208

Dar MS, Wooles WR (1984): The effect of acute ethanol on dopamine metabolism in the striatum of mice. *J Neural Transm* 60:283-294

Davis VE, Walsh MJ (1970): Alcohol, amines, and alkaloids: a possible biochemical basis for alcohol addiction. *Science* 167:1005-1007

DeWit H, Wise RA (1977): Blockade of cocaine reinforcement in rats with the dopamine receptor blocker pimozide, but not with the noradrenergic blockers phentolamine and phenoxybenzamine. *Can J Psychol* 31:195-203

DiChiara G, Corsini GU, Mereu GP, Tissari A, Gessa GL (1979): Self-inhibitory dopamine receptors: their role in the biochemical and behavioral effects of low doses of apomorphine. In: *Advances in Biochemical Pharmacology.* Roberts PJ, Woodruff GN, Iversen LL, eds. New York: Raven Press

DiChiara G, Imperato A (1988): Preferential stimulation of dopamine release in mesolimbic systems: a common feature of drugs of abuse. In: *Neurotransmitter Interactions in the Basal Ganglia.* Sandler M, Feuerstein C, Scatton B, eds. New York: Raven Press

Dole VP (1986): On the relevance of animal models to alcoholism in humans. *Clin Exp Res* 10:361-363

Duncan C, Dietrich RA (1980): A critical evaluation of tetrahydroisoquinolines-induced ethanol preference in rats. *Pharmacol Biochem Behav* 13:265-281

Eriksson K (1969): Factors affecting voluntary alcohol consumption in the albino rat. *Ann Zool Fenn* 6:227-265

Ettenberg A, Koob GF, Bloom FE (1981): Response artifact in the measurement of neuroleptic-induced anhedonia. *Science* 213:357-359

Ettenberg A, Pettit HO, Bloom FE, Koob GF (1982): Heroin and cocaine intravenous self-administration in rats: mediation by separate neural systems. *Pharmacol Biochem Behav* 13:729-731

Faber DS, Klee MR (1977): Actions of ethanol on neuronal membrane properties and synaptic transmission. In: *Alcohol and Opiates,* Blum K, ed. New York: Academic Press

Fadda F, Mosca E, Colombo G, Gessa GL (1989): Effects of spontaneous ingestion of ethanol on brain dopamine metabolism. *Life Sci* 44:281-287

Falk JL (1961): Production of polydipsia in normal rats by an intermittent food schedule. *Science* 133:195-196

Falk JL, Samson HH, Tang M (1973): Chronic ingestion techniques for the production of physical dependence on ethanol. In: *Alcohol Intoxication and Withdrawal.* Gross MM, ed. New York: Plenus Press

Falk JL, Samson HH, Winger G (1972): Behavioral maintenance of high concentrations of blood ethanol and physical dependence in the rat. *Science* 177:811-813

Ferko AP, Bobyock E (1979): Rates of ethanol disappearance from blood and hypothermia following acute and prolonged ethanol inhalation. *Toxicol Appl Pharmacol* 50:417-427

Fertel RH, Greenwald JE, Schwarz R, Wong L, Binanchine J (1980): Opiate receptor binding and analgesic effects of the tetrahydroisoquinolines salsinol and tetrahydropapaveroline. *Res Commun Chem Pathol Pharmacol* 27:3-16

Fibiger HC (1978): Drugs and reinforcement mechanisms: a critical review of the catecholamine theory. *Annu Rev Pharmacol Toxicol* 18:37-56

Frenk H, Rogers GH (1979): The suppressant effects of naloxone on food and water intake in the rat. *Behav Neural Biol* 26:23-40

Frey H-H, Magnussen MP, Kaergaard H, Nielsen C (1970): The effect of p-chloroamphetamine on the consumption of ethanol by rats. *Arch Int Pharmacodyn Ther* 183:165-172

Froehlich JC, Harts J, Lumeng L, Li T-K (1987): Naloxone attenuation of voluntary alcohol consumption. *Alcohol Suppl* 1:333-337

Geller I (1973): Effects of para-chlorophenylalanine and 5-hydroxytryptophane on alcohol intake in rats. *Pharmacol Biochem Behav* 1:361-365

Genazzani AR, Nappi G, Facchinetti F, Mazella GL, Parrin D, Sinforiani E, Petraglia F, Savoldi F (1982): Central deficiency of β-endorphin in alcohol addicts. *J Clin Endocrinol Metab* 55:583-586

Gianoulakis C (1989): The effect of ethanol on the biosynthesis and regulation of opioid peptides. *Experientia* 45:428-435

Gill K, Amit Z (1987): Effects of serotonin uptake blockade on food, water and ethanol consumption in rats. *Alcohol Clin Exp Res* 11:444-449

Goeders NE, Smith JE (1983): Cortical dopaminergic involvement in cocaine reinforcement. *Science* 221:773-775

Gongwer MA, Murphy JM, McBride WJ, Lumeng L, Li TK (1989): Regional brain contents of serotonin, dopamine and their metabolites in the selectively bred high- and low-alcohol drinking lines of rats. *Alcohol* 6:317-320

Gothoni P, Ahtee L (1980): Chronic ethanol administration decreases 5-HT and increases 5-HIAA concentration in rat brain. *Acta Pharmacol Toxicol* 46:113-120

Grant KA, Samson HH (1985): Induction and maintenance of ethanol self-administration without food deprivation in the rat. *Psychopharmacology* 86:475-479

Grupp LA, Perlanski E, Steward RB (1989): Angiotensin II-induced suppression of alcohol intake and its reversal by the angiotensin antagonist Sar-1 Thr-8 Angiotensin II. *Pharmacol Biochem Behav* 31:813-816

Ho AKS, Tsai CS, Chen RCA, Begleiter H, Kissin B (1974): Experimental studies on alcoholism I. Increase in alcohol preference by 5.6-dihydroxytryptamine and brain acetylcholine. *Psychopharmacologia* 40:101-107

Holman RB, Snape BM (1985a): Effects of ethanol on 5-hydroxytryptamine release from rat corpus striatum *in vivo*. *Alcohol* 2:249-253

Holman RB, Snape BM (1985b): Effects of ethanol *in vitro* and *in vivo* on the release of endogenous catecholamines from specific regions of the rat brain. *J Neurochem* 44:357-363

Holtzman SG (1979): Suppression of appetitive behavior in the rat by naloxone: lack of effect of prior morphine dependence. *Life Sci* 24:219-226

Hubner CB, Koob GF (1990): Bromocriptine produces decreases in cocaine self-administration in the rat. *Neuropsychopharmacology* 3:101-108

Hunt WA, Majchrowicz E (1974): Rates and steady-state levels of brain serotonin in alcohol-dependent rats. *Brain Res* 72:181-184

Hunt WA, Majchrowicz E (1983): Studies of neurotransmitter interactions after acute and chronic ethanol administration. *Pharmacol Biochem Behav* 18:371-374

Hynes MA, Gallagher M, Yacos KV (1981): Systemic and intraventricular naloxone administration: effects on food and water intake. *Behav Neural Biol* 32:334-342

Imperato A, DiChiara G (1986): Preferential stimulation of dopamine release in the nucleus accumbens of freely moving rats by ethanol. *J Pharmacol Exp Ther* 239:219-239

Kalant H (1983): Animal models of alcohol and drug dependence: some questions, answers, and clinical implications. In: *Etiologic Aspects of Alcohol and Drug Abuse.* Gottheil E, Druley KA, Skoloda TE, Waxman HM, eds. Springfield, Ill.: Charles C. Thomas

Kelly PH, Seviour PW, Iversen SD (1975): Amphetamine and apomorphine responses in the rat following 6-OHDA of the nucleus accumbens septi and corpus striatum. *Brain Res* 94:507-522

Khanna JM, Kalant H, Le AD, Mayer J, LeBlanc AE (1979): Effect of modification of brain serotonin (5-HT) on ethanol tolerance. *Alcohol Clin Exp Res* 3:353-358

Khanna JM, Le AD, Kalant H, LeBlanc AE (1980): Role of serotonin (5-HT) in tolerance to ethanol and barbiturates. In: *Biological Effects of Alcohol.* Begleiter H, ed. New York: Plenum Press

Khatib SA, Murphy JM, McBride WJ (1988): Biochemical evidence for activation of specific monoamine pathways by ethanol. *Alcohol* 5:295-299

Kiianmaa K, Fuxe K, Jonson G, Ahtee L (1975): Evidence for involvement of central NA neurons in alcohol intake. Increased alcohol consumption after degeneration of the NA pathway in the cortex cerebri. *Neurosci Lett* 1:41-45

Kiianmaa K (1976): Alcohol intake in the rat after lowering brain 5-hydroxytryptamine content by electrolytic midbrain raphe lesions, 5,6-hydroxytryptamine or p-chlorophenylalanine. *Med Biol* 54:203-209

Kiianmaa K, Andersson K, Fuxe K (1979): On the role of ascending dopamine systems in the control of voluntary ethanol intake and ethanol intoxication. *Pharmacol Biochem Behav* 10:603-608

Koob GF, Goeders N (1988): Neuroanatomical substrates of drug self-administration. In: *Neuropharmacological Basis of Reward.* Liebman JM, Cooper SJ, eds. Oxford: Oxford University Press

Koob GF, Vaccarino FJ, Amalric M, Swerdlow NR (1987): Neural substrates for cocaine and opiate reinforcement. In: *Cocaine: Clinical and Biobehavioral Aspects*. Fischer S, Raskin A, Uhlenhuth EH, eds. New York: Oxford University Press

Korpi ER, Sinclair JD, Malminen O (1987): Dopamine D2 receptor binding in striatal membranes of rats selected for differences in alcohol-related behaviors. *Pharmacol Toxicol* 61:94-97

Kulonen E (1983): Ethanol and GABA. *Med Biol* 61:147-167

Lawrin MO, Naranjo CA, Sellers EM (1986): Identification of new drugs for modulating alcohol consumption. *Psychopharmacol Bull* 22:1020-1025

Le AD, Khanna JM, LeBlanc AE (1981): Effect of modification of brain serotonin (5-HT), norepinephrine (NE) and dopamine (DA) on ethanol tolerance. *Psychopharmacology* 75:231-235

Lester D, Freed EX (1973): Criteria for an animal model of alcoholism. *Pharmacol Biochem Behav* 1:103-107

Li T-K, Lumeng L, McBride WJ, Waller MB, Murphy JM (1986): Studies on animal model of alcoholism. In: *National Institute on Drug Abuse Research Monograph, Genetic and Biological Markers in Drug Abuse and Alcoholism*. Braude E, Chao HM, eds. Rockville: NIDA

Liljeqvist S (1978): Changes in the sensitivity of dopamine receptors in the nucleus accumbens and in the striatum induced by chronic ethanol administration. *Acta Pharmacol Toxicol* 43:19-28

Liljequist S, Engel J (1979): The effect of chronic ethanol administration on central neurotransmitter mechanisms. *Med Biol* 57:199-210

Linseman MA (1986): Alcohol consumption in free-feeding rats—procedural and genetic factors. *Soc Neurosci Abstr* 12:279-279

Linseman MA (1987): Alcohol consumption in free-feeding rats: procedural, genetic and pharmacokinetic factors. *Psychopharmacology* 92:254-261

Lucchi L, Lupini M, Govoni S, Covelli V, Spano PF, Trabucchi M (1983): Ethanol and dopaminergic systems. *Pharmacol Biochem Behav* 18(Suppl 1):379-382

Lumeng L, Li T-K (1986): The development of metabolic tolerance in the alcohol-preferring P-rats: comparison of forced and free-choice drinking of ethanol. *Pharmacol Biochem Behav* 25:1013-1020

Lumeng L, Waller MB, McBride WJ, Li T-K (1982): Different sensitivities to ethanol in alcohol-preferring and non-preferring rats. *Pharmacol Biochem Behav* 16:125-130

Lyness WH, Friedle NM, Moore KE (1979): Destruction of dopaminergic nerve terminals in the nucleus accumbens: Effect on d-amphetamine self-administration. *Pharmacol Biochem Behav* 11:556-563

Lyon M, Robbins TW (1975): The action of central nervous system stimulant drugs: a general theory concerning amphetamine effects. In: *Current Developments in Psychopharmacology, vol. 2*. Essman W, Valzelli L, eds. New York: Spectrum Publications

Marfaing-Jallat P, Miceli D, LeMagnen J (1983): Decrease in ethanol consumption by naloxone in naive and dependent rats. *Pharmacol Biochem Behav* 18:5355-5395

McBride WJ, Murphy JM, Lumeng L, Li T-K (1988): Effects of Ro-15-4513, fluoxetine and desipramine on the intake of ethanol, water and food by the alcohol-preferring (P) and non-preferring (NP) lines of rats. *Pharmacol Biochem Behav* 30:1045-1050

Meisch RA (1977): Ethanol self-administration: infrahuman studies. In: *Advances in Behavioral Pharmacology, vol. 1.* Thompson T, Dews PB, eds. New York: Academic Press

Meisch RA (1982): Animal studies of alcohol intake. *J Psychiatr Res* 141:113-120

Meisch RA (1984): Alcohol self-administration in experimental animals. In: *Research Advances in Alcohol and Drug Problems.* Smart RG, Glaser FB, Israel Y, Cappel H, Kalant H, Schmidt W, Sellers EM, eds. New York: Plenum Press

Meisch RA, Henningfield JE (1977): Drinking of ethanol by rhesus monkeys: experimental strategies for establishing ethanol as a reinforcer. *Adv Exp Med Biol* 85:443-463

Meisch RA, Thompson T (1971): Ethanol intake in the absence of concurrent food reinforcement. *Psychopharmacologia* 22:72-79

Mello NK (1973): A review of methods to induce alcohol addiction in animals. *Pharmacol Biochem Behav* 1:89-101

Mello NK (1976): Animal models for the study of alcohol addiction. *Psychoneuroendocrinology* 1:347-357

Morinan A (1987): Reduction in striatal 5-hydroxytryptamine turnover following chronic administration of ethanol to rats. *Alcohol* 22:56-60

Murphy JM, McBride WJ, Lumeng L, Li T-K (1982): Regional brain levels of monoamines in alcohol-preferring and non-preferring lines of rats. *Pharmacol Biochem Behav* 16:145-149

Murphy JM, McBride WJ, Lumeng L, Li T-K (1987): Contents of monoamines in forebrain regions of alcohol-preferring (P) and non-preferring (NP) lines of rats. *Pharmacol Biochem Behav* 26:389-392

Murphy JM, Waller MB, Gatto GJ, McBride WJ, Lumeng L, Li T-K (1988): Effects of fluoxetine on the intragastric self-administration of ethanol in the alcohol-preferring P line of rats. *Alcohol* 5:283-286

Myers RD (1978a): Psychopharmacology of alcohol: a review. *Pharmacol Toxicol* 18:125-144

Myers RD (1978b): Tetrahydroisoquinolines in the brain: the basis of an animal model of alcoholism. *Clin Exp Res* 2:145-154

Myers RD (1989): Isoquinolines, beta-carbolines and alcohol drinking: involvement of opioid and dopaminergic mechanisms. *Experientia* 45:436-443

Myers RD, Critcher EC (1982): Naloxone alters alcohol drinking induced in the rat by tetrahydropapaveroline (THP) infused ICV. *Pharmacol Biochem Behav* 16:827-836

Myers RD, Martin GE (1973): The role of cerebral serotonin in the ethanol preference of animals. *Ann NY Acad Sci* 215:135-144

Myers RD, Melchior CL (1975): Alcohol drinking in the rat after destruction of serotonergic and catecholaminergic neurons in the brain. *Res Commun Chem Pathol Pharmacol* 10:363-378

Myers RD, Privette TH (1989): A neuroanatomical substrate for alcohol drinking: identification of tetrahydropapaveroline (THP)-reactive sites in rat brain. *Brain Res Bull* 22:899-911

Myers RD, Veale WL (1968): Alcohol preference in the rats: reduction following depletion of brain serotonin. *Science* 160:1469-1471

Naber D, Soble MG, Pickar D (1981): Ethanol increases opioid activity in plasma of normal volunteers. *Pharmacopsychiatry* 14:160-161

Nachman M, Lester D, LeMagnen J (1970): Alcohol aversion in the rat: behavioural assessment of noxious drug effects. *Science* 168:1244-1246

Opitz K (1969): Beobachtungen bei Alkohol trinkenden Ratten-Einfluss von Fenfluramin. *Pharmacopsykiat Neurospychopharmakol* 2:202-205

Ostrowski NL, Foley TL, Lind MD, Reid LD (1980): Naloxone reduces fluid intake: effects of food and water deprivation. *Pharmacol Biochem Behav* 12:431-435

Parker LF, Radow BL (1976): Effects of parachlorophenylalanine on ethanol self-selection in the rat. *Pharmacol Biochem Behav* 4:535-540

Patel VA, Pohorecky LA (1989): Acute and chronic ethanol treatment on beta-endorphin and catecholamine levels. *Alcohol* 6:59-63

Pekkanen L, Rusi M (1979): The effects of niacin and riboflavin on voluntary ethanol intake and metabolism in rats. *Pharmacol Biochem Behav* 11:575-579

Pfeffer A, Seizinger BR, Herz A (1981): Chronic ethanol inhibition interferes with delta-, but not with mu-opiate receptors. *Neuropharmacology* 20:1229-1232

Pfeffer AO, Samson HH (1985): Oral ethanol reinforcement in the rat: effects of acute amphetamine. *Alcohol* 2:693-697

Pfeffer AO, Samson HH (1985): Oral ethanol reinforcements: interactive effects of amphetamine, pimozide and food restriction. *Alcohol Drug Res* 6:37-48

Pfeffer AO, Samson HH (1986): Effect of pimozide on home cage ethanol drinking in the rat: dependence on drinking session length. *Drug Alcohol Depend* 17:47-55

Pfeffer AO, Samson HH (1988): Haloperidol and apomorphine effects on ethanol reinforcement in free-feeding rats. *Pharmacol Biochem Behav* 29:343-350

Pohorecky LA, Newman B, Sun J, Baile WH (1978): Acute and chronic ethanol ingestion and serotonin metabolism in the rat brain. *J Pharmacol Exp Ther* 224:424-432

Pulvirenti L, Kastin AJ (1988): Naloxone, but not Tyr-MIF-1, reduces volitional ethanol drinking in rats: correlation with degree of spontaneous preferences. *Pharmacol Biochem Behav* 31:129-129

Rassnick S, Pulvirenti L, Koob GF (1989): Effects of a novel dopamine agonist, Sandoz 205-152, on ethanol self-administration. *Soc Neurosci Abstr* 15:251

Reid LD, Hunter GA (1984): Morphine and naloxone modulate intake of ethanol. *Alcohol* 1:33-37

Richter CP, Campbell KH (1940): Alcohol taste thresholds and concentrations of solution preferred by rats. *Science* 91:507-508

Robbins TW, Roberts TCS, Koob GF (1983): The effects of d-amphetamine and apomorphine upon operant behavior and schedule-induced licking in rats with 6-hydroxydopamine lesions of the nucleus accumbens. *J Pharmacol Exp Ther* 224:662-673

Roberts DCS, Koob GF, Klonoff P, Fibiger HC (1980): Extinction and recovery of cocaine self-administration following 6-hydroxydopamine lesions of the nucleus accumbens. *Pharmacol Biochem Behav* 12:781-787

Roberts SCS, Koob GF (1982): Disruption of cocaine self-administration following 6-hydroxydopamine lesions of the ventral tegmental area in rats. *Pharmacol Biochem Behav* 17:901-904

Rockman GE, Amit Z, Brown W, Bourque C, Ogren SO (1982): An investigation of the mechanisms of action of 5-hydroxytyptamine in the suppression of ethanol intake. *Neuropharmacology* 21:341-347

Rockman GE, Amit Z, Carr G, Brown ZW, Ogren SO (1979): Attenuation of ethanol by 5-hydroxytryptamine blockade in laboratory rats. I. Involvement of brain 5-hydroxytryptamine in the mediation of positive reinforcing properties of ethanol. *Arch Int Pharmacodyn Ther* 241:245-259

Roehrs TA, Samson HH (1982): Relative responding on concurrent schedules: indexing ethanol's reinforcing efficacy. *Pharmacol Biochem Behav* 16:393-396

Samson HH (1986): Initiation of ethanol reinforcement using a sucrose-substitution procedure in food- and water-sated rats. *Alcohol Clin Exper Res* 10:436-442

Samson HH (1987): Initiation of ethanol-maintained behavior: a comparison of animal models and their implication to human drinking. In: *Neurobehavioral Pharmacology, vol. 6: Advances in Behavioral Pharmacology*. Thompson T, Dews P, Barret J, eds. New Jersey: Erlbaum Associates

Samson HH, Doyle TF (1985): Oral ethanol self-administration in the rat: effects of naloxone. *Pharmacol Biochem Behav* 22:91-99

Sandi C, Borell J, Guzaz C (1988): Naloxone decreases ethanol consumption within a free choice paradigm in rats. *Pharmacol Biochem Behav* 29:39-43

Sandler M, Carter SB, Hunter KR, Stern GM (1973): Tetrahydroisoquinoline alkaloids: in vivo metabolites of L-dopa in man. *Nature* 241:439-443

Sandler M, Glover V, Armando I, Clow A (1982): Pictet-Spengler condensation products, stress and alcoholism: some clinical overtones. *Prog Clin Biol Res* 90:215-226

Sanger DL, McCarthy PS (1982): A comparison of the effects of opiate antagonists on operant and ingestive behavior. *Pharmacol Biochem Behav* 16:1013-1015

Schaefer GJ (1988): Opiate antagonists and rewarding brain stimulation. *Neurosci Bio behav Rev* 12:1-17

Schaefer GJ, Michael RP (1984): Drug interactions on spontaneous locomotor activity in rats: neuroleptics and amphetamine-induced hyperactivity. *Neuropharmacology* 23:909-914

Schultz R, Wuster M, Duka T, Herz A (1980): Acute and chronic ethanol treatment changes endorphin levels in brain and pituitary. *Psychopharmacology* 68:221-227

Seizinger BR, Bovermann K, Moysinger D, Hollt V, Herz A (1983): Differential effect of acute and chronic ethanol treatment on particular opioid peptide systems in discrete regions of the rat brain and pituitary. *Pharmacol Biochem Behav* 18:361-369

Signs SA, Yamamoto BK, Schechter MD (1987): In vivo electrochemical determination of extracellular dopamine in the caudate of freely moving rats after a low dose of ethanol. *Neuropharmacology* 26:1653-1656

Sinclair JD, Senter RJ (1967): Increased preference for ethanol in rats following alcohol deprivation. *Psychon Sci* 8:11-12

Stapleton JM, Ostrowski NL, Merriman VJ, Lind MD, Reid LD (1979): Naloxone reduces fluid consumption in deprived and nondeprived rats. *Bull Psychon Soc* 13:237-239

Stein JM, Wayner MJ, Tilson HA (1977): The effect of parachlorophenylalanine on the intake of ethanol and saccharin solutions. *Pharmacol Biochem Behav* 6:117-122

Steward RB, Grupp LA (1984): A simplified procedure for producing ethanol self-administration in rats. *Pharmacol Biochem Behav* 21:255-258

Stewart RB, Perlanski E, Grupp LA (1988): Ethanol as a reinforcer for rats: factors of facilitation and constraint. *Alcoholism Clin Exp Res* 12:599- 608

Tabakoff B (1977): Neurochemical aspects of ethanol dependence. In: *Alcohol and Opiates*. Blum K, ed. New York: Academic Press

Tabakoff B, Boggan WO (1974): Effects of ethanol on serotonin metabolism in brain. *J Neurochem* 22:759-764

Tabakoff B, Hoffman PL (1983): Alcohol interaction with brain opiate receptors. *Life Sci* 32:197-204

Tabakoff B, Ritzmann RF, Boggan WO (1975): Inhibition of the transport of 5-hydroxyindoleacetic acid from brain by ethanol. *J Neurochem* 24:1043-1051

Ushijima I, Mizuki Y, Yamada M (1988): The mode of action of bromocriptine following pretreatment with reserpine and a-methyl-p-tyrosine in rats. *Psychopharmacology* 95:29-33

Van de Kar LD, Wilkinson CW, Ganong WF (1981): Pharmacological evidence for a role of brain serotonin in the maintenance of plasma renin activity in unanaesthetized rats. *J Pharmacol Exp Ther* 219:85-90

Veale WL (1973): Ethanol selection in the rat following forced acclimation. *Pharmacol Biochem Behav* 1:233-235

Veale WL, Myers RD (1970): Decrease in ethanol intake in rats following administration of p-chlorophenylalanine. *Neuropharmacology* 9:317-326

Volpicelli R, Davis MA, Olgin JE (1986): Naltrexone blocks the post-shock increase of ethanol consumption. *Life Sci* 38:841-847

Waller MB, Murphy JM, McBride WJ, Lumeng L, Li T-K (1986): Effect of low-dose ethanol on spontaneous motor activity in alcohol-preferring and nonpreferring rats. *Pharmacol Biochem Behav* 24:617-623

Wallgren H, Barry HIII (1970): *Actions of Alcohol.* Amsterdam: Elsevier Publishing Corporation

Wayner MJ, Greenberg I (1972): Effects of hypothalamic stimulation, acclimation and periodic withdrawal on ethanol consumption. *Physiol Behav* 9:737-740

Wayner MJ, Greenberg I, Tartaglione R, Nolley D, Fraley S, Cott A (1972): A new factor affecting the consumption of ethyl alcohol and other sapid fluids. *Physiol Behav* 8:345-362

Weiss F, Mitchiner M, Bloom FE, Koob GF (1990): Free-choice responding for ethanol versus water in alcohol-preferring (P) and unselected Wistar rats is differentially altered by naloxone, bromocriptine and methysergide. *Psychopharmacology* 101:178-186

Wise RA (1973): Voluntary ethanol intake in rats following exposure to ethanol on various schedules. *Psychopharmacology* 29:203-210

Wise RA (1978): Catecholamine theories of reward: a critical review. *Brain Res* 152:162-175

Wise RA (1980): Action of drugs of abuse on brain reward systems. *Pharmacol Biochem Behav* 13(Suppl 1):213-232

Wise RA (1982): Neuroleptics and operant behavior: the anhedonia hypothesis. *Behav Brain Sci* 5:39-88

Wise RA (1984): Neural mechanisms of the reinforcing actions of cocaine. In: *NIDA Research Monograph Cocaine: Pharmacology, Effects, and Treatment of Abuse.* Grabowski, ed. Rockville: NIDA

Wise RA, Bozarth MA (1982): Action of drugs of abuse on brain reward systems: an update with specific attention to opiates. *Pharmacol Biochem Behav* 17:239-243

Yokel RA, Wise RA (1975): Increased lever pressing for amphetamine after pimozide in rats: Implications for a dopamine theory of reward. *Science* 187:547-549

162   Weiss and Koob

Yokel RA, Wise RA (1976): Attenuation of intravenous amphetamine reinforcement by central dopamine blockade in rats. *Psychopharmacology* 48:311-318
York JL (1978): A comparison of the discriminative stimulus properties of ethanol, barbital, and phenobarbital in rats. *Psychopharmacology* 60:19-23
Yoshimoto K, Komura S (1987): Re-examination of the relationship between alcohol preference and brain monoamines in inbred strains of mice including senescence-accelerated mice. *Pharmacol Biochem Behav* 27:317-322
Yoshimoto K, Komura S, Mizohata K (1985): Alcohol preference and brain monoamines in five inbred strains of mice. *IRCS Med Sci* 13:1192-1193
Zabik JE, Blinkerd K, Roache JD (1985): Serotonin and ethanol aversion in the rat. In: *Research Advances in New Psychopharmacological Treatments of Alcoholism*. Naranjo CA, Sellers EM, eds. New York: Excerpta Medica
Zimmerman H, Ganong WF (1980): Pharmacological evidence that stimulation of central serotonergic pathways increases renin secretion. *Neuroendocrinology* 30:101-107

Alcohol Effects on Brain-Stimulation Reward: Blood Alcohol Concentration and Site Specificity

Michael J. Lewis

Ethanol produces pleasant subjective effects for many who consume alcoholic beverages. There is little doubt that these effects reinforce drinking of alcoholic beverages, play a significant role in alcohol abuse and may contribute significantly to the development of alcohol dependence. There are, however, different views about the nature of the reinforcing effects that ethanol produces. Anxiety or stress reduction has frequently been suggested as an important effect of ethanol. The anxiolytic actions of ethanol have been demonstrated experimentally employing anticonflict tests (Dalterio et al., 1988; Koob et al., 1984).

Alternatively, or perhaps in addition to, ethanol may produce euphoria or strongly positive affective states as other drugs of abuse (e.g., cocaine). Experimental evidence on ethanol euphoria has been contradictory. Oral and intravenous self-administration studies have often produced variable results. Electrical brain-stimulation reward (BSR; also known as intracranial self-stimulation) studies, which have been used to measure the euphoric properties of drugs such as cocaine and morphine, have also produced variable results when ethanol is tested (Esposito and Kornetsky, 1978; Kornetsky et al., 1988). Recently, more positive results have been found with this experimental paradigm (Bain and Kornetsky, 1989). This chapter focuses on the role of stimulation at specific brain sites and testing at different times along the blood alcohol curve (BAC) as two important factors in ethanol's enhancement of BSR performance.

BSR THRESHOLD AND RESPONSE RATE MEASUREMENT

BSR has been used to investigate the rewarding properties of drugs since its discovery by Olds and Milner (1954). Olds and his collaborators (Olds, 1958; Olds et al., 1956; Olds et al., 1957) did some of the first investigations of the effects of drugs on BSR. Generally, studies of BSR have primarily employed simple measurement of response rate as the indication of reward strength. Although this method provides a simple and quantifiable measure, it is impossible to differentiate the effects of a given drug or other manipulations on brain reward properties from those on motor functioning. The problem is probably most apparent with drugs that decrease motor activity such as opioids and barbiturates. Several procedures have been employed to interpret changes in response rate after drug administration (see Liebman, 1983, for review). Other methods, however, have been developed that represent attempts to measure more directly changes in reward properties. Various techniques determine BSR threshold to directly have been shown to provide sensitive and reliable measures of drug effects on brain reward mechanisms (Liebman, 1983). Generally, drugs of abuse have been found to decrease reward threshold, whereas drugs that are not abused either have no effect or increase the reward threshold (Kornetsky et al., 1979) .

The effects of ethanol on BSR discussed in this chapter are based on a multifunctional on-line BSR system that provides BSR threshold as well as BSR response rate. Some of these data on the BSR system have been presented before (Lewis and June 1990; Lewis and Phelps, 1987). The determination of threshold is by the classic psychophysical method of limits using a technique that permits the evaluation of stimulation intensities below and above threshold without extinction of responding. This ingenious technique was developed by Huston and Mills (1971) and was further developed by Cassens et al. (1975) and Phelps and Lewis (1982). Huston and Mills (1971) measured BSR threshold with a psychophysical procedure based on the observation that performance under a fixed-ratio (FR) schedule is different from that under a continuous reinforcement (CRF) schedule (Ferster and Skinner, 1957). In this procedure rats press a lever for rewarding stimulation on an FR schedule and, concurrently, on a CRF schedule, using a single lever. This combined schedule with the FR fixed at a suprathreshold level maintains the lever-pressing response at any CRF current intensity.

As previously mentioned, the method of determining threshold is based on the difference between responding under CRF and FR schedules of reinforcement. Typically, animals performing on a FR schedule alone exhibit post-reinforcement pauses (PRP). Under the concurrent CRF-FR schedule, as current intensity is increased from zero, FR pauses become shorter and eventually disappear. Therefore, the rat's performance shifts from that which is characteristic of an FR schedule with many PRPs to that which is characteristic of CRF with no PRPs. Threshold is determined by the appearance or disappearance of these pauses as the CRF current intensity is varied. Huston and Mills (1971) reported that threshold determination was independent of the size of the FR and of the suprathreshold FR current intensity.

Threshold determination is rate-independent in that PRPs are defined based on each animals response pattern. A PRP is a pause in responding after the completion of the FR that is two standard deviations greater than the preceding interresponse interval (IRI) of the responding under the CRF schedule of reinforcement. A fixed number of FR reinforcements are presented at each CRF current level. Threshold is defined as the current level that produces PRPs half of the time; hence, a PRP/FR ratio of 0.50. Threshold is determined by evaluating PRP/FR ratios over a preselected CRF current range and then by interpolating the current value at a PRP/FR of 0.50.

Stimulation is produced by lever presses that produce a 0.2-second train of 100 Hz biphasic rectangular pulses of 1.0 msec duration (current intensity varies, as previously discussed). A detailed discussion of the constant current stimulator, computer equipment, and software is provided in Phelps and Lewis (1982).

In these studies, rats were implanted with electrodes aimed at either the lateral hypothalamus (LH) or mesencephalic ventral noradrenergic bundle (VNB) (Fig.1). The latter is a site that is within an ascending norepinephrine pathway described by Ungerstedt (1971) and Jacobowitz (1978). It lies posterior to the mesencephalic nuclei, which give rise to forebrain dopamine terminals.

After recovery from surgery, animals were first shaped to press a lever for BSR on a continuous reinforcement schedule. The rat then acquires the response on a FR-15 schedule of reinforcement using the method of Huston (1968). This procedure involves decreasing CRF current intensities gradually while maintaining FR current intensities at suprathreshold intensities. After this initial training, rats were tested on the concurrent CRF/FR schedule. The length of time to complete an operant session was variable, depending on the rate of lever pressing by the animal. Animals with implant in the LH typically complete a session in approximately 15 or 20 minutes. After stable performance was attained, all rats received three intraperitoneal (IP) injections of saline and ethanol (0.1, 0.25, 0.50, 0.75, and 1.50 g/kg in saline) 5 minutes before BSR sessions.

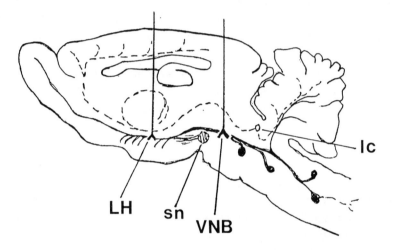

Figure 1.   Midsaggital section of the rat brain indicating the location of two sites from which the effects of ethanol on BSR was examined. Abbreviations: LH - lateral hypothalamus; VNB - ventral noradrenergic bundle; lc - locus coeruleus; sn = substantia nigra.

EFFECTS OF ETHANOL ON BSR PERFORMANCE

BSR threshold was reduced after the administration of the 0.25, 0.5, and 0.75 g/kg ethanol doses at the LH site (Fig. 2) (Lewis and Phelps, 1987). This enhancement of BSR appeared dose-dependent. The 1.50 g/kg produced no significant effect on threshold at the lateral hypothalamus, although there was a trend toward a reduction in doses up to 0.75 g/kg. The 1.50 g/kg dose so disrupted performance at the VNB site that threshold could not be determined despite frequent priming.

Overall, BSR response rate was unchanged at the 0.10, 0.25, and 0.50 g/kg doses of ethanol at the LH brain site (Fig. 3, panel B). There was, however, a trend toward an increase in responding at the 0.25 and 0.50 g/kg doses at this site. Closer inspection of individual data showed that response rate during the first CRF current level was increased by 0.25 and 0.50 doses in many LH animals (Fig. 3, panel A), although statistical significance was not attained. This lack of significance was due to high variability, which was generally seen with the response rate measure. No enhancement of response rate or trends in that direction were found at the VNB site. There was a significant reduction in performance at the 1.50 doses at both brain loci. The 0.75 dose showed no significant difference from saline baseline, although most VNB animals showed a slight reduction in rate at this dose.

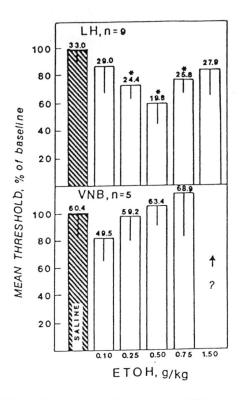

Figure 2. Effects of five doses of ethanol on BSR threshold expressed as the percentage of baseline. Numbers above each bar are absolute threshold values in microamperes. Vertical lines within each bar are the SEM. Asterisks indicate significant differences from baseline (p<0.05). Reprinted with permission of Pergamon Press Inc. from Lewis and June (1990): Neurobehavioral studies of ethanol reward and activation. *Alcohol* 7:213-219.

The performance of individual animals over multiple sessions shows that the decrease in threshold and the increase in response rate in the LH was reliable (Fig. 4). This facilitation did not show a decline with repeated testing over the three sessions tested. These findings suggest that the enhancement in performance may not exhibit tolerance. Of course, more research on this point is necessary; if reliable, however, this phenomenon would be in common with opioids, which also do not exhibit tolerance to the threshold lowering effects of IP administration (Esposito and Kornetsky, 1977).

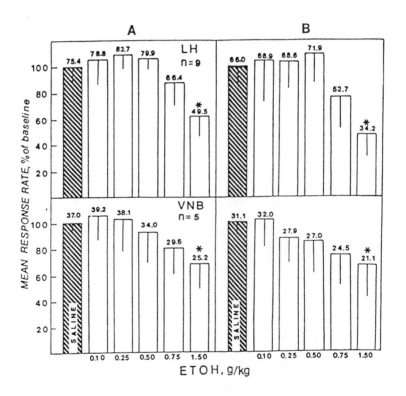

Figure 3.   Effects of five doses of ethanol on BSR response rate during the first 300 responses (A) and the entire operant session (B). Values are expressed as the percentage of baseline. Numbers shown above each bar are the absolute response rates in responses per minute. Vertical lines within each bar are the SEM. Asterisks indicate significant differences from baseline (p<0.05). Reprinted from Lewis and June with permission of Pergamon Press Inc. (1990): Neurobehavioral studies of ethanol reward and activation. *Alcohol* 7:213-219.

To investigate further the site specificity of the effects of ethanol, animals with double implants (one electrode in the LH and the other contralateral in the VNB) were tested on two different occasions with a 0.5 g/kg dose of ethanol. Threshold was lowered and response rate was slightly increased at the LH site by ethanol, whereas performance for stimulation at the VNB site was unaffected (Lewis and June, 1990).

As is the case in published literature on the effects of ethanol on BSR, research in our laboratory has often produced variable effects with ethanol. In addition to site specificity, we have explored the possibility that the time of testing after IP injection may be an important determinant of ethanol's effects. Prior testing at various times produced evidence that the earlier the testing after administration, the more positive the results. In the studies described above, testing began within 5 minutes after

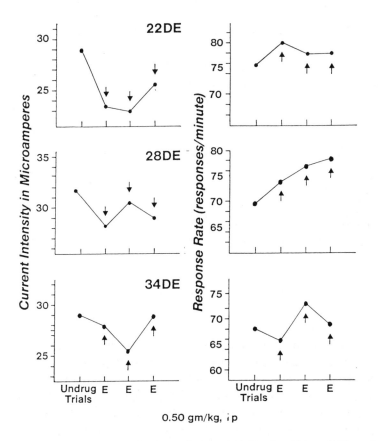

Figure 4. Effects of three injections of ethanol (0.50 g/kg, IP) on BSR performance of three representative rats with LH electrode implants.

injection and was usually completed within 20 minutes. To determine ethanol's effects with a more prolonged delay in testing, animals with single electrode LH implants that had shown threshold reduction and increased response rate to ethanol injection were tested beginning at 30 min after an injection of 0.50 g/kg (Lewis and June, 1990). These animals generally completed the session by 50 min. No change in threshold or response rate was observed in these animals. Additional testing of animals with VNB implants also showed that, as is the case during the first 20-minutes testing, no effects of ethanol were found 30 to 50 minutes after IP injection (Lewis and June, 1990).

BLOOD ALCOHOL CONCENTRATION
AND ETHANOL EFFECTS ON BSR

After administration, ethanol concentration increases in the blood to a peak and then slowly decreases after a well-known time function. Activity measurement has been found to differ depending on when it is observed during that blood alcohol curve BAC (Lewis and June, 1990). Because of the obvious possibility that the difference observed in BSR performance when animals are tested 5 minutes rather than 30 minutes after ethanol injection, could be due to events related to the BAC, measurement of blood alcohol concentration at the dose range that was employed in our BSR experiments was performed. Blood samples were taken from the tip of the tail every 5 minutes from three rats given 0.50, 0.75 and 1.00 g/kg of ethanol (IP). Ethanol concentration was determined by a modification of the ethanol dehydrogenase method (Poklis and Mackell, 1982). The BAC rose progressively to a peak at about 20 minutes (Fig. 5) and decreased slowly during the remainder of the 90-minute test period with all three doses. These data show that ethanol concentrations are increasing during the period when ethanol facilitates BSR performance at LH sites. Moreover, the concentrations are decreasing when tested at 30 to 50 minutes.

To evaluate further the possibility that ethanol facilitation of BSR performance depends on events that occur during the ascending limb of the BAC, the effects of ethanol administered intragastrically were examined in rats with LH implants. After oral administration, ethanol absorption would be slower and therefore the rise in the BAC would be expected to be prolonged. Animals previously tested with ethanol IP were given 0.50 g/kg by gavage, then tested at 0 to 20, 20 to 40, and 40 to 60 minutes (Lewis and June, 1990). Threshold and/or response rate were reduced during the first time period for all four animals and three of four animals during the second twenty minutes. No effect was observed during the 40 to 60 minute time period. The facilitation of BSR responding appeared to have been prolonged when ethanol was administered via the alimentary canal.

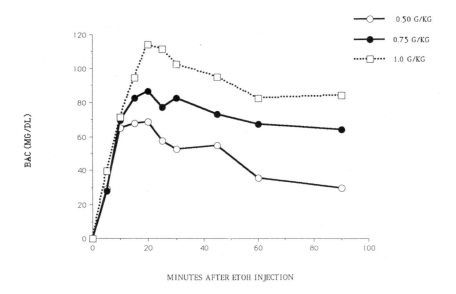

Figure 5. BAC of three animals given 0.50, 0.75, and 1.00 g/kg of ethanol intraperitoneally. Reprinted with permission of Pergamon Press Inc. from Lewis and June (1990): Neurobehavioral studies of ethanol reward and activation. *Alcohol* 7: 213-219.

POSSIBLE DOPAMINE MEDIATION
OF ETHANOL FACILITATION OF BSR

The differential effects of low doses of ethanol on BSR responding when tested 5 minutes versus 30 minutes after injection are most likely due to events in the brain that occur during the ascending portion of the BAC and not during the descending portion of this well known curve. Because of the extensive research on the role of dopamine (DA) in mediating reward (Wise, 1978; Wise and Bozarth, 1981), investigation of brain DA seems warranted. Several studies have shown that ethanol has significant effects on this neurotransmitter system (Engel and Liljequist, 1983; Engel et al., 1988; Fadda et al., 1989; Gessa et al., 1985). An important study by Imperato and Di Chiara (1986) suggests that these ethanol effects on BSR may involve DA release in the nucleus accumbens (NA). They employed a transcerebral dialysis technique to measure the release of DA and its principal metabolites from the NA and dorsal caudate regions of the brain of freely moving animals. They report (Fig. 6) that with low doses of ethanol (0.25 and 0.50 g/kg, IP) there is a selective rise in DA and a slight rise in 3,4-dihydroxyphenylacetic acid (DOPAC) (0.50 dose) within the nucleus accumbens. This effect is of relatively short duration,

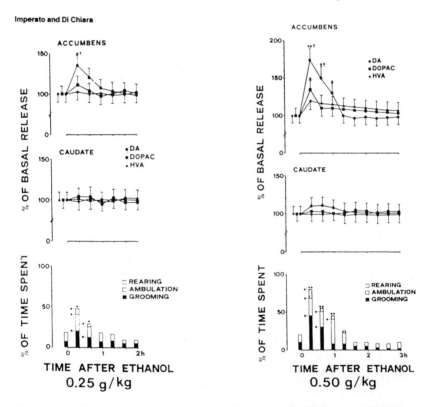

Figure 6. Effects of 0.25 and 0.50 g/kg, IP of ethanol on behavior and dopamine, DOPAC, and HVA release from the nucleus accumbens and the caudate. Reprinted with permission of the American Society of Pharmacology and Experimental Therapeutics from Imperato and Di Chiara (1986): Preferential stimulation of dopamine release in the nucleus accumbens of freely moving rats by ethanol. *Pharmacol* 239:219-228.

reaching its peak at about 20 minutes and returning to baseline levels at approximately 1 hour after administration. No change was found in the striatal DA at these doses. With higher doses (1.0 to 5.0 g/kg), however, there is an increase in release in DA in the nucleus accumbens, but a much larger release in the striatum, which persisted for a much longer duration.

In the same research, Imperato and Di Chiara (1986) concurrently measured several types of activity (Fig. 7) during the measurement of DA release. They found that the 0.25 and 0.50 g/kg doses of ethanol increased all measures of activity during the first 20 minutes and this increase correlated with the release of DA from the NA. With high doses of ethanol, activity was reduced for 2 hours or more and corresponded with a large increase in striatal DA. These data agree with recent data from our lab indicating that low doses of ethanol increase horizontal and vertical activity of Charles River (Sprague-Dawley) rats that have been either habituated to the open field environment or selected for low activity. This increase occurs during the ascending, but not the descending limb of the BAC.

DISCUSSION AND CONCLUSIONS

The neurobehavioral actions of ethanol are complex and have proved to be perhaps the most challenging of all drugs. The extensive research on alcohol reinforcement is consistent with this complexity. The effects of ethanol on BSR are conflicting. Facilitation of BSR has been observed by several investigators (Carlson and Lydic, 1976; DeWitte and Bada, 1983; Lewis and Phelps, 1987; Musgrave et al., 1989; St. Laurent, 1972; St. Laurent and Olds, 1967; Vrtunski, 1973) and either no effect or only inhibition of BSR has been found by others (Routtenberg, 1981; Schaefer and Michael, 1987; Unterwald et al., 1984;). These varied effects may indeed be due to differences in methodology that have been employed to measure BSR. Most studies have used the simple rate of lever-pressing as the sole dependent measure of the effect of ethanol. Others have attempted to determine whether ethanol produces any change in the subjective effects of the stimulation without the confound of psychomotor effects. Methods to determine these effects have included duration of stimulation as well as various threshold techniques. The research discussed in this chapter examined the effects of ethanol on both threshold for BSR and lever-pressing rate.

The lowering of BSR threshold induced by ethanol given IP is in disagreement with the findings of Carlson and Lydic (1976), Schaefer and Michael (1987), and Unterwald et al., (1984). Many procedural details differ between their research and ours, the most notable being threshold determination. Moreover, although none of these investigators measured ethanol concentration, it appears from the procedures that BSR testing was not restricted to the ascending limb of the BAC. De Witte and Bada (1983) found that IP injection of low doses of ethanol increased time receiving stimulation as well as response rate. This effect began at 5 minutes after injection and curiously lasted at least 2 hours. Although Carlson and Lydic (1976) found no effect on threshold using a simple rate-dependent method, they did find that 0.6 g/kg IP did increase response rate. As with most of the early studies, the lack of details make it difficult to determine at what point along the BAC testing took place.

Recently, Musgrave et al. (1989) reported that the rate of response in a shuttle task, but not time of stimulation, was increased by intra-gastric ethanol. The time of testing was for 30 minutes after adminis-tration, which agrees with the data presented here after gavage. Bain and Kornetsky (1989) reported that response rate and threshold (see this volume) are facilitated by low doses of ethanol if the animals orally self-administer ethanol. IP injection did not facilitate performance. While self-administration may be the key as these investigators suggest, it is also possible that their more positive results are due to slower rise in the BAC with self-administration, which may permit a longer period of time to observe the facilitation of BSR. De Witte and Bada (1983) found that both oral and IP ethanol facilitated response rate and time spent receiving stimulation.

The differential effects of ethanol on BSR between LH and VNB sites is consistent with early reports (St. Laurent, 1972; St. Laurent and Olds, 1967) showing site-specific effects. Most studies have examined LH sites. (Lewis et al., 1976). We investigated VNB sites. The data presented here suggest that ethanol may produce reinforcement via neural activity at specific brain sites. The LH contains a heterogeneous group of ascending and descending fiber tracks including the monoamines norepinephrine, DA, and serotonin. The VNB contains diffuse ascending noradrenergic fibers and other neurotransmitters including ascending and descending serotonergic neurons (Jacobowitz, 1978). In addition, this region contains enkephalin neurons (Uhl et al., 1979). Previous research (Lewis, 1980,

1981) showed that low doses of the opioid antagonist naloxone decreases BSR performance at VNB sites, but not LH sites. It appears that there are substantial differences in the brain systems that mediate the reward properties of ethanol and opioids.

In conclusion, these data show that ethanol, similar to other substances of abuse, enhances BSR performance when given in low to moderate doses. These effects were dependent on site of stimulation and whether BSR was determined during the ascending or descending limb of the BAC. We recently found (Lewis and June, 1990) correspondence between the facilitation of BSR and behavioral activation, both of which appear to occur only during the ascending limb. These effects appear to involve brain DA systems that are widely believed to be involved with the rewarding properties of other drugs, since DA release from these systems also shows increases that correspond to the ascending portion of the BAC. The enhancement of BSR is consistent with human data, indicating that the euphoria experienced after drinking alcohol occurred during the ascending portion of the BAC (Lukas et al., 1986; Lukas and Mendelson, 1988; see also Lukas et al. and Mendelson et al., this volume). The lack of consensus in previous BSR research concerning ethanol's effects may be attributed to differences on site implantation, differences in time on the BAC, and differences in dose of alcohol. There is a fair amount of agreement that high doses of ethanol inhibit BSR performance. Of course it is important to point out that methodologies have differed widely in these studies. Route of ethanol administration, type of electrode, and wave form, frequency, and train duration of electrical stimulation have varied substantially from study to study. Although such differences have not made consensus difficult with other drugs, they may contribute to the variability of a drug that has either weak or brief euphoric properties.

Future research should be undertaken with care. Particular attention should be given to determining the BAC when reinforcing effects are occurring. Most importantly, considerable attention should be directed at the undoubtedly complex neurochemical events that occur in the brain, particularly those which occur during the ascending limb of the BAC. It appears, based on an increasing body of data, that DA is involved with behavioral activation and is the most likely in the rewarding effects of ethanol, given the complexity of ethanol behavioral effects. However, it is certain that other neurochemical systems play a significant role.

REFERENCES

Bain GT, Kornetsky C (1989): Ethanol oral self-administration and rewarding brain stimulation. *Alcohol* 6 (6):499-503

Carlson RH, Lydic R (1976): The effects of ethanol upon threshold and response rate for self-stimulation. *Psychopharmacology* 50:61-64

Cassens G, Mills A (1973): Lithium and amphetamine: opposite effects on threshold of intracranial reinforcement. *Psychopharmacologia* 30:283-290

Cassens GP, Shaw C, Dudding KE, Mills AW (1975): On-line brain stimulation: measurement of threshold of reinforcement. *Behav* 7:145-150

Dalterio SL, Wayner MJ, Geller I, Hartmann RJ (1988): Ethanol and diazepam interactions on conflict behavior in rats. *Alcohol* 5(6):471-476

DeWitte P, Bada MF (1983): Self-stimulation and alcohol administered orally or intraperitoneally. *Exp Neurol* 8:675-682

Engel J, Liljequist S (1983): The involvement of different central neurotransmitters in mediating stimulatory and sedative effects of ethanol. In: *Stress and Alcohol Use*. Pohorecky L, Brick J, eds. New York: Elsevier, pp 153-169

Engel JA, Fahlke C, Hulthe P, Hard E, Johannessen K, Snape B, Svensson L (1988): Biochemical and behavioral evidence for an interaction between ethanol and calcium channel antagonists. *J Neural Trans* 74:181-193

Esposito RU, Kornetsky C (1977): Morphine lowering of self-stimulation thresholds: lack of tolerance with long term administration. *Science* 195:189-191

Esposito RU, Kornetsky C (1978): Opioids and rewarding brain stimulation. *Neurosci Biobehav Rev* 2:115-122

Fadda F, Mosca E, Colombo G, Gessa GL (1989): Effect of spontaneous ingestion of ethanol on brain dopamine metabolism. *Life Sci* 44:281-287

Ferster M, Skinner B (1957): *Schedule of reinforcement*. New York: Appleton-Century-Crofts

Gessa GL, Muntoni G, Collu M, Vargiu L, Mereu G (1985): Low doses of ethanol activate dopaminergic neurons in the ventral tegmental area. *Brain Res* 348:201-203

Huston J (1968): Reinforcement reduction: a method for training ratio behavior. *Science* 159:444

Huston JP, Mills AW (1971): Threshold of reinforcing brain stimulation. *Comm Behav Biol* 5:331-340

Imperato A, Di Chiara G (1986): Preferential stimulation of dopamine release in the nucleus accumbens of freely moving rats by ethanol. *J Pharmacol Exp Ther* 239(1):219-228

Jacobowitz DM (1978): Monoaminergic pathways in the central nervous system. In: *Psychopharmacology: A generation of progress*. Lipton MA, DiMascio A, Killam KF, eds. New York: Raven Press, pp 119-129

Koob GF, Thatcher-Britton K, Roberts DCS, Bloom FE (1984): Destruction of the locus coeruleus or dorsal noradrenergic bundle does not alter release of punished responding by ethanol and chlordiazepoxide. *Physiol Behav* 33:479-485

Kornetsky C, Bain GT, Unterwald EM, Lewis MJ (1988): Brain stimulation reward: effects of alcohol. *Alcoholism: Clinical and Experimental Research* 12(5):609-616

Kornetsky C, Esposito RU, McLean S, Jacobson JO (1979): Intracranial self-stimulation thresholds: a model for the hedonic effects of drugs of abuse. *Arch Gen Psych* 38:289-292

Lewis MJ (1980): Naloxone suppression brain stimulation reward in the VNB but not in MFB. *Soc Neurosci Abstr* 6:367

Lewis MJ (1981): Effects of naloxone on brain stimulation reward threshold in the VNB and MFB. *Soc Neurosci Abstr* 7:165

Lewis MJ, Costa JL, Jacobowitz DM, Margules DL (1976): Tolerance, physical dependence, and opioid-seeking behavior: dependence on norepinephrine. *Brain Res* 107:156-167

Lewis MJ, June HL (1990): Neurobehavioral studies of ethanol reward and activation. *Alcohol* 7:213-219

Lewis MJ, Phelps RW (1987): A multifunctional on-line brain stimulation system: investigation of alcohol and aging. In: *Methods of Assessing the Reinforcing Properties of Abused Drugs*. Bozarth MA, ed. New York: Springer-Verlag, pp 463-478

Liebman JM, (1983): Discriminating between reward and performance: a critical review of intracranial self-stimulation methodology. *Neurosci Biobehav Rev* 7:45-72

Lukas SE, Mendelson JH, Benedikt RA, Jones B (1986): EEG alpha activity increases during transient episodes of ethanol-induced euphoria. *Pharmacol Biochem Behav* 25:889-895

Lukas SE, Mendelson JH (1988): Electroencephalographic activity and plasma ACTH during ethanol-induced euphoria. *Biol Psychiatry* 23:141-148

Musgrave MA, Randolph AD, Nelson LF (1989): Antagonism of selected ethanol-enhanced brain stimulation properties by Ro15-4513. *Alcohol* 6:65-70

Olds J (1958): Self-stimulation experiments and differentiating reward systems. In: *Reticular formation of the brain*. Jasper HH, Proctor LD, Knighton RS, Noshay WC, Costello RT, eds. Boston: Little Brown, pp 671-687

Olds J, Killam KF, Bach-Rita P (1956): Self-stimulation of the brain used as a screening method for tranquilizing drugs. *Science* 124:265-266

Olds J, Killam KF, Eiduson S (1957): Effects of tranquilizers on self-stimulation of the brain. In: *Psychotropic Drugs*. Garrantini S, Ghetti V, eds. New York: Elsevier, pp 234-243

Olds J, Milner P (1954): Positive reinforcement produced by electrical stimulation of septal area and other regions. *J Comp Physiol Psychol* 47:419-427

Phelps R, Lewis MJ (1982): A multifunctional on-line brain stimulation system. *Behav Res Meth Instrum* 14:323-328

Poklis A, Mackell MA (1982): Evaluation of a modified alcohol dehydrogenase assay for the determination of ethanol in blood. *Clin Chem* 28(10):2125-2127

Routtenberg A (1981): Drugs of abuse and the endogenous reinforcement system: the resistance of intracranial self-stimulation behavior to the inebriating effects of ethanol. *Ann NY Acad Sci* 362:60-66

Schaefer GJ, Michael RP (1987): Ethanol and current thresholds for brain self-stimulation in the lateral hypothalamus of the rat. *Alcohol* 4:209-213

St. Laurent J (1972): Brain centers of reinforcement and the effects of alcohol. In: *Biology of Alcoholism*. Kissin B, Begleiter H, eds. New York: Plenum Press, pp 85-106

St. Laurent J, Olds J (1967): Alcohol and brain centers of positive reinforcement. In: *Alcoholism-Behavioral Research, Therapeutic Approaches*. Fox R, ed. New York: Springer-Verlag pp 80-101

Uhl G, Kuhar MJ, Goodman RR, Snyder SH (1979): Histochemical localization of the enkephalins. In: *Endorphins in Mental Health Research*. Usdin WE, Bunney Jr, Kline NS, eds. New York: Oxford University, pp 74-83

Ungerstedt U (1971): Stereotaxic mapping of the monoamine pathways in the rat brain. *Acta Physiol Scandi* 82:(Suppl 367) 1-48

Unterwald EM, Clark JA, Bain G, Kornetsky C (1984): The effects of ethanol on rewarding intracranial stimulation: rate and threshold measures. *Soc Neurosci Abstr* 10:572

Vrtunski P, Murray R, Wolin LR (1973): The effect of alcohol on intracranially reinforced response. *Q J Stud Alcohol* 34:718-725

Wise RA (1978): Catecholamine theories of reward: a critical review. *Brain Res* 152:215-247

Wise RA, Bozarth MA (1981): Brain substrates for reinforcement and drug self-administration. *Prog Neuropsychopharmacology* 5:467-474

Ethanol and Rewarding Brain Stimulation

Conan Kornetsky, Marjorie Moolten and George Bain

INTRODUCTION

When a substance is repeatedly used it is reasonable to assume that in some way its use is reinforcing. It may be that it is necessary for life, it has a taste or smell worth seeking, or its use may lead to acceptance by peers. During periods of depression or anxiety, self-administration of an abused substance may relieve anxiety or depression.

Although many abused substances are used for hedonic pleasure, it has not been clearly demonstrated that alcohol causes a drug-induced euphoria that is not due to the alleviation of some underlying depression or anxiety, or to an inhibition of various control systems resulting in an apparent stimulation. This stimulation may result in aggressive behavior that is not unlike aggressive behavior precipitated by some but not all abused substances.

There have been many theories proposed that attempt to explain the nonmedical use of drugs, including alcohol. Like the theories on other abused substances, those that attempt to explain the abuse liability of ethanol run the gamut from environmental to genetic explanations (Pickens and Svikis, 1988). Implicit in many theories is the underlying premise that there is a defect in the individual and the substance is used to restore the individual to a normal state. This hypothesis that abused substances are primarily used to restore the individual to some normal state suggests that the pharmacotherapeutic drugs would be highly abused. Except for the anxiolytic agents, this is not the case. In some individuals at risk, anxiolytic compounds may be abused on this basis. For some individuals the reinforcing effects of ethanol may be only on the basis of its anxiolytic action. However, ethanol's widespread use, and the large number of people who use it without abuse, suggest that there are reinforcing effects that cannot be explained by a simple restorative model. It is highly unlikely that any substance would be extensively abused if it did not in some way cause some rewarding or hedonic effect whether or not it also caused some pharmacotherapeutic effect.

Most abused substances, in addition to being self-administered by animals, will also increase the sensitivity of animals to rewarding brain stimulation, often called intracranial self-stimulation or brain stimulation reward (BSR) (see Lewis, this volume). This increased sensitivity to the stimulation has been used as a model for the study of the underlying neuronal events that are responsible for drug-induced euphoria. Experiments on the effects of ethanol on BSR have been directed to determining what extent the rewarding effects of ethanol are mediated by similar neuronal events as seen with such abused substances as psychomotor stimulants or opiates.

The phenomenon that rats would work in order to receive intracranial electrical stimulation was a serendipitous finding by Olds and Milner (1954). This discovery suggested that there was a functional reward system in the brain. It was immediately seen as a method that would be useful for the study of the effects of drugs on brain function with the first drug study by Olds et al. in 1956 and the first report on the effect of abused substances on BSR by Killam et al. in 1957. Killam et al. (1957) reported that 10 mg/kg of pentobarbital slightly increased the rate of responding in an operant paradigm for rewarding brain stimulation in rats with electrodes in some areas of the hypothalamus. Amphetamine increased response rate as well as lowered the threshold for stimulation. The inference was that as rate of response increased the threshold for stimulation was lowered and the stimulation became more rewarding. Although these early papers suggested that the technique might be a useful model for the study of drug-induced euphoria, this model was not pursued to any great extent until the 1970s. During the last 15 years there has been a plethora of reports of the effects of abused substances, including ethanol, on BSR (Broekkamp et al., 1975, 1979; Caudarella et al., 1982; Esposito et al., 1978; Lewis and Phelps, 1987).

Although the effects of psychomotor stimulants and opiate drugs on BSR are generally consistent and robust, this has not been the case with ethanol. Part of the problem may be that the rewarding effects of ethanol may be more complicated than the effects of the psychomotor stimulants and opiates. Ethanol's rewarding effects may depend on such factors as taste, the physiological and psychological state of the organism, and the amount of exposure to ethanol. Finally, some of the reasons that ethanol is so popular as a beverage may be quite different from the reasons that the substance is abused. These include the concomitant reinforcers of social drinking behavior that are, at least in part, independent of ethanol's pharmacological action.

With the exception of reports by Lorens and Sainati in 1978 and DeWitte and Bada in 1983, most investigators report small effects of ethanol on BSR with short duration of action. When facilitation has been observed, it was usually at doses below 1.0 g/kg (Carlson and Lydic, 1976; DeWitte and Bada, 1983; Lewis et al., 1984; Lewis and Phelps, 1987; Lorens and Sainati, 1978; Vrtrunski et al., 1973). However, a number of investigators have failed to find facilitation at any dose (Arregui-Aguirre et al., 1987; Routtenberg, 1981; Schaeffer and Michael, 1987; Smith et al., 1982; Unterwald et al., 1984). Most investigators, even those who failed to find that lower doses facilitated BSR, reported that doses higher than 1.0 g/kg decreased rate of response for BSR.

The mixed results obtained by various investigators may be, as suggested by some investigators (St. Laurent, 1972), a function of the brain site stimulated. Although results of some investigators, including Lewis and Phelps (1987; Lewis, this volume) have shown clear differences in effects as a function of brain site, comparisons across experiments in our laboratory showed no consistent pattern of effects as a function of where the animal is stimulated (Kornetsky et al., 1988).

We believe that some of the variability of results obtained between investigators and often within a single laboratory might be due to the marked motor effects of ethanol. Thus, we studied the effects of ethanol on the threshold for BSR using a rate-independent, discrete trial procedure method for determining the threshold for BSR. This procedure makes few demands on the psychomotor ability of the animal and is not generally affected by direct psychomotor stimulation.

METHODS

Fig. 1 shows a cartoon of the experimental chamber and a schematic representation of the two possible outcomes during a single trial of the BSR procedure. In the first example (I) the subject is presented with a non-reinforcing stimulus (S1), after which it does not respond during the 7.5-second available response time. The animal's failure to respond has no scheduled consequences and a new trial begins after a 5-second intertrial interval. In the second example (II), a reinforcing stimulus (S1) is presented and the subject responds by turning the wheel manipulandum within the 7.5-second available response interval and receives a second stimulus (S2) of the same intensity as the S1.

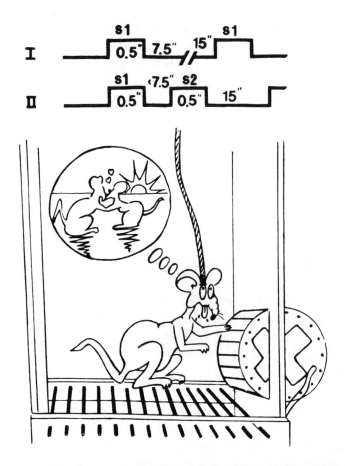

Figure 1. Cartoon of the experimental chamber with the wheel manipulandum. Although we are not sure what the animal feels when it receives BSR, areas of the brain that are activated by stimulation are those that subserve natural reinforcers. Shown at the top is the schematic of the sequence of the stimulation paradigm. Example I shows the sequence when the noncontingent stimulus is delivered (S1) and the animal fails to respond. Example II shows the sequence when the animal responds with 7.5 sec and receives the contingent stimulus (S2) that is identical to the S1.

Fig. 2 shows examples of the percent trials at each intensity that a rat turned the wheel manipulandum and received the S2 stimulation pre- and post-administration of morphine. As shown, these are a sigmoid-shaped curve with threshold defined as that intensity in which the animal responded 50% of the time.

If the obtained threshold is converted to a z score based on the mean and standard deviations of all the saline treatments for an individual animal, a probability can be assigned to the threshold value obtained after a drug treatment for that individual animal. In our experiments we rejected the null hypothesis when the z score equals or exceeds ± 2.0 (the 95% confidence limits). Fig. 3 shows a mean z score dose-response curve for the effects of morphine. This U-shaped curve is characteristic of all drugs that lower the threshold for BSR when a full range of doses is tested.

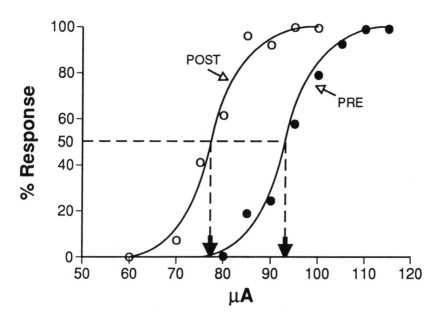

Figure 2. The percent of trials at each intensity that an animal responded after the delivery of the noncontingent sample pre- and post-administration of 4 mg/kg of morphine. Reprinted from Kornetsky (1985): Brain stimulation reward: a model for the neuronal basis for drug induced euphoria. In: *Neuroscience Methods in Drug Abuse Research*, National Institute on Drug Abuse Research Monograph, Washington, DC.

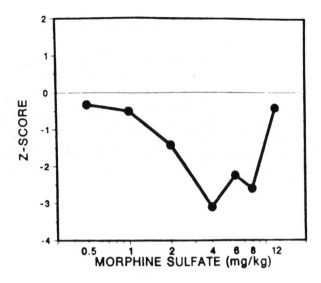

Figure 3. A mean dose-response curve for the effects of morphine on BSR. The ordinate indicates the mean z score based on the mean and standard deviation of the individual animal's response to saline. Reprinted with permission of Springer-Verlag, New York, from Bain and Kornetsky (1990): Opioids modification of central reward processes. In: *Opioids, Bulimia and Alcohol Abuse and Alcoholism*, Reid L, ed.

ETHANOL EFFECTS: INTRAPERITONEAL ADMINISTRATION

Unterwald et al. (1984) and Kornetsky et al. (1988) determined the effect of ethanol on both the above described threshold procedure and rate of response on a continuous operant reinforcement schedule after the intraperitoneal (IP) administration of 20% ethanol. The electrodes in these animals were in the medial forebrain bundle at the level of the lateral hypothalamus. In the experiment in which the animals were tested on the effect of ethanol on rate of response for rewarding brain stimulation, the manipulandum was a lever rather than the cylinder shown in Fig. 1. The results of this experiment are shown in Fig. 4.

As can be seen there was no evidence of facilitation in either rate of response or change in threshold after IP ethanol at any dose. What is shown is that doses of ethanol that had no effect on threshold produced a decrease in rate of response, suggesting that at higher doses ethanol was impairing motor functioning but had little effect on the sensitivity of the animals to the BSR. The comparison of the threshold method with the rate of response method indicates that threshold was independent of motor effects.

Given these results, or lack of results, we were convinced that ethanol had no effect on the sensitivity of animals to BSR that could not be accounted for by its effects on motor systems. As mentioned, the threshold procedure we used was a discrete trial procedure that made minimum motor demands on the subject (Esposito and Kornetsky, 1977). In repeated experiments we have found that changes in threshold caused by drugs can be obtained without altering latency to respond (Bird and Kornetsky, 1990). Although other threshold procedures have been used, almost all make considerable motor demands on the subject and rate of response is an integral part of the procedure.

Although our results suggested that the rewarding system in the brain was unaffected by ethanol we believe that some of the differences obtained between investigators and our failure to find effects on the threshold for rewarding brain stimulation might be due to the stress resulting from IP or gavage administration of ethanol. To determine whether the

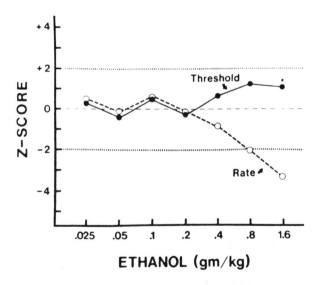

Figure 4. Mean dose-response curves (z score) for the effects of ethanol on the threshold for BSR and rate of response for BSR. The asterisk indicates that not all the animals could complete the task at this dose. Horizontal lines indicate the 95% confidence limits. Reprinted with permission of Springer-Verlag, New York, from Kornetsky et al. (1988): Brain stimulation reward: effects of ethanol. *Alcohol Clin Exp Res* 12(5):609-616.

lack of consistent effects was a function of the aversive nature of the methods used to administer ethanol, we determined the effects of orally self-administered ethanol on BSR. The use of the self-administered ethanol also raised the possibility that if there was a facilitation of BSR after self-administered ethanol, it may be the result of the control the animal had over the administration of the drug and not just the consequence of a less stressful route of administration.

SELF-ADMINISTRATION OF ETHANOL

Ethanol Effects on Rate of Response

In the first such experiment (Bain and Kornetsky, 1989) we elected to determine if self-administration of ethanol would result in facilitation in rate of response for BSR. Six male F-344 rats were prepared with stimulating electrodes in the medial forebrain bundle (MFB) or the ventral tegmental area (VTA) and animals were trained to respond by pressing on a lever manipulandum rather than the previously described wheel. Each lever press resulted in the delivery of a 500-msec train of biphasic symmetrical pulses. The intensity of stimulation in uA used for the experiment was that intensity that resulted in a response rate that was 75% of the individual animal's maximal rate.

After stable baselines were obtained, animals were trained on a limited access ethanol oral self-administration procedure. Animals were water deprived for 22 hours, then tested in the operant chamber and placed in their home cages where they were allowed 30 minutes' access to ethanol solution (12% ethanol, 5% sucrose), control solution (5% sucrose), or tap water before testing. Animals were then placed in the experimental chamber and tested for 35 minutes. During the 35 minute test session animals were presented with four 5-minute on periods (chamber illuminated) where a response on the lever resulted in delivery of BSR. Also interspersed during the testing session were 3 off periods (chamber darkened) when animals were not rewarded for any lever pressing. Forty-five minutes after testing was completed animals were allowed a 30-minute access to tap water. The results of this experiment were contrary to those obtained in the previous experiments in which ethanol was intraperitoneally administered. In all six experimental animals ethanol increased rate of response for BSR.

Due to variation in the volume of ethanol-sucrose solutions consumed from one test session to another, volumes or doses of similar magnitude were grouped together. For example, if before three different testing sessions a subject drank 1.90, 2.0. and 2.1 g/kg respectively, the rates of responding were averaged and the dose then labeled as 2.0 g/kg. This method of data reduction allowed for a reasonable comparison of dose-effect curves between the subjects. It is clear that as doses increased beyond 0.96 g/kg the rate of response declined, so that at the highest doses some of the animals had rates of response that were lower than that seen after the vehicle. An example of this is shown in Fig. 5. The decrease in response rate observed may be the result of the sedative effects of ethanol at doses above 0.96 g/kg and not due to an actual decrease in the rewarding value of the BSR. The increase in response rate at lower doses might not reflect the effect of ethanol on the rewarding value of the stimulation but simply the result of a nonspecific stimulation effect of ethanol on rate of response. In our previously described experiment in which we administered ethanol at these doses using IP route of administration we had not found such facilitation, suggesting that the difference observed between this and the previous experi-

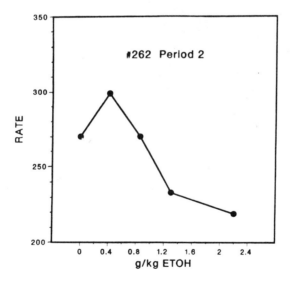

Figure 5. Dose-effect curve for an individual animal. Period 2 indicates the rate for 10-15 min after cessation of ethanol drinking. Adapted with permission of Pergamon Press, Inc. from Bain and Kornetsky (1989): Ethanol oral self-administration and rewarding brain stimulation. *Alcohol* 6:499-503.

ment is related to the less aversive nature of self-administration, which allowed for the expression of either the rewarding and/or general stimulation properties of low dose ethanol.

Since animals determined the amount of ethanol ingested it was possible to plot a frequency polygon of the preferred dose; that is, doses most often consumed by the animals. This is shown in Fig. 6, which is the mean percent of times the animals selected each of the described range of doses. The doses most often selected were similar to those that caused the greatest facilitation in rate of response.

Ethanol Effect on the Threshold for BSR

Although these results using rate of response were encouraging, we had still not truly demonstrated that the animals were more sensitive to BSR.

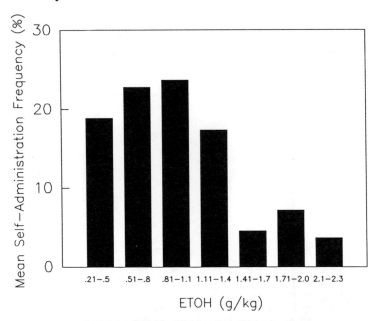

Figure 6. This frequency polygon showing the mean frequency (%) of self-administration of various doses of ethanol on BSR test days was constituted as follows: Animals were allowed free access to ethanol for a 30-min period and then tested on BSR. Since the rats were allowed free access the amount consumed would vary from session to session. The frequency of selection of dose in each of the defined dose range were determined and then converted to percent of total number of test days.

Since an increase in rate of response may not necessarily reflect an increase sensitivity but a function of nonspecific low dose stimulation, we repeated the above experiment using threshold as our measure (Moolten and Kornetsky, 1990). The method of inducing drinking was the same as in the previous experiment except the vehicle was always the water-sucrose vehicle. Animals were allowed a 30-minute access to the sucrose-ethanol solution followed by immediate testing of BSR for 30 minutes. On alternate days animals were allowed to drink the vehicle alone.

Although the dose-effect curve for each individual animal was U-shaped, there was sufficient difference between subjects in the dose causing the greatest sensitivity as well as the form of the U-shaped curve so that an adjusted mean dose-response curve was calculated based on the dose of maximum lowering for each animal. This is shown in Fig. 7, which indicates that the mean maximum lowering of the threshold was obtained at 1.2 ± 0.2 g/kg. Each of the five animals making up the mean showed a significant lowering of the threshold (z score: -2.1 to -2.8). It

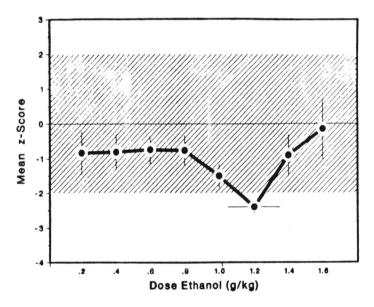

Figure 7. Mean adjusted dose-response curve $\pm$SEM based on the maximum lowering of the threshold for each individual animal for orally self-administered ethanol on the threshold for BSR. Reprinted with permission of Pergamon Press, Inc., from Moolten and Kornetsky (1990): Oral self-administration of ethanol and not experimenter administered ethanol facilitates rewarding electrical brain stimulation. *Alcohol Clin Exp Res* 7:221-225.

is important to note that the results shown in Fig. 7 were not generated until after the animals had experienced approximately 15 ethanol test days over a six week period.

As in the previous experiment (see Fig. 6) the frequency polygon of preferred doses of the animal in this experiment are shown in Fig. 8. As can be seen the preferred dose reflected those doses in which there was the greatest lowering of the threshold in these animals.

As shown (Fig. 7), the threshold is lowered after self-administered ethanol. These two experiments, however, do not answer the question of whether the self-administration is simply a less aversive procedure allowing for ethanol to manifest its effects on brain-stimulation, or if it is the result of the self-administration itself playing a major role in the increased sensitivity of ethanol to brain stimulation. To the extent that increased sensitivity to BSR is a model for drug-induced euphoria, then these results suggest that for ethanol the nonpharmacological factor of control of the voluntary drinking is an important component of the reinforcing effects of ethanol.

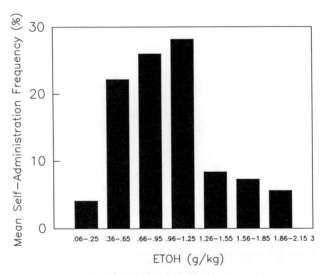

Figure 8. This frequency polygon was constructed in a similar fashion as in Fig. 6. The only difference was that animals were tested for changes in threshold, not rate of response for BSR after ethanol consumption. Reprinted with permission of Pergamon Press, Inc. from Moolten and Kornetsky (1990): Oral self-administration of ethanol and not experimenter administered ethanol facilitates rewarding electrical brain stimulation. *Alcohol Clin Exp Res* 7:221-225.

Contingent Versus Noncontingent Ethanol Administration

To test the role of the control over the drinking of ethanol we compared animals allowed to drink an ethanol-sucrose solution with yoked control animals that received ethanol at the same rate and dose via an indwelling gastric cannula (Moolten and Kornetsky, 1990). Five pairs of animals were studied in this experiment. The procedure for self-administration of ethanol was similar to that in the previously described experiment. The yoked animals were prepared with an indwelling gastric cannula and except for the passive administration of ethanol these animals were tested in exactly the same manner as the animals contingently receiving ethanol. All animals received ethanol 2 to 3 times weekly and the sucrose-water vehicle on the remaining days.

Fig. 9 shows a comparison of the mean percent of the number of times in the first 24 experimental days that the self-administering and the yoked ethanol group had a threshold value at any dose that was lower than the mean threshold value after vehicle administration. As shown there was no significant difference between the groups during the first 24 experimental days. During the second 24 experimental days the self-administering animals showed an increase in the number of days that the threshold was lower than saline, whereas the yoked animals showed a decrease. A paired t test comparing the self-administering (contingent) to the yoked animals (noncontingent) on days 24 to 48 (based on a number of days and not percent) yielded a significant difference ($t = 3.14$, $p<.03$). A comparison of the first 24 days versus the second 24 days gave a $t = 2.30$ ($p<.1$) for the contingent and $t = 1.72$ (p, n.s.) for the noncontingent animals. These findings suggest that not only is self-administration of ethanol important in causing increased sensitivity to brain stimulation but failure to show increased sensitivity during the first 24 experimental days indicates that experience with both ethanol and the procedure may be necessary. The actual adjusted dose-response curves for the yoked and non-yoked animals are shown in Fig. 10. These curves, as in previous dose-response curves of the self-administering animals, indicate that ethanol under these conditions of experience and contingent administration increases the animal's sensitivity to BSR. In these 5 animals the individual z scores were -1.9 to -2.2. Comparisons of blood levels between the contingent and its paired noncontingent animal yield no significant differences ($t = 0.2$, n.s.).

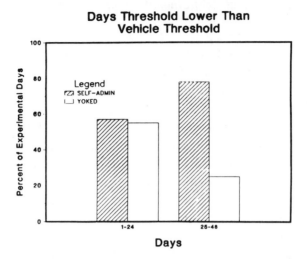

Figure 9. Percent of the first 24 and second 24 ethanol administration days in which the threshold for BSR after ethanol was lower than after saline.

DISCUSSION

The results of these experiments suggest that the reinforcing effects of ethanol are in part the result of activation of some of the same neuronal systems involved in the reinforcing effects of other abused substances. Although it is beyond the scope of this chapter, there is considerable evidence implicating the mesolimbic-cortical dopamine system in BSR and the rewarding effects of the psychomotor stimulants and the abused opiate drugs (Fibiger et al., 1987). Evidence is given by Engel and Liljequist (1976), who reported that ethanol increases the sensitivity of animals to dopamine in discrete brain regions that are associated with the anatomy of the reward system. Acute injections of ethanol will increase dopamine turnover in the striatum (Lai et al., 1979; Reggiani et al., 1980). When iontophoretically applied, ethanol will increase the firing rate of neurons in the lateral hypothalamic area of the brain (Wayner et al., 1975).

The results of the experiments of ethanol on BSR suggest that although there is activation of the reward system by ethanol, it clearly is not the result of only a direct pharmacological action. The role of experience as well as the control of the administration of ethanol seems to play

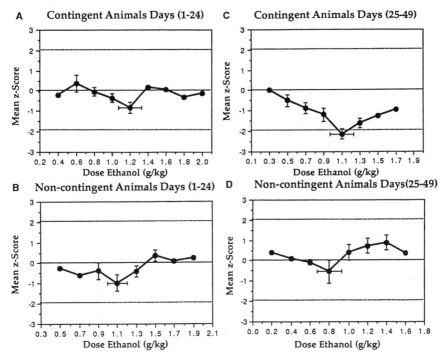

Figure 10. Mean adjusted dose-response curve for the orally self-administered ethanol group (contingent) and their noncontingent yoked controls on the threshold for BSR. A & B indicate the results of the first 24 experimental days, whereas C & D indicate the results for the second 24 experimental days. Reprinted with permission of Pergamon Press, Inc., from Moolten and Kornetsky (1990): Oral self-administration of ethanol and not experimenter administered ethanol facilitates rewarding electrical brain stimulation. *Alcohol Clin Exp Res* 7:221-225.

an imporant role in ethanol's reinforcing effects. There is considerable evidence indicating that when the subject has the contingencies of reinforcement under its control, different behavioral results may be expected. One of the classic examples of this is in experiments of learned helplessness (Seligman, 1972). In this animal model of depression, animals that can terminate electric shock show little effect of the painful stimulation. Initially the animal will display stress behavior such as defecating, urinating, and whining; however, once it discovers the response necessary to terminate the shock it will immediately learn to avoid subsequent shocks and show little evidence of what is termed "learned helplessness." Yoked animals receiving the same amount of shock but who cannot terminate it show all the behavioral signs of learned helplessness and when given the opportunity to terminate the shock, they fail to exhibit normal avoidance directed behavior. Even if they accidentally perform the necessary procedure they are unable to make the association between their actions and termination of the shock; thus, they will continue to bear the shock.

There is no magic in such findings. It is likely that such environmental manipulation results in changes in the brain chemistry of the subject so that when given a drug it is now acting on a different brain. Smith et al. (1982) demonstrated significant differences in brain neurotransmitter turnover as a function of whether morphine was experimenter-administered to the subject or was self-administered by the animal. The areas of the brain implicated in self-administration were the hippocampus, nucleus accumbens, septum, stratium, amygdala, and frontal-pyriform cortex. They concluded in their paper that,

> The neurotransmitter turnover rate changes resulting from contingent administration suggest that the drug administration environment is an important factor that should be considered in the studies of interactions between drugs and neuronal system.

In a recent report by Dworkin et al. (1988), data were presented showing that there was significantly less toxicity of cocaine in animals that self-administered the drug when compared to animals that were passively administered it. The conditions of the environment during which an abused drug is administered is also important for the maintenance of drug-seeking behavior. Hospital patients who receive morphine for its analgesic purposes do not display drug-seeking behavior when released (Haertzen and Hooks, 1969). This remains true despite the fact that the individuals may have received large enough doses to cause physiological dependence. The mindset of these patients receiving the drug for medicinal purposes is obviously different from those individuals who actively self-administer morphine or other opiates. As a consequence of this difference in the environment, circumstances and the mindset of the patient versus the street user, addiction and drug-seeking behavior rarely occur in those receiving opiates for medical reasons (Rayport, 1954). Further support that there are differences in the brains of animals that have control of the stimulation as compared to those that do not is given by the report of Porrino et al. (1984). In this experiment measurements of local cerebral glucose utilization in specific brain sites in animals that self-administered BSR and in animals that were experimentally administered equivalent stimulation showed marked differences in metabolic activity in the terminal fields of the VTA.

SUMMARY AND CONCLUSIONS

To the extent that a drug increases the sensitivity of an animal to BSR is a model for drug-induced euphoria, the results of the ethanol self-administration experiments support the hypothesis that ethanol's reinforcing properties are a function of activation of those pathways that subserve reward. As stated earlier, some abuse substances increase the sensitivity of an animal to BSR the first time the animal receives the drug. It seems to be relatively irrelevant whether it is contingently or noncontingently administered if the dose is appropriate. Failure of ethanol, however, to increase sensitivity to BSR except after contingent ethanol administration suggests that the effect is not obligatory. It is probably necessary to activate those areas of the brain that subserve reward for a drug to be reinforcing; however, direct activation may not be a sufficient action.

The hedonic effects responsible for the reinforcing properties of cocaine and probably to a slightly lesser extent heroin are determined for the most part by a direct pharmacological action on those areas of the brain that subserve reward. Thus, if the dose is appropriate these rewarding effects are almost obligatory. This is not true for ethanol and probably not true for other sedative-hypnotics, for example, the benzodiazepines, which depend much more on nonpharmacological factors interacting with pharmacological action to achieve their hedonic effects.

This theoretical schema of the relative contribution of pharmacological effects and nonpharmacological factors in the rewarding effects of cocaine, heroin, benzodiazepines, and ethanol as depicted in Fig. 11. As indicated, cocaine's rewarding effects are mainly a function of direct pharmacological factors, such as previous drug experience and personality of the subject, and the environment in which the drug is used, interact with pharmacological actions, resulting in the final rewarding effect of the drug.

In summary, the described experiments suggest that the rewarding effects of ethanol, although mediated by some of the same systems that affect other abuse substances, are influenced to a major extent by nonpharmacological factors. Although we do not know the specific mechanism by which nonpharmacological factors contribute to the rewarding effects of ethanol, we suggest that these contingencies change the chemical and neural network of the brain in a manner that may be necessary for the drug to be reinforcing.

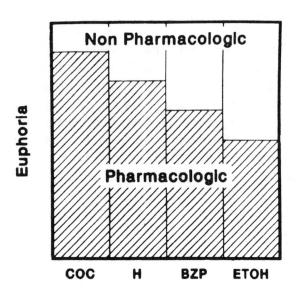

Figure 11. Schematic representation of relative role of pharmacological and nonpharmacological factors contributing to the reinforcing effects of cocaine (COC), heroin (H), benzodiazepines (BZP), ethanol (ETOH). Reprinted with permission of Springer-Verlag, New York, from Bain and Kornetsky (1990): Opioids modification of central reward processes. In: *Opioids, Bulimia and Alcohol Abuse and Alcoholism*, Reid L, ed.

ACKNOWLEDGMENTS

Supported in part by grants AA05950 and NIDA Research Scientist Award DA00099 to CK.

REFERENCES

Arregui-Aguirre A, Claro-Izaguirre F, Goni-Garrido MJ, Zarate-Oleaga JA, Morgado-Bernal I (1987): Effects of acute nicotine and ethanol on medial prefrontal cortex self-stimulation in rats. *Pharmacol Biochem Behav* 27(1):15-20
Bain GT, Kornetsky C (1989): Ethanol oral self-administration and rewarding brain stimulation. *Alcohol* 6:499-503
Bain GT, Kornetsky C (1990): Opioids modification of central reward processes.

In: *Opioids, Bulimia and Alcohol Abuse and Alcoholism*. Reid L, ed. New York: Springer-Verlag, pp 73-87

Bird M, Kornetsky C (1990): Dissociation of the attentional and motivational effects of pimozide on the threshold for rewarding brain stimulation. *Neuropsychopharmacology* 3:33-40

Broekkamp CL, Phillips AG, Cools AR (1979): Facilitation of self-stimulation behavior following intracerebal microinjections of opioids into the ventral tegmental area. *Pharmacol Biochem Behav* 11:289-295

Broekkamp CL, Pijnenburg AJ, Cools AR, Van Rossum JM (1975): The effect of microinjections of amphetamine into the neostriatum and the nucleus accumbens on self-stimulation behavior. *Psychopharmacologia* 42(2):179-183

Carlson RH, Lydic R (1976): The effects of ethanol upon threshold and response rate for self-stimulation. *Psychopharmacology* 50:61-64

Caudarella M, Campbell KA, Milgram NW (1982): Differential effects of diazepam (Valium) on brain stimulation reward sites. *Pharmacol Biochem Behav* 16:17-21

DeWitte P, Bada MF (1983): Self-stimulation and alcohol administered orally or intraperitoneally. *Exp Neurol* 8:675-682

Dworkin SM, Volkner C, Dworkin SI (1988): Toxic consequences of cocaine are augmented by non-contingent drug administration. *Abstr Soc Neurosci* 14:961

Engel J, Liljequist S (1976): The effect of long-term ethanol treatment on the sensitivity of the dopamine receptors in the nucleus accumbens. *Psychopharmacology* 49:253-257

Esposito R, Kornetsky C (1977): Morphine lowering of self-stimulation thresholds: lack of tolerance with long-term administration. *Science* 195:189-191

Esposito RU, Motola AH, Kornetsky C (1978): Cocaine: acute effects on reinforcement thresholds for self-stimulation behavior to the medial forebrain bundle. *Pharmacol Biochem Behav* 8:437-439

Fibiger HC, LePiane FG, Jakobovic A, Phillips AG (1987): The role of dopamine in intercranial self-stimulation of the ventral tegmental area. *J Neurosci* 7:3888-3896

Haertzen CA, Hooks NT (1969): Changes in personality and subjective experience associated with the chronic administration and withdrawal of opiates. *J Nerv Ment Dis* 148:606-614

Killam KF, Olds J, Sinclair J (1957): Further studies on the effects of centrally acting drugs on self-stimulation. *J Pharmacol Exp Ther* 119:157

Kornetsky C (1985): Brain-stimulation reward: a model for the neuronal bases for drug induced euphoria. In: *Neuroscience Methods in Drug Abuse Research*. National Institute on Drug Abuse Research Monograph, Supt. of Docs., U.S. Govt Printing Office, Washington DC, p 30

Kornetsky C, Bain GT, Unterwald EM, Lewis MJ (1988): Brain stimulation reward: effects of ethanol. *Alcoholism: Clin Exp Res* 12(5): 609-616

Lai H, Makous WL, Horita A, Leung H (1979): Effects of ethanol on turnover and function of striatal dopamine. *Psychopharmacology* 61:1-9

Lewis MJ, Andrade JR, Mebane C, Phelps R (1984): Differential effects of ethanol and opiates on BSR threshold. *Soc Neurosci Abstr* 10:960

Lewis MJ, Phelps RW (1987): A multifunctional on-line brain stimulation system: investigation of alcohol and aging effects. In: *Methods of Assessing the Reinforcing Properties of Abused Drugs*. Bozarth MA, ed. New York: Springer-Verlag, p 463

Lorens SA, Sainati SM (1978): Naloxone blocks the excitatory effect of ethanol and chlordiazepoxide on lateral hypothalamic self-stimulation behavior. *Life Sci* 23:1359-1364

Moolten M, Kornetsky C (1990): Oral self-administration of ethanol and not experimenter administered ethanol facilitates rewarding electrical brain stimulation. *Alcohol Clin Exp Res* 7:3

Olds J, Killam KF, Bach-y-Rita P (1956): Self-stimulation of the brain used as a screening method for tranquilizing drugs. *Science* 124:265-266

Olds J, Milner P (1954): Positive reinforcement produced by electrical stimulation of septal area and other regions of the rat brain. *J Comp Physiol Psychol* 47(6):419-427

Pickens RW, Svikis DS (1988): Genetic vulnerability to drug abuse. In: *Biological Vulnerability to Drug Abuse*. Pickens RW, Svikis DS, eds. NIDA Research Monograph 89, Supt. of Docs., US Govt Printing Office, Washington, DC, pp 1-7

Porrino LJ, Esposito RU, Seeger TF, Crane AM, Pert A, Sokoloff L (1984): Metabolic mapping of the brain during rewarding self-stimulation. *Science* 224:306-309

Rayport M (1954): Experience in the management of patients medically addicted to narcotics. *JAMA* 156:684-691

Reggiani A, Barbaccia ML, Spano PF, Trabucchi M (1980): Dopamine metabolism and receptor function after acute and chronic ethanol. *J Neurochem* 35:34-37

Routtenberg A (1981): Drugs of abuse and the endogenous reinforcement system: the resistance of intracranial self-stimulation behavior to the inebriating effects of ethanol. *Ann NY Acad Sci* 362:60-66

Schaefer GJ, Michael RP (1987): Ethanol and current thresholds for brain self-stimulation in the lateral hypothalamus of the rat. *Alcohol* 4:209-213

Seligman MEP (1972): Learned helplessness. In: *Annual Review of Medicine*. DeGraff AC, Creger WP, eds. California: Annual Reviews Inc, 23:407-412

Smith JE, Co C, Freeman ME, Lane JD (1982): Brain neurotransmitter turnover correlated with morphine-seeking behavior of rats. *Pharmacol Biochem Behav* 16:509-519

St. Laurent J (1972): Brain centers of reinforcement and the effects of alcohol. In: *The Biology of Alcoholism, Volume 2: Physiology and Behavior*. Kissen B, Begleiter H, eds. New York: Plenum Press, pp 85-106

Unterwald EM, Clark JA, Bain G, Kornetsky C (1984): The effects of ethanol on rewarding intracranial stimulation: rate and threshold measures. *Abstr Soc Neurosci* 10:572

Vrtunski P, Murray R, Wolin LR (1973): The effect of alcohol on intracranially reinforced response. *Q J Stud Alcohol* 34:718-725

Wayner MJ, Ono T, Nolley D (1975): Effects of ethyl alcohol on central neurons. *Pharmacol Biochem Behav* 3:499-506

Electrophysiological Correlates
of Ethanol Reinforcement

Scott E. Lukas, Jack H. Mendelson, Leslie Amass,
Richard A. Benedikt, John N. Henry, Jr. and Elena M. Kouri

INTRODUCTION

Previous studies using visual inspection and spectral analysis procedures have found that ethanol increases the voltage and slows the predominant frequency of the resting electroencephalogram (EEG) (Abramson 1945; Begleiter and Platz, 1972; Davis et al., 1941; Docter et al., 1966; Ekman et al., 1963, 1964; Engel and Rosenbaum, 1945; Lukas et al., 1986a,c,d; Myrsten et al., 1975; Warren and Raynes, 1972). Although the results from these studies are fairly consistent, they were based on recordings from only a few EEG electrode sites, usually located over the occipital and parietal cortex. A re-examination of ethanol's effects on brain electrical activity has been prompted by recent technical advances in quantitative analysis of the topographic distribution of EEG activity using far more recording sites than conventional EEG studies.

Computerized analysis of EEG activity uses high-speed computers to digitize the original analog EEG activity, transform the data with a Fast Fourier Transformation (Walter, 1963), and generate a power spectrum containing numerical values for the amount of power in specific frequency bands. Thus, quantification of brain electrical activity using power spectral analysis provides concomitant measures of power and frequency independent of sample length. Topographic mapping of brain electrical activity employs the same basic technology used in power spectral analysis, but expands on them to configure the topographic information. These mapping techniques are useful because standard EEG recordings contain more information than can be assimilated readily by the human brain. Thus, computerized assistance of the analysis may reveal information that is missed by visual scoring (Duffy, 1989; Duffy et al., 1979, 1981). Topographic mapping procedures assemble information from multiple EEG leads by simultaneously creating power spectral arrays from all electrode sites. The values between electrode sites are computed with linear interpolation algorithms using the activity from the nearest three or four electrodes. The data are then combined into a composite color-coded (cf. Duffy et al., 1979, 1981) or gray-level (Buchsbaum et al., 1982) map that provides an overall view of brain electrical activity at the moment the map is generated. This technique has been used recently in the differential diagnosis of brain dysfunctions (John et al., 1988). An extensive discussion of the principles and the clinical and research applications of topographic mapping of brain electrical activity has been published recently (Duffy, 1986).

Measures of brain electrical activity have been useful in characterizing various naturally occurring behavioral states such as sleep and wakefulness, but EEG correlates of drug-induced euphoria, anxiety, or dysphoria have been difficult to obtain. One major problem associated with determining the relationship between brain electrical activity and drug-induced mood changes is the procedural difficulty associated with accurately measuring changes in subjective mood states without introducing EEG artifacts. The use of questionnaires and visual analog scales alters levels of alertness that in turn affect the EEG (Matousek and Petersen, 1983; Otto, 1967). Therefore, the use of a nonverbal method for recording drug-induced changes in mood is necessary to avoid disturbing the subject's level of alertness and thus altering EEG activity. Such a device has been employed in recent years (cf. Lukas, 1991; Lukas et al., 1986a,c).

For the past 5 years we have been studying the immediate effects of acute ethanol challenges in an attempt to evaluate more carefully the behavioral profile of ethanol intoxication and to quantify its electrophysiological correlate. It is hypothesized that the unique alterations in brain electrical activity that occur during the initial phases of ethanol-induced intoxication, particularly when blood ethanol levels are rising rapidly, are related to the reinforcing effects of ethanol. This hypothesis is supported by the results from a number of studies demonstrating that drugs that produce rapid changes in behavior are more likely to be abused than drugs that have a delayed onset of action.

METHODS

Subjects

All studies were conducted using healthy adult male and female volunteers (ages 21-35 years). Subjects were recruited via newspaper advertisements and were paid for their participation. After a full explanation of the nature of the study, all subjects provided informed consent for participation. All subjects received a complete physical examination, including an electrocardiogram, blood chemistry, and urinalysis evaluations. In addition, female subjects were tested for beta subunit human chorionic gonadotropic hormone levels 1 to 2 days before the study to ensure that they were not pregnant. Subjects with any neurological, psychiatric, or alcohol- or drug abuse-related problems were excluded. Selection criteria also included a lean body mass of between 0.3 and 0.4 kg/cm to ensure minimal variability in ethanol volume of distribution (Reed, 1978). Subjects were not currently taking any prescription medication (including oral contraceptives), and urine screens for recreational drugs were conducted on each study day–all results were negative. Analysis of the recruiting questionnaires revealed that all subjects described themselves as social drinkers who consumed, on average, the equivalent of 1 to 3 glasses of wine per week. All but one subject reported a negative family history for alcohol abuse or dependence based on DSM-III criteria.

Subjective State Assessments-Instrumental Joystick Device

These studies were designed to determine the covariance between ethanol-induced intoxication, EEG activity, and plasma ethanol levels. Continuous measures of ethanol-induced intoxication were obtained using a nonverbal instrumental joystick device. This device was used in lieu of frequent verbal questioning to avoid distracting the subjects because such interference could alter EEG activity and prevent the acquisition of spontaneous EEG activity during the transitions between behavioral states.

A customized instrumental joystick device was constructed using the shell of a standard computer game joystick (Lukas et al., 1986a,c). The stock "fire" buttons were removed and were replaced with three, low tension, momentary-on buttons. These buttons require less than 1 N of force for operation. Movement of the joystick in one of three directions (forward, sideways, backward) activated a different microswitch that completed a circuit to a pen on the polygraph, providing a written record of the subject's response immediately below the EEG tracings (Fig. 1). The joystick was spring-loaded to return to the neutral center position upon release. Subjects were instructed to keep their left hand on the joystick at all times. Installed on one side of the joystick shell was a photosensor that was covered by the subject's hand and transmitted a signal to the EEG technician if the subject completely released the joystick.

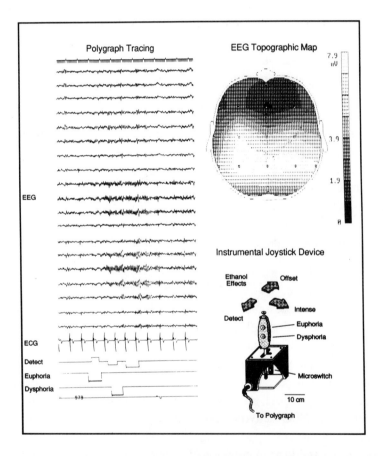

Figure 1. Representative polygraphic recording of EEG activity, electrocardiographic activity, and subject's responses on the instrumental joystick device (*left panel*). Details of the joystick device are shown in the lower right panel. The corresponding EEG topographic map (shown using a gray scale) is depicted in the upper right panel.

Subjects were instructed in the operation of the joystick device and were then told to move the joystick according to the following instructions:

Forward:	"when you feel intoxicated or under the influence of alcohol"
Sideways:	"when you feel that these effects are getting stronger"
Backward	"when the alcohol effects disappear"
Top button	"when you experience a feeling of intense well-being or euphoria"
Bottom button	"when you experience a bad feeling or dysphoria"

Self-reports of intoxication were obtained verbally from some subjects for comparison with the joystick response data. A questionnaire was administered every 15 minutes in which the subject was asked to rate him- or herself on a scale of 0 to 10, with a 0 signifying "completely sober," a 5 signifying "moderately intoxicated," and a 10 signifying "extremely intoxicated."

Experimental Design and Procedure

Each subject served as his or her own control and participated in the study on two or three occasions, 1 to 7 days apart. Female subjects were scheduled such that the first study day occurred on the day after the last day of menses. All subjects were told that they might receive either placebo or ethanol on each study day. Each subject actually received one or two doses of ethanol and placebo on each day in a randomized counterbalanced design. The ethanol drink contained either 0.35 or 0.70 g/kg of beverage grade ethyl alcohol [86 proof vodka] mixed in chilled fresh orange juice. The placebo drink contained only orange juice. The total volume of both drinks was 350 ml. To help mask the drink's content, a 10-ml reservoir within the straw was filled with 3 ml of vodka and 7 ml of orange juice to provide a strong initial ethanol taste before both placebo and active drinks were consumed (Mendelson et al., 1984). Subjects were informed of this procedure in order to discourage them from using taste as a discriminating cue.

Both beverages were administered via a peristaltic pump (located outside the experimental room) (Lukas et al., 1986a,c,d) that delivered fluid at a rate of 23 ml/min. The tubing and mouthpiece were supported by a flexible metal arm to permit hands-free drinking and allow the subjects to keep their eyes closed and one hand on the joystick device during the drinking procedure. The pump was activated for 3 minutes followed by a 1-minute rest period. This procedure was repeated until the drink was consumed (19 minutes).

Subjects arrived at the laboratory at 9:00 am and reported that they had refrained from eating or drinking (except water) since midnight the night before. Thirty minutes of baseline EEG activity was collected before ethanol or placebo was administered. Since the goal of the experiment was to study the early effects of ethanol, all measures were recorded for only 90 minutes after the drink was consumed.

Blood Sample Collections

Blood samples for analysis of integrative plasma ethanol concentrations were withdrawn continuously during the entire study. A 183-cm Kowarski-Dakmed Thromboresistant Blood Withdrawal Butterfly Needle and Tubing Set (Dakmed Inc., Buffalo, NY) was used for blood sampling. The extra long length was necessary so that blood could be drawn from outside the chamber. Blood was withdrawn from the right antecubital vein. The end of the catheter was attached to a 10-ml syringe mounted on a syringe pump (Harvard Apparatus, Cambridge, MA), which was calibrated to withdraw blood at a rate of 1 ml/minute. Syringes were changed at 5 minute intervals to measure rapid changes in blood ethanol levels.

Plasma Ethanol Level Assay

Blood samples were immediately spun and the plasma frozen for subsequent batch analysis for ethanol concentration. Initial samples were analyzed using the spectrophotometric method of Lèric et al. (1970). Intra- and interassay coefficient of variation (CV) were 3.0% and 7.4%, respectively. Subsequent samples were analyzed via gas chromatography using a modification of the methods of Freund (1967) and Gentry et al. (1983). Briefly, plasma samples were thawed and then centrifuged at 4°C to remove fibrin clots. The vials were resealed with septum caps, mixed, and placed in an autosampler turntable. An external standard curve, covering the range of 1 to 300 mg/dl ethanol concentration, was prepared in a similar manner. Analyses were carried out using a

Hewlett-Packard Model 5890 Gas Chromatograph, equipped with an automatic liquid sample injector and a Model 3393A Integrator/Recorder. A 6-foot coiled glass column (2 mm inner diameter, 6.4 mm outer diameter) packed with Chromosorb 101, 80/100 mesh, was used. The carrier gas was nitrogen and the column oven and injection port temperatures were 130 and 175°C, respectively. Ethanol was detected using a flame ionization detector (hydrogen and air) maintained at 200°C.

EEG Recording Procedure

All recordings were obtained while subjects sat in a reclining chair and housed in a sound- and light-attenuated electrically-shielded chamber. Subjects were prepared with 6 scalp electrodes (C3, C4, P3, P4, O1, and O2) affixed with cream paste and referenced to linked earlobes. Temporalis muscle electrodes were used to record muscle tension, a thermocouple electrode attached to the subject's nostril provided respiratory data, and a fingertip photoelectric transducer recorded pulse data. All EEG and physiologic recordings were made on a Model 78D polygraph (Grass Instrument Co., Quincy, MA). The EEG activity was also recorded on FM magnetic tape for off-line power spectral analysis using a Pathfinder signal-averaging microprocessor (Nicolet Biomedical Instrument Co., Madison, WI). A digital time code was also recorded on one channel of the magnetic tape to facilitate identification of specific epochs of EEG activity during off-line computerized EEG analysis.

Topographic EEG Mapping Procedure

Subjects were prepared with 25 scalp electrodes affixed with collodion using the International 10-20 system of electrode application (Jasper, 1958). In addition, bilateral neck electrodes were attached to record muscle activity and two electrodes were placed above and below the left eye to monitor eye movements. Subjects were seated in a dimly lit room and the recording polygraph was located in an adjacent room. Unipolar activity from leads F3, F4, C3, C4, P3, P4, O1, O2, FP1, FP2, F7, F8, T3, T4, T5, T6, Fz, Cz, Pz, Oz, linked eyes, left zygomatic, right zygomatic, and linked bilateral electrodes placed over the fifth cervical vertebrate were referenced to linked earlobes and collected during eyes closed conditions.

Topographic mapping of EEG activity was conducted using Grass
12A5S amplifiers at a bandpass of 1 to 300 Hz and a Brain Electrical Activity Mapping (BEAM™) system (Nicolet Biomedical Instrument,
Madison, WI). Additional mapping studies were conducted using a Nicolet Model A198 polygraph and a Brain Atlas II system (Bio-logic Inc.,
Mundelein, IL). EEG activity was recorded continuously on a paper chart
driver during the study. Two to three-minute epochs of EEG activity were
recorded on the mapping systems every 10 minutes for subsequent analysis. Additional epochs of EEG activity were recorded during joystick
responding events using the synchronized time code as a reference.

Data Analysis

Pulse rate, muscle tension and respiratory rate data were quantified at
one-minute intervals during the first 60 minutes after drinking and at
five-minute intervals for the remainder of the experiment. Movements of
the joystick indicating ethanol detection and episodes of euphoria were
directly recorded on the polygraph; these behavioral data were manu-
ally retrieved from the polygraphic recordings and the latency to onset,
duration, and number of events were tabulated in synchrony with the
digital time code that was recorded with the EEG data. Mean latency
to detection, intense intoxication, and termination of ethanol effects as
well as number and duration of euphoric and dysphoric episodes were
determined after placebo and ethanol treatments.

Discrete two-minute, artifact-free epochs of EEG activity were selected every 15 minutes for power spectral analysis using frequency analysis software developed by Nicolet. The program digitized the analog
waveforms at a rate of 256 Hz, performed a Fast Fourier Transformation,
and then generated a compressed spectral array representing EEG power
as a function of frequency. The corresponding power ($\mu V^2/Hz$) and peak
frequency (Hz) in the 0.25 to 4.0 Hz, 4.0 to 8.0 Hz, 8 to 13 Hz, and 13
to 30 Hz bands were quantified at 20-second intervals.

Topographic maps were generated as follows: Two-minute epochs
of brain electrical activity maps were collected during the control period
and at 10-minute intervals after drinking began. Additional samples of
EEG activity were recorded when subjects pushed the button to report
euphoria. Digitized epochs of EEG activity were edited on a blind basis
for eye and head movement artifact (abrupt deflections of 50 μV). Since
the buttons on the joystick require only 1 N of force to operate, move-

ment artifact was minimal or nonexistent; when present, only a one to two-second epoch of EEG activity required editing. Using the BEAM™ system software, Fast Fourier Transformations were performed on the remaining EEG activity. Brain electrical activity between electrode sites was calculated using a three-point interpolation algorithm, and the resultant spectral arrays were color-coded on the basis of power in each of the following frequency bands: delta (0.5-3.5 Hz), theta (4.0-7.5 Hz), slow alpha (7.5-9.5 Hz), fast alpha (9.5-12.5 Hz), beta$_1$ (12.0-15.5 Hz), beta$_2$ (16.0-19.5 Hz), and beta$_3$ (20.0-23.5 Hz). To avoid false interpretations due to truncation, the range of absolute values (μV) and corresponding color codes were used for data analysis but then were scaled identically across all time points and subjects for graphic display.

Topographic maps were compared to a nontreated control database consisting of data from thirty 20 to 29-year-old right-handed women by using significant probability mapping (SPM) techniques (Duffy et al., 1981). SPM is a procedure that constructs z scores for the voltage and frequency values at each data point. Brain electrical activity in each region of a subject's scalp is then displayed on a color scale that is calibrated in the number of standard deviations the subject's activity is from the control group. Because of the controversy surrounding the validity of techniques that employ multiple post hoc comparisons (Duffy et al., 1986; Kahn et al., 1988; Oken and Chiappa, 1986), an alternative approach to quantifying the topographic maps was developed.

The color-coded BEAM™-generated maps were collected and stored as gray-scale images using a high-resolution digitizer/flat bed optical scanner (Datacopy, Mountain View, CA) and a Macintosh™ microcomputer (Apple Computer, Inc., Cupertino, CA). The digitized images were then read into a drafting program (MacDraft™, Innovative Data Design, Inc., Concord, CA). The contours of individual colors on each BEAM™-generated map were traced using an autotrace feature in Illustrator™ '88, Adobe, Mountainview, CA). A quantitative measure of the distribution of alpha activity over the scalp was obtained by determining the area (in mm^2) of the various color-coded regions using the *Show Area* command of the MacDraft™ graphics program. The area of each color was then multiplied by its corresponding voltage value provided by the absolute scale supplied with each topographic map. Values for each voltage range were then added together to yield a measure of alpha density for each topographic map (Fig. 2).

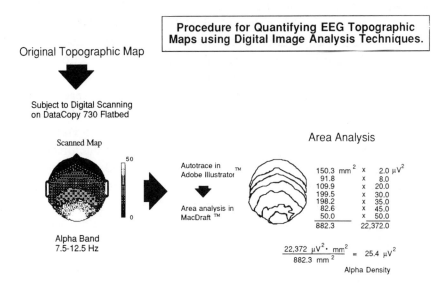

Figure 2.   Procedure for quantifying EEG topographic maps using digital image analysis techniques. Color-coded maps are converted to their corresponding alpha density using a series of image processing techniques.

RESULTS

Verbal Self-reports of Intoxication

This study was conducted to compare verbal reports of intoxication with spontaneously emitted responses on the joystick device. Fig. 3 shows average verbal self-rating scores (top panel) and corresponding plasma ethanol levels (bottom panel) after placebo, low-dose ethanol, and high-dose ethanol. Subjects who received placebo reported significantly lower levels of intoxication than ethanol-treated subjects ($f = 1.845$, $df = 20$, $p < 0.025$). The two ethanol groups reported equivalent levels of intoxication during the two hour session ($f = 0.140$, $df = 10$, n.s). Intoxication levels peaked at 45 minutes after drinking began when plasma ethanol levels were in the 50 to 55 mg/dl range. Thus, although the two ethanol doses did differ from placebo, the verbal reports were not sensitive to the differences in ethanol dose.

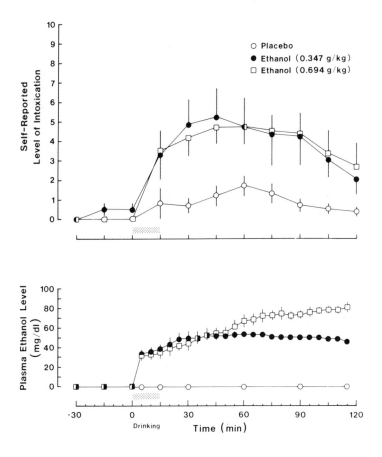

Figure 3. Self-reported levels of intoxication and plasma ethanol levels after either placebo, low-dose ethanol (0.35 g/kg), or high-dose ethanol (0.7 g/kg). Subjects were asked to rate themselves every 15 min on a scale of 0-10, with 0 representing a completely sober state, 5 representing a moderately intoxicated state, and 10 representing an extremely intoxicated state. Data represent mean ±SEM for six subjects per treatment. Reprinted with permission of Springer-Verlag, New York, from Lukas et al. (1986): Instrumental analysis of ethanol-induced intoxication in human males. *Psychopharmacology* 89:8-13.

Instrumental Self-reports of Intoxication

Acute ethanol administration produced obvious behavioral changes but did not alter pulse, muscle tension, or respiratory rate (see Lukas et al., 1986c). Representative behavioral profiles of three subjects who had received either placebo, low-dose ethanol, or high-dose ethanol are shown in Fig. 4. The placebo response was characterized by a delayed onset and a shorter duration than the ethanol-treated subjects. Subjects who received the high-dose ethanol experienced a slightly quicker onset and longer duration of effects than those who received the low dose. However, the high-dose ethanol subjects experienced multiple paroxysmal episodes of euphoria (Fig. 4, top panel). Joystick responding on the top button, which indicated euphoria, was fairly consistent in all subjects who received high-dose ethanol and in about one fifth of the subjects who received low-dose ethanol. No subject who received placebo reported euphoria.

The relationship between the onset of ethanol-induced behavioral effects and plasma ethanol levels is shown in Fig. 5. The onset of detection and peak effects after both ethanol doses occurred at similar times and plasma ethanol levels. In general, euphoria was reported sooner than

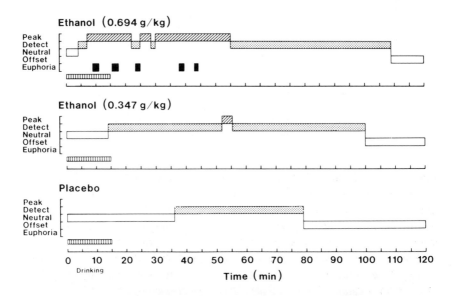

Figure 4. Representative behavioral profiles of three different subjects' response to drinking either placebo, or low-dose (0.35 g/kg) or high-dose (0.7 g/kg) ethanol. Behaviors were recorded instrumentally using a joystick device. Reprinted with permission of Springer-Verlag, New York, from Lukas et al. (1986): Instrumental analysis of ethanol-induced intoxication in human males. *Psychopharmacology* 89:8-13.

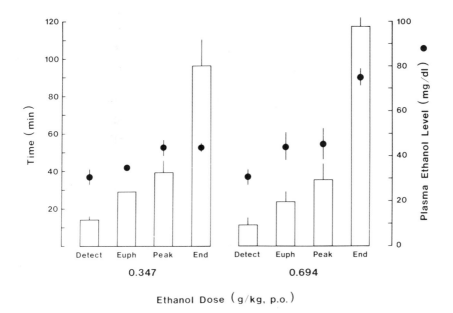

Figure 5. Correlations between ethanol-induced changes in behavioral states and plasma ethanol levels. Data represent mean ±SEM for six subjects per treatment. Behavioral responses were recorded using an instrumental joystick device. Reprinted with permission of Springer-Verlag, New York, from Lukas et al. (1986): Instrumental analysis of ethanol-induced intoxication in human males. *Psychopharmacology* 89:8-13.

"peak" effects, but this difference was not statistically significant. Finally, plasma ethanol levels remained elevated even though subjects reported that the effects had subsided.

Ethanol-induced EEG Effects

Fig. 6 shows the temporal relationship between the behavioral responses, plasma ethanol levels, and EEG changes in one subject who received 0.7 g/kg of ethanol. This subject detected ethanol effects 14 minutes after he began drinking when his plasma ethanol level was 42 mg/dl. Changes in EEG alpha and theta power also paralleled the behavioral effects. Alpha power was initially increased after ethanol, but returned to control levels about 1 hour after drinking. Theta power gradually increased during the experiment.

214   Lukas et al.

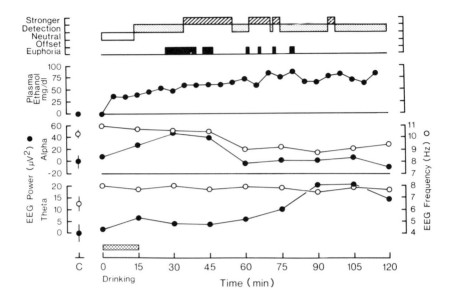

Figure 6. Time course of behavioral changes, plasma ethanol levels, and EEG activity in one subject after drinking 0.7 g/kg ethanol. Behavioral measures were obtained continuously using an instrumental joystick device. Two min artifact-free epochs of EEG activity were analyzed every 15 min using power spectral analysis. Control values represent mean ±SD of five 2-min samples obtained during the 30-min control session. Reprinted with permission of Pergamon Press, Inc. from Lukas et al. (1986): EEG alpha activity increases during transient episodes of ethanol-induced euphoria. *Pharmacol Biochem Behav* 25:889-895.

Fig. 7 depicts the temporal pattern of EEG changes in theta (4–8 Hz) and alpha (8–13 Hz) power, plasma ethanol levels, and the incidence of euphoric episodes for all ethanol-treated subjects. No changes in either theta or alpha power occurred after placebo administration. Low-dose ethanol failed to affect EEG alpha power, but did significantly increase theta activity 60 to 90 minutes after drinking began. High-dose ethanol significantly increased theta activity over a time course that paralleled the plasma ethanol curve. This relationship was found to be linear $(y = 0.34x - 11.70; r^2 = 0.93)$ and the correlation coefficient (r) of 0.97 confirmed this relationship. Alpha power was significantly increased 15, 30, and 45 minutes after subjects consumed the high-dose ethanol beverage. Low-dose ethanol had no effect on alpha power. The high-dose ethanol-induced increase in EEG alpha power declined to control levels by 55 minutes after drinking began. The incidence of episodes of euphoria paralleled this bimodal change in alpha power (y = 0.49x + 5.61; r^2 = 0.89) and was highly correlated (r = 0.95).

Whereas the absolute plasma ethanol levels after both doses did not

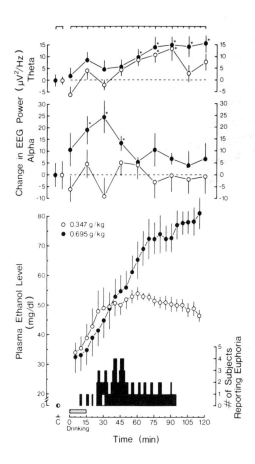

Figure 7. Time course of changes in theta (4-8 Hz) and alpha (8-13 Hz) EEG activity, plasma ethanol levels, and reported episodes of euphoria after low dose (o) and high dose (•) ethanol administration. Values represent means ±SEM for six subjects except for the reported episodes of euphoria which are plotted as actual events. The single episode produced by low dose ethanol is indicated by the small white block at 30-31 min. Reprinted with permission of Pergamon Press, Inc. from Lukas et al. (1986): EEG alpha activity increases during transient episodes of ethanol-induced euphoria. *Pharmacol Biochem Behav* 25:889-895.

differ up to 45 minutes after drinking began, the slopes of the plasma ethanol curves were significantly different during the 25 to 50 minute period when the greatest incidence of reported episodes of euphoria occurred. The slopes and 95% confidence intervals of the plasma ethanol curves after high dose and low dose were 0.599 (0.432-0.767) and 0.153 (0.091-0.214) mg/dl/minutes, respectively. These two curves were not parallel (calculated t (8)=6.943, $p<0.01$).

The nature of the general increases in EEG alpha activity observed in the previous analysis was difficult to assess. To determine the profile of this response the electrophysiological correlates of ethanol-induced euphoria were more precisely measured by subjecting 20-second epochs of EEG activity to power spectral analysis. Fig. 8 shows a representative series of power spectra from one subject during euphoria (shaded area) that occurred 34 minutes after consuming 0.70 g/kg of ethanol. Pro-

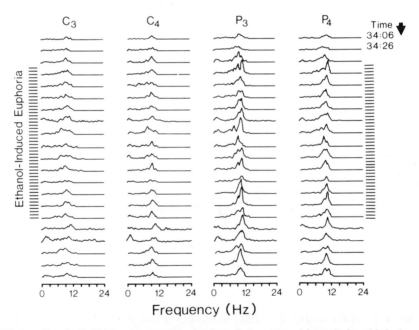

Figure 8. Individual power spectral plots from one subject during high-dose ethanol-induced euphoria. Each plot represents 20 sec of EEG activity from electrode sites C3, C4, P3, and P4. Shaded area indicates joystick responding by the subject indicating that he felt euphoric. Time elapses from top to bottom. Reprinted with permission of Pergamon Press, Inc. from Lukas et al. (1986): EEG alpha activity increases during transient episodes of ethanol-induced euphoria. *Pharmacol Biochem Behav* 25:889-895.

nounced increases in EEG alpha activity are apparent in leads P3 and P4. The increase in alpha activity persisted one to two minutes after the joystick was released. This increase in alpha was not observed during simulated control joystick responses obtained during the first 30 minutes of the study.

Group EEG data from leads C4 and P4 recorded before, during the first 40 seconds of, and after reported episodes of euphoria are shown in Fig. 9. Data are from all episodes of euphoria reported by subjects who received high dose ethanol. Each histogram represents 20 seconds of EEG activity and is divided into the amount of power in the various frequency bands. Alpha power in lead P4 was significantly increased during euphoria and returned to pre-euphoria levels after the joystick button had been released.

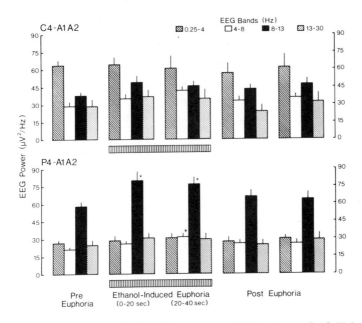

Figure 9. Group delta (0.25-4 Hz), theta (4-8 Hz), alpha (8-13 Hz) and beta (13-30 Hz) EEG activity 20 sec before, during the first 40 sec of euphoria, and 40 sec after high-dose ethanol-induced euphoria (indicated by horizontal bar). Data represent mean ±SEM of 20-sec epochs of EEG activity recorded from C4 (**top panel**) and P4 (**bottom panel**) electrode sites. * Denotes values significantly different from pre-euphoria values at $p<0.05$. Reprinted with permission of Pergamon Press, Inc. from Lukas et al. (1986): EEG alpha activity increases during transient episodes of ethanol-induced euphoria. *Pharmacol Biochem Behav* 25:889-895.

Topographic EEG Activity After Ethanol Administration

Data from the previous studies suggested that whereas EEG alpha activity was increased in some scalp leads, information regarding the distribution of such increases was lacking. Topographic maps of each frequency band (e.g., delta, theta, alpha, beta) obtained during the pre-drink control period exhibited distribution patterns normally found during an eyes closed/quiet awake state (Gibbs and Gibbs, 1951; Niedermeyer, 1987). This included a localization of alpha activity over the occipital poles, midline theta and frontal delta. Ethanol-induced behavioral reports of intoxication were associated with alterations in brain electrical activity in the subjects with a *negative* family history (FHN) for alcoholism. Fig. 10 depicts this relationship for both a representative FHN subject and the one family history positive (FHP) subject. In the FHN subjects, topographic mapping of alpha activity after ethanol revealed that the distribution of high-amplitude alpha activity (white areas) extended bilaterally to encompass parietal, temporal, and frontal areas that were rostral to the central

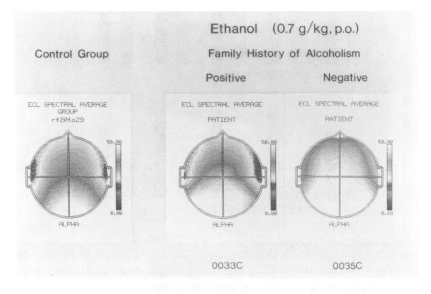

Figure 10. Topographic maps of EEG alpha activity from a control database **(left map)**, and from two subjects who received ethanol. Subjects differed in their family history of alcoholism. Maps were generated using a BEAM™ system during the control period and 15 min after the completion of drinking ethanol (0.7 g/kg). Maps are plotted using identical scaling factors (0-50 μV) to aid in visual comparisons. Subjects' eyes were closed during data collection.

sulcus (electrodes C3=Cz=C4). EEG alpha activity was only slightly increased after ethanol in the FHP subject even though her plasma ethanol level (62 mg/dl measured via expired air analysis) was in the same range as the FHN subject's at the time these maps were generated.

The results of the area analysis of alpha activity are shown in Fig. 11. The overall ANOVA showed a significant effect of ethanol on EEG alpha activity F (3,20) = 20.757, $p<.001$. Scheffe F test follow-up tests revealed significance ($p<.05$) after ethanol in both slow and fast alpha activity of the FHN subjects during the first 15 minutes after the drink

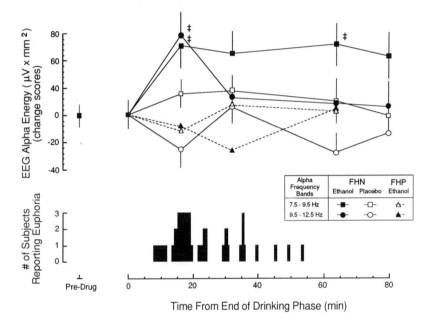

Figure 11. Quantitative area analysis of slow and fast EEG alpha activity at various times before and after drinking ethanol (0.7 g/kg) or placebo in five FHN subjects and the one (dotted lines) FHP subject. The number and distribution of subjective reports of euphoria are plotted along the time axis for direct comparison. All five FHN subjects reported euphoria while the FHP subject did not. EEG alpha energy was quantified using a contour area analysis procedure. ‡Denotes significance at $p<0.05$ level using ANOVA. Reprinted with permission of Alcohol Research Documentation, Inc., Rutgers Center of Alcohol studies, New Brunswick, NJ. from Lukas et al. (1989): Topographic distribution of EEG alpha activity during ethanol-induced intoxication in women. *J Stud Alcohol* 50:176-185.

was consumed, whereas the placebo did not significantly alter the topographic distribution of EEG alpha activity. The association between subjective reports of euphoria and increased alpha distribution was quite high ($r=0.61$, $p<.01$ for slow alpha and $r=0.74$, $p<.01$ for fast alpha); no subject reported euphoria after receiving placebo. Slow alpha activity continued to remain elevated while fast alpha activity returned to control levels. The one FHP subject displayed a marginal decrease in both slow and fast alpha activity and reported only mild ethanol effects.

SPM techniques were applied to track the changes in alpha activity during the course of reported feelings of sobriety, intoxication, and euphoria. Results from a representative FHN subject are shown in Fig. 12. The scale in these topographic maps represents the difference between this subject and the other subjects' results in the control database in units of standard deviations. The increased EEG alpha activity in frontal areas is evident by 30 minutes after ethanol—the same time this subject reported an intense pleasurable feeling. The last panel of this figure demonstrates that alpha power over the frontal cortex has increased by 4 standard deviations (white area) during button pushing behavior that signified that the subject was experiencing euphoria.

DISCUSSION

The neural mechanisms underlying ethanol-induced changes in feeling states and behavior remain to be determined. Most social drinkers, as well as persons who abuse ethanol, report changes in feeling states shortly after initiation of drinking. It is likely that these alterations in mood states induced by ethanol are reinforcing since ethanol abusers continue to drink even though dysphoric responses develop during protracted drinking episodes. This series of studies represents an attempt to determine if such a relationship exists, and if so, to quantify its effects. We found that acute administration of ethanol produced EEG and behavioral changes that were most prominent during the ascending limb of the plasma-ethanol curve. The EEG changes were limited to the theta and alpha bands and were positively correlated with plasma ethanol levels and discrete episodes of euphoria.

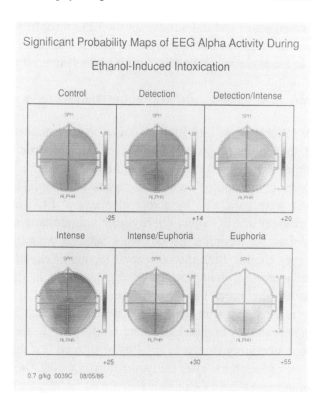

Figure 12. Significant probability maps of EEG alpha activity from one FHN subject during the progression from a sober state to ethanol intoxication. Reference bars to the right of each map are calibrated in units of standard deviations of the control sample population (20 to 29-year-old right-handed women) in the BEAM™ system database. Reprinted with permission of Alcohol Research Documentation, Inc., Rutgers Center of Alcohol studies, New Brunswick, NJ. from Lukas et al. (1989): Topographic distribution of EEG alpha activity during ethanol-induced intoxication in women. *J Stud Alcohol* 50:176-185.

Exhilaration, elation, or euphoria after consuming ethanol have been measured using various questionnaires and have been associated with talkativeness, raised spirits, higher pitched voice and increased feelings of contentment and relaxation (Abramson, 1945; Alha, 1951; Bjerver and Goldberg, 1950; Howells, 1956; King, 1943; Pihkanen, 1957). In this series of studies subjects were required to report ethanol intoxication and euphoria using an instrumental joystick device. By avoiding structured questionnaires, the subjects were free to report spontaneous changes in subjective mood states and did not disrupt the EEG recordings. It is this unique procedure (i.e., the use of a joystick) that permitted us to measure alterations in brain electrical activity during ethanol-induced euphoria.

EEG Changes After Ethanol: Behavioral Correlates

All subjects reliably moved the joystick device to indicate that they were intoxicated. In addition, subjects who received the high-dose ethanol reported that they experienced brief periods of intense pleasure or euphoria during ethanol intoxication. Subjective reports of ethanol intoxication and euphoria were paralleled by abrupt increases in EEG alpha activity. These changes in EEG alpha activity were not normally seen during control, quiet awake recording periods when subjects were instructed to keep their eyes closed. Both the behavioral reports of euphoria and the concomitant increased alpha density were paroxysmal in nature. The relatively brief duration of the euphoric episodes is difficult to explain. However, it is consistent with the notion that substances that produce relatively rapid alterations in mood states are reinforcing. In fact, previous data from our laboratory (Lukas et al., 1986b) showed that reports of intense pleasure and euphoria after marijuana smoking were also associated with abrupt increases in EEG alpha activity.

Pleasurable, free-floating, and extremely relaxed states are associated with increased EEG alpha activity (Brown, 1970; Lindsley, 1952; Matejcek, 1982; Wallace, 1970) and similar levels of alpha enhancement are seen in individuals who practice transcendental meditation (Wallace, 1970). The covariance between increased EEG alpha activity and subjective reports of euphoria after ethanol suggests that this neurophysiologic response may be associated with ethanol's reinforcing properties. Berger (1931) reported a similar increase in alpha activity after cocaine administration. Herning et al. (1985) replicated Berger's findings, but noted that the alpha increases did not persist for extended periods of time. It is quite possible that the reason for this rather modest alpha response was because the subjects in the Herning et al. (1985) study were required to perform a sequential subtraction task. It is well known that baseline EEG alpha activity is markedly reduced or even eliminated in individuals who are engaged in such task performance. Therefore, it is plausible that increased EEG alpha activity may be associated with drug-induced reinforcement in general, and may not be selective for a single drug class. This interpretation is consistent with the notion that drug-seeking behavior is a form of stimulus self-administration that produces a change (regardless of the direction) in subjective state (Mello, 1977, 1983).

Topography of Ethanol-induced EEG Alpha Activity

Ethanol-induced increases in alpha activity have been reported by a number of laboratories (Begleiter and Platz, 1972; Davis et al., 1941; Docter et al., 1966; Engel and Rosenbaum, 1944; Lukas et al., 1986c,d; Newman, 1959). High-amplitude alpha activity is normally localized about the occipital area in the area of electrode leads O1, O2, P3, and P4 and is usually most prominent when the eyes are closed. This study (where topographic mapping techniques were used to analyze EEG activity after ethanol administration) showed a unique pattern of increased alpha activity developing over the entire scalp; this pattern was not observed during nonintoxicated states. While low-amplitude, slow-frequency alpha activity can be recorded over the entire scalp, it is noteworthy that high-amplitude, fast-frequency alpha activity is not normally recorded over the frontal cortex; these studies (Lukas et al., 1989) are the first to document an ethanol-induced alteration in the topographic distribution of EEG alpha activity.

The observed increases in EEG alpha activity were not the result of neurophysiologic processes associated with intentional or voluntary movement such as that which would occur during movement of the joystick. Control recordings obtained during simulated joystick responding failed to produce observable changes in EEG alpha activity. Voluntary movements can activate cortical recordings, particularly over the sensorimotor cortex, but these effects are observed only when the movement is repetitive in nature and is paced over a specific time interval (Harner, 1986; Pfurtscheller, 1986). Joystick responding in this study was limited to single movements of the wrist or either the index or middle finger. Furthermore, voluntary movements actually reduce central beta activity (Jasper and Andrews, 1938; Pfurtscheller, 1981), and exogenous stimulation or increased attentiveness to the environment actually attenuates or "blocks" alpha activity (Morrell, 1966).

The source of EEG alpha activity is still a matter of some controversy (Neidermeyer, 1987). Data from ablation studies suggest that the thalamus acts as a generator for 8 to 13 Hz rhythmic activity recorded from cortex (Bremer, 1958). However, the use of precise cortical recording procedures has revealed that the cerebral cortex can generate alpha activity on its own (Lopes da Silva and Storm van Leeuwen, 1977). The significance of the source of EEG alpha activity is twofold: First, it may help determine if ethanol-induced alpha activity is simply an increase in the basal alpha activity that is usually present during resting states or if it represents a unique neurophysiological process. A similar issue regarding the similarities and differences between alpha rhythms and barbiturate-induced spindles has suggested that these are distinct waveforms (Lopes da Silva et al., 1973). Such information might prove helpful in treatment strategies for alcoholics patients where they are taught to relax using alpha biofeedback techniques. They may be better served by being taught to use alpha biofeedback as a substitute for ethanol intoxication instead of simply for relaxation. Second, it is thought that thalamic and cortical sites are independent of one another during alpha generation in naturalistic settings. Ethanol may cause a synchronization of the thalamo-cortical connections, thus causing an increase in alpha amplitude and a reduction in the variability of the predominant frequency. As will be discussed in the next section, the fact that both alcoholism and EEG alpha activity have been found to exhibit genetic-related profiles suggests that the relationship between spontaneous alpha rhythms and ethanol-induced alterations of alpha may provide further evidence for a link between alpha activity and alcoholism. Such a relationship might then be incorporated into a alcoholism prevention program.

EEG Indices of the Genetic Component of Alcoholism

Studies from other laboratories have demonstrated that subjects with a positive family history of alcoholism have a differential sensitivity to ethanol effects in comparison to subjects without this history. The observed differences are reflected as an attenuated response in the FHP subjects as compared to FHN subjects and include measures of body sway (Hegedus et al., 1984; Schuckit, 1985), subjective reports of intoxication (Pollock et al., 1986; Schuckit, 1984), motor control (O'Malley and Maisto, 1985), spontaneous electromyographic activity (Schuckit et al., 1981), and spontaneous EEG activity (Pollock et al., 1983). Attenuated behavioral and electrophysiological responses to ethanol have also been associated with a positive family history of alcoholism (Lukas et al., 1989).

One laboratory that found a greater response in subjects with a family history of alcoholism also reported that men with an alcoholic father exhibited alpha activity at a slower frequency than individuals without this history (Pollock et al., 1983). It appears that the effects of ethanol on alpha frequency are somewhat dependent on the subject's baseline alpha frequency (Engel and Rosenbaum, 1945; Varga and Nagy, 1960). Propping et al. (1980) demonstrated that ethanol elicited a more pronounced alpha rhythm in control subjects who have very little spontaneous EEG alpha activity. Additional evidence supporting a genetic component to ethanol's effects comes from studies with young boys who have a positive family history of alcoholism. Both spontaneous EEG activity (Gabrielli et al., 1982) and visual P300 evoked response potentials (Begleiter et al., 1984) differentiated these boys from control subjects without a family history of alcoholism. These data are particularly striking because the alterations in EEG and evoked response potentials were observed without ethanol administration. Thus, it is likely that the absolute direction and magnitude of the EEG differences between FHP and FHN subjects in a natural setting may be just as important as the differences observed after ethanol challenge.

Similar data obtained with adults are not as conclusive as those observed in children since visual (O'Connor et al., 1987) but not auditory (Polich and Bloom, 1986, 1987) P300 evoked potential amplitudes were lower in adult male subjects with a positive family history of alcoholism. Since spontaneous EEG activity is genetically related (Propping et al., 1980; Vogel, 1970; Vogel et al., 1979), it would appear that genetic predispositions to ethanol-related problems may be reflected in certain measures of brain electrical activity

Analysis of Topographic Mapping Data

Abrupt increases in alpha activity can also be quantified using a statistical tool—(SPM). Because of limitations of the BEAM™ system, which prevented the creation of a separate database, the SPM comparisons were made against the resident BEAM™ database (30 adult, right-handed female, women between the ages of 20 and 29 years). The validity of using SPM techniques as a diagnostic tool to classify a patient as either normal or possessing a specific disease has been challenged recently (Oken and Chiappa, 1986). Additional concerns regarding the care exercised during the collection process have been voiced because of the complexity of the topographic data obtained (Kahn et al., 1988). Duffy et al. (1986) defend SPM as being an exploratory procedure and emphasize that it is designed to localize regional differences in brain electrical activity, not to make diagnoses (Duffy, 1982; Duffy et al., 1984). Oken and Chiappa (1986) argue that the use of "significant difference" tests for evaluating differences between control groups and patients must be based on planned comparisons between the control group and the patient.

One method of circumventing the problem addressed above is to subject the topographic data to analyses that are especially appropriate for such graphic-oriented data–contour area analysis. Lukas et al. (1989) employed such a procedure that is based on digitized image reproduction using a microcomputer-based system. Although it is clearly more desirable to use the actual data points generated by the BEAM™ system, these data are not easily obtained using the currently available software. Thus, area analysis of EEG topographic maps, represents a compromise between the precision of the algorithms in the BEAM™ program that generate the maps, and interpretable differences in area that yielded clear distinctions between treated and non-treated conditions as well as between FHP and FHN subject

Results presented here from EEG and topographic mapping studies demonstrate that alpha activity is increased over the **entire** scalp after ethanol administration and that these changes parallel subjective reports of intoxication. Discovery of this relationship was made possible because subjective reports of euphoria were obtained using an instrumental joystick device and not through the use of verbal questionnaires. Taken together, these data suggest that ethanol-induced increases in EEG alpha activity may correlate with its reinforcing properties. Earlier reports from this laboratory (Lukas et al., 1986c; Lukas and Mendelson, 1988) made this suggestion based on data from only a limited number of electrode sites. With the advent of topographic mapping procedures, a more detailed and descriptive analysis of this phenomenon was possible. Since the ethanol-induced increases in EEG alpha activity were associated with pronounced pleasurable subjective effects, it is possible that this neurophysiological alteration may be related to processes that maintain continued ethanol-seeking behavior despite the aversive consequences associated with its chronic use and abuse (Alterman et al., 1975; McGuire et al., 1966; Mello, 1983; Mello and Mendelson, 1978).

ACKNOWLEDGMENTS

These studies were supported in part by grants: DA 00115, DA 00064, DA 03994, and DA 04059 from the National Institute on Drug Abuse and AA 06252 from the National Institute on Alcohol Abuse and Alcoholism.

REFERENCES

Abramson HA (1945): The effect of alcohol on the personality inventory (Minnesota): a preliminary report. *Psychosom Med* 7:184-185

Alha AR (1951): Blood alcohol and clinical inebriation in Finnish men. *Ann Acad Sci Fenn [A]* 26:1-92

Alterman AI, Gottheil E, Crawford DH (1975): Mood changes in an alcoholism treatment program based on drinking decisions. *Am J Psychiat* 132:1032-1037

Begleiter H, Platz A (1972): The effects of alcohol on the central nervous system in humans. In: *The Biology of Alcoholism, vol. 2.* Kissin B, Begleiter H, eds. New York: Plenum Press, pp 293-343

Begleiter H, Porjesz B, Bihari B, Kissin B (1984): Event-related brain potentials in boys at risk for alcoholism. *Science* 225:1493-1496

Berger H (1931): Uber das E.E.G. des menschen. [On the electroencephalogram of man: third report]. *Arch Psychiat Nervenkr* 94:16-30. Translated in: P. Gloor, ed. (1969) Hans Berger on the electroencephalogram of man. *Electroenceph Clin Neurophysiol* (Supplement 28): 95-132, Amsterdam: Elsevier

Bjerver K, Goldberg L (1950): Effects of alcohol ingestion on driving ability. *Q J Stud Alcohol* 11:1-30

Bremer F (1958): Cerebral and cerebellar potentials. *Physiol Rev* 38:357-388

Brown BB (1970): Recognition of aspects of consciousness through association with EEG alpha activity represented by a light signal. *Psychophysiology* 6:442-452

Buchsbaum MS, Rigal F, Coppola R, Cappelletti J, King C, Johnson J (1982): A new system for gray-level surface distribution maps of electrical activity. *Electroenceph Clin Neurophysiol* 53:237-242

Davis PA, Gibbs FA, Davis H, Jetter WW, Trowbridge LS (1941): The effects of alcohol upon the electroencephalogram (brain waves). *Q J Stud Alcohol* 1:626-637

Docter RF, Naitoh P, Smith JC (1966): Electroencephalographic changes and vigilance behavior during experimentally induced intoxication with alcoholic subjects. *Psychosom Med* 28:605-615

Duffy FH, ed. (1986): *Topographic Mapping of Brain Electrical Activity,* Boston: Butterworths

Duffy FH (1989): Comments on quantified neurophysiology–Problems and advantages. *Brain Topogr* 1:153-155

Duffy FH (1982): Topographic display of evoked potentials: Clinical applications of brain electrical activity mapping (BEAM™). In: *Evoked Potentials*, Bodis-Wollner I, ed. *Ann NY Acad Sci* 388:183-196

Duffy FH, Albert MS, McAnulty G, Garvey AJ (1984): Age-related differences in brain electrical activity of healthy subjects. *Ann Neurol* 16:430-438

Duffy FH, Bartels PH, Burchfiel JL (1981): Significance probability mapping: An aid in the topographic analysis of brain electrical activity. *Electroenceph Clin Neurophysiol* 51:455-462

Duffy FH, Bartels P H, Neff R (1986): A response to Oken and Chiappa. *Ann Neurol* 19:494-496

Duffy FH, Burchfiel JL, Lombroso CT (1979): Brain electrical activity mapping (BEAM™): a method for extending the clinical utility of EEG and evoked potential data. *Ann Neurol* 5:309-321

Ekman G, Frankenhaeuser M, Goldberg L, Bjherver K, Jarpe G, Myrsten A-L (1963): Effects of alcohol intake on subjective and objective variables over a five-hour period. *Psychopharmacologia* 4:28-38

Ekman G, Frankenhaeuser M, Goldberg L, Hagdahl R, Myrsten A-L (1964): Subjective and objective effects of alcohol as functions of dosage and time. *Psychopharmacologia* 6:399-409

Engel GL, Rosenbaum M (1944): Studies of the electroencephalogram in acute alcoholic intoxication. *Proc Cent Soc Clin Res* 17:62-63

Engel GL, Rosenbaum M (1945): Delirium III. Electroencephalographic changes associated with acute alcohol intoxication. *Arch Neurol Psychiat* 53:44-50

Freund G (1967): Exchangeable injection port cartridge for gas chromatographic determination of volatile substances in aqueous fluids. *Anal Chem* 39:545-546

Gabrielli WF, Mednick SA, Volavka J, Pollock VE, Schulsinger F, Itil TM (1982): Electroencephalograms in children of alcoholic fathers. *Psychophysiology* 19:404-407

Gentry RT, Rappaport MS, Dole VP (1983): Serial determination of plasma ethanol concentrations in mice. *Physiol Behav* 31:529-532

Gibbs FA, Gibbs EL (1951): *Atlas of Electroencephalography, Voume 1, Methodology and Controls*. Reading, MA: Addison-Wesley

Harner RN (1986): Clinical application of computed EEG topography. In: *Topographic Mapping of Brain Electrical Activity*. Duffy FH, ed. Boston: Butterworths, pp 347-356

Hegedus AM, Tarter RE, Hill S, Jacob T, Winsten NE (1984): Static ataxia: a possible marker for alcoholism. *Alcoholism: Clin Exp Res* 8:580-582

Herning RI, Jones RT, Hooker WD, Mendelson J, Blackwell L (1985): Cocaine increases EEG beta: a replication and extension of Hans Berger's historic experiments. *Electroenceph Clin Neurophysiol* 60:470-477

Howells DE (1956): Nystagmus as a physical sign in alcoholic intoxication. *Br Med J* 1:1405-1406

Jasper HH (1958): The 10-20 electrode system of the International Federation. *Electroenceph Clin Neurophysiol* 10:371-375

Jasper HH, Andrews HL (1938): Electroencephalography. III. Normal differentiations of occipital and precentral regions in man. *Arch Neurol Psychiat* 39:96-115

John ER, Prichep LS, Fridman J, Easton P (1988): Neurometrics: computer-assisted differential diagnosis of brain dysfunctions. *Science* 239:162-169

Kahn EM, Weiner RD, Brenner RP, Coppola R (1988): Topographic maps of brain electrical activity: pitfalls and precautions. *Biol Psychiat* 23: 628-636

King AR (1943): Tunnel vision. *Q J Stud Alcohol* 4:362-367

Lèric H, Kaplan JC, Broun G (1970): Dosage enzymatique de l'alcool sanguin par microméthode colorimétrique. *Clin Chim Acta* 29:523-528

Lindsley DB (1952): Psychological phenomena and the electroencephalogram. *Electroenceph Clin Neurophysiol* 4:443-456

Lopes da Silva FH, Storm van Leeuwen W (1977): The cortical source of the alpha rhythm. *Neurosci Letts* 6:237-241

Lopes da Silva FH, van Lierop THMT, Schrijer CF, Storm van Leeuwen W (1973): Essential differences between alpha rhythms and barbiturate spindles: Spectra and thalamo-cortical coherences. *Electroenceph Clin Neurophysiol* 35:641-645

Lukas SE (1991): Brain electrical activity as a tool for studying drugs of abuse. In: *Advances in Substance Abuse, Behavioral and Biological Research, vol. 4.* Mello NK, ed. London: Jessica Kingsley Publishers, pp 1-88

Lukas SE, Mendelson J H (1988): Electroencephalographic activity and plasma ACTH during ethanol-induced euphoria. *Biol Psychiat* 23:141-148

Lukas SE, Mendelson JH, Benedikt RA (1986a): Instrumental analysis of ethanol-induced intoxication in human males. *Psychopharmacol* (Berlin) 89:8-13

Lukas SE, Mendelson JH, Amass L, Smith R (1986b): Plasma delta-9-tetra-hydrocannibinol (THC) levels during marijuana-induced EEG and behavioral effects in human subjects. *Pharmacologist* 28:191

Lukas SE, Mendelson JH, Benedikt RA, Jones B (1986c): EEG alpha activity increases during transient episodes of ethanol-induced euphoria. *Pharmacol Biochem Behav* 25:889-895

Lukas SE, Mendelson JH, Benedikt RA, Jones B (1986d): EEG, physiologic and behavioral effects of ethanol administration. In: *Problems of Drug Dependence 1985*, NIDA Research Monograph 67, DHHS Publication No. (ADM)86-1448, Harris LS, ed. Washington, DC: U.S. Government Printing Office, pp 209-214

Lukas SE, Mendelson JH, Woods BT, Mello NK, Teoh SK (1989): Topographic distribution of EEG alpha activity during ethanol-induced intoxication in women. *J Stud Alcohol* 50:176-185

Matejcek M (1982): Vigilance and the EEG: psychological, physiological and pharmacological aspects. In: *EEG in Drug Research,* Hermann WM, ed. Stuttgart: Gustav Fischer, pp 405-508

Matousek M, Petersen I (1983): A method for assessing alertness fluctuations from EEG spectra. *Electroenceph Clin Neurophysiol* 55:108-113

McGuire MT, Stein S, Mendelson JH (1966): Comparative psychosocial studies of alcoholic and nonalcoholic subjects undergoing experimentally-induced ethanol intoxication. *Psychosom Med* 28: 13-26

Mello NK (1977): Stimulus self-administration: Some implications for the prediction of drug abuse liability. In: *Predicting Dependence Liability of Stimulant and Depressant Drugs.* Thompson T, Unna KR, eds. Baltimore: University Park Press, pp 243-260

Mello NK (1983): A behavioral analysis of the reinforcing properties of alcohol and other drugs in man. In: *The Pathogenesis of Alcoholism, Biological Factors,* vol. 7, Kissin B, BegleiterH, eds. New York: Plenum Press, pp 133-198

Mello NK, Mendelson JH (1978): Alcohol and human behavior. In: *Handbook of Psychopharmacology, Section III, Chemistry, Pharmacology, and Human Use.* Iversen LL, Iversen SD, Snyder SH eds. New York: Plenum Press, pp 235-317

Mendelson JH, McGuire M, Mello NK (1984): A new device for administering placebo alcohol. *Alcohol* 1:417-419

Morrell LK (1966): Some characteristics of stimulus-provoked alpha activity. *Electroenceph Clin Neurophysiol* 21:552-561

Myrsten A-L, Hollstedt C, Holmberg N (1975): Alcohol-induced changes in mood and activation in males and females. *Scan J Psychol* 16:303-310

Niedermeyer E (1987): *Electroencephalography* 2nd ed., New York: Urban and Schwarzenberg

Newman HW (1959): The effect of alcohol on the electroencephalogram. *Stanford Med Bull* (South Stacks) 17:55-60

O'Connor S, Hesselbrock V, Tasman A, DePalma N (1987): P3 amplitudes in two distinct tasks are decreased in young men with a history of paternal alcoholism. *Alcohol* 4:323-330

Oken BS, Chiappa KH (1986): Statistical issues concerning computerized analysis of brainwave topography. *Ann Neurol* 19:493-494

O'Malley SS, Maisto SA (1985): Effects of family drinking history and expectancies on responses to alcohol in men. *J Stud Alcohol* 46:289-297

Otto E (1967): The effect of instructions influencing the level of alertness on the EEG activity. In: *Mechanisms of Orienting Reaction in Man.* Nedecky I, ed. Bratislave: Slovak Academy of Science Publishing House, pp 351-365

Pfurtscheller G (1981): Central beta rhythm during sensorimotor activities in man. *Electroenceph Clin Neurophysiol* 51:253-264

Pfurtscheller G (1986): Event-related desynchronization mapping. In: *Topo-*

graphic Mapping of Brain Electrical Activity, Duffy FH ed. Boston: Butterworths, pp 99-111

Pihkanen TA (1957): Neurological and physiological studies on distilled and brewed beverages. *Ann Med Exp Biol Fenn* 35 (Suppl 9):1-152

Polich J, Bloom FE (1986): P300 and alcohol consumption in normals and individuals at risk for alcoholism. *Prog Neuro-Psychopharmacol Biol Psychiat* 10:201-210

Polich J, Bloom FE (1987): P300 from normals and adult children of alcoholics. *Alcohol* 4:301-305

Pollock VE, Teasdale TW, Gabrielli WF, Knop J (1986): Subjective and objective measures of response to alcohol among young men at risk for alcoholism. *J Stud Alcohol* 47:297-304

Pollock VE, Volavka J, Goodwin DW, Mednick SA, Gabrielli WF, Knop J, Schulsinger F (1983): The EEG after alcohol administration in men at risk for alcoholism. *Arch Gen Psychiatry* 40:857-861

Propping P, Kruger J, Janah A (1980): Effect of alcohol on genetically determined variants of the normal electroencephalogram. *Psychiat Res* 2:85-98

Reed TE (1978): Racial comparisons of alcohol metabolism: background, problems, and results. *Alcoholism* 2:83-87

Schuckit MA (1984): Subjective responses to alcohol in sons of alcoholics and control subjects. *Arch Gen Psychiat* 41:879-884

Schuckit MA (1985): Ethanol-induced changes in body sway in men at high alcoholism risk. *Arch Gen Psychiat* 42:375-379

Schuckit MA, Engstrom D, Alpert R, Duby J (1981): Differences in muscle-tension response to ethanol in young men with and without family histories of alcoholism. *J Stud Alcohol* 42:918-924

Varga B, Nagy T (1960): Analysis of alpha-rhythms in the electroencephalogram of alcoholics. *Electroenceph Clin Neurophysiol* 12:933

Vogel W (1970): The genetic basis of the normal human electroencephalogram. *Humangenetik* 10:91-114

Vogel W, Schalt E, Kruger J, Propping P, Lehnert KF (1979): The electroencephalogram (EEG) as a research tool in human behavior genetics: psychological examinations in healthy males with various inherited EEG variants. *Hum Genet* 47:1-45

Wallace RK (1970): Physiological effects of transcendental meditation. *Science* 167:1751-1754

Walter DL (1963): Spectral analysis for electroencephalogram: mathematical determination of neurophysiological relationships from records of limited duration. *Exp Neurol* 8:155-181

Warren GH, Raynes AE (1972): Mood changes during three conditions of alcohol intake. *Q J Stud Alcohol* 33:979-989

Neuroendocrine Concomitants of Alcohol Reinforcement

Jack H. Mendelson, Nancy K. Mello, Scott E. Lukas,
Siew K. Teoh, William R. Phipps, James Ellingboe,
Isaac Schiff, and Susan Palmieri

INTRODUCTION

The specific neural mechanisms underlying alcohol-induced changes in mood and feeling states are unknown. Although experimental animal studies have shown that many biologic processes in the brain are affected by ethanol, it appears unlikely that any single neurochemical or neurophysiologic system uniquely determines its reinforcing properties. At present, we postulate that multiple physiological, psychological and sociocultural factors enhance or reduce the probability for initiation and perpetuation of alcohol abuse by humans.

In this chapter we discuss the role of neuroendocrine systems for mediating the reinforcing properties of alcohol in men and women. Our primary database for review of this topic has been derived from observations of alcohol effects on the hypothalamic-pituitary-gonadal and the hypothalamic-pituitary-adrenal axis in men and women studied on a clinical research facility (for reviews, see Mello, 1988 and Mello et al., 1989). Our studies with humans were stimulated in part by research findings of ethanol-induced changes in neuroendocrine function in experimental animals. The interested reader may wish to consult several comprehensive reviews in this area (Cicero, 1980, 1981; Van Thiel et al., 1982, 1988) for details of important data that cannot be described thoroughly in the following overview which focuses on human studies.

ACUTE EFFECTS OF ETHANOL ON THE
HYPOTHALAMIC-PITUITARY-ADRENAL AXIS IN MEN:
SIGNIFICANCE FOR ETHANOL REINFORCEMENT

The effects of ethanol on mood may be paradoxical, as relaxation and pleasurable effects of moderate intoxication may rapidly change to dysphoria and anxiety as drinking progresses. In the chronic ethanol abuser, anxiety and depression are often the sequelae of high-dose intoxication (Mello, 1972; Mendelson, 1964; Nathan et al., 1970). Although it has been postulated that the way in which ethanol perturbates neural function to alter mood during the ascending phase of the blood ethanol curve may differ from ethanol's effects during the peak and descending phases of the blood ethanol curve (Goldberg, 1943; Jones, 1973; Mendelson, 1970), it has been difficult to analyze this sequence of events and to establish concordance between physiological processes and mood changes.

We have assessed the covariance of neurophysiological, neuroendocrine and behavioral events in human subjects during the first 2 hours after ingesting ethanol or ethanol placebo administered under controlled double-blind conditions (Lukas and Mendelson, 1988). Analysis of plasma adrenocorticotropic hormone (ACTH) and cortisol levels at 5-minute intervals and electroencephalogram (EEG) power spectral analysis in multiple 2-minute epochs permitted examination of the biobehavioral correlates of intoxication. Data obtained establish that ethanol induces rapid changes in brain electrical activity and ACTH secretion from the pituitary that are correlated with subjective perceptions of positive changes in mood (Lukas and Mendelson, 1988).

Methods

Twelve adult male volunteers, ages 21 to 35 years (57-98 kg), provided informed consent for participation in this study. Subjects were recruited via newspaper advertisements and were given a complete medical evaluation, including an electrocardiogram, blood chemistry studies and urinalysis. Subjects with ethanol or drug abuse-related problems were not permitted to participate in the study. All subjects described themselves as social drinkers who, on the average, consumed ethanol 1 to 3 times/week.

Electrophysiological Recording and Blood Withdrawal Procedures

Subjects were studied while they were seated in a recliner chair, in a sound- and light-attenuated, electrically shielded chamber, with their eyes

closed (Fig. 1). Scalp EEG electrodes were applied using the International
10-20 System (Jasper, 1958) over sites C3, C4, P3, and P4. Electrodes
were referenced to linked earlobes. A Kowarski-Cormed butterfly nee-
dle/catheter was inserted into an antecubital vein of the right arm and
threaded through the chamber wall. The end was attached to a syringe,
mounted on a syringe pump and adjusted to exfuse blood continuously at
a rate of 1.0 ml/minute. Blood samples were collected at 5-minute intervals to obtain integrative plasma levels of ACTH, cortisol and ethanol.

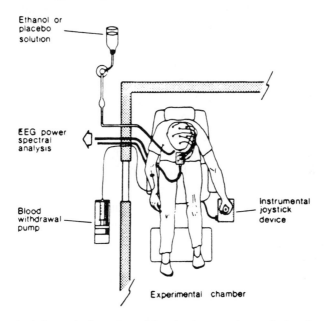

Figure 1.   Artist's rendering of a subject in the experimental chamber, demonstrating the multiple components of the study.   Movement of the instrumental
joystick device is recorded on the polygraph, along with electroencephalographic
activity. Reprinted with permission from Lukas SE, Mendelson JH (1988): Electroencephalographic activity and plasma ACTH during ethanol-induced euphoria.
Biol Psychiatry 23:141-148.

Subjective Reports of Intoxication

As verbal or written reports of perceived mood state changes may compromise the accuracy of EEG measures (Matousek and Petersen, 1983;
Otto, 1967), a custom-made instrumental joystick device was used to obtain mood status reports. Movement of the handle or depression of the
button resulted in a deflection of an event pen located on the polygraph.

Thus, behavioral responses were monitored continuously with EEG activity. Details of the device are presented in Lukas et al. (1986a,b). These behavioral measures of mood status do not confound recording of electroencephalographic activity or influence pituitary secretion of ACTH. Subjects were instructed to use their left hand to move the instrumental joystick device as follows: forward when they detected an ethanol effect, left when the effects became intense, and backward when the effects disappeared. In addition, they were instructed to press a small button located on the top of the joystick during periods when they perceived feelings of intense pleasure or euphoria.

Experimental Procedure

After 30 minutes of baseline recordings, subjects drank either a placebo or ethanol (0.695 g/kg) solution at a constant rate over a 15-minute interval. A total of 350 ml was delivered via a drinking tube/peristaltic motor device, which permitted the subjects to drink without opening their eyes or moving their hands. The placebo solution contained only grapefruit juice, whereas the ethanol solution was made with 40% beverage ethanol (vodka). For both doses, a 10-ml reservoir located between the pump and the mouthpiece was filled with 3 ml of vodka to provide a strong initial taste to mask the two treatments. This practice is an effective placebo that does not produce measurable plasma ethanol levels (Mendelson et al., 1984). EEG activity and behavioral responses were monitored continuously for the next 2 hours. Multiple 2-minute epochs were digitized at a rate of 256/second, followed by a fast Fourier Transformation using a Pathfinder II signal processor (Nicolet Biomedical Instrumentation Co., Madison, WI). EEG power in the 0.25 to 4, 4 to 8, 8 to13 and 13 to 30 Hz bands was determined and block averaged over 2-minute intervals. Consecutive 5-minute integrated plasma samples were removed without disturbing the subject for the duration of the study.

Results

After placebo administration, subjects did not report episodes of euphoria, and there were no significant changes in plasma ACTH, cortisol levels or EEG alpha power. In contrast, after ethanol administration, subjects reported several paroxysmal episodes of euphoria that began within 10 minutes after drinking and continued for an additional 40 minutes. Plasma ethanol levels were 32.85 ± 5.35 gm/dl within 10 minutes after drinking began and peaked at 81.79 ± 5.35 mg/dl at 115 minutes after drinking.

Plasma ACTH levels increased an average 20 pg/ml within 10 to 20 minutes after drinking began and subsequently declined. Plasma cortisol levels gradually increased and peaked at 30 minutes when blood ethanol levels averaged 44.98±6.14 mg/dl.

Fig. 2 shows regression lines for the linear portion of the time-effect curves for plasma ACTH, cortisol and ethanol levels, EEG alpha power and the incidence of reported euphoria after placebo (top) and ethanol (bottom) administration. Tests for parallelism (Tallarida and Murray, 1981) revealed that EEG alpha power, subjective reports of euphoria,

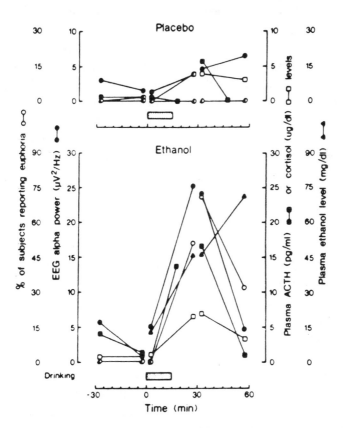

Figure 2. Regression analysis of changes in plasma ACTH, cortisol, and ethanol levels, EEG alpha power, and incidence of reported euphoria after placebo (top) and ethanol (bottom) administration. Data are derived from 6 subjects per group. Reprinted with permission from Lukas SE, Mendelson JH (1988): Electro-encephalographic activity and plasma ACTH during ethanol-induced euphoria. *Biol Psychiatry* 23:141-148.

plasma ACTH levels and plasma ethanol levels were parallel, and all increased linearly during the first 30 minutes after ethanol consumption ($p < 0.05$). Increases in plasma cortisol were not statistically significant. All physiological and behavioral measures decreased linearly within 35 to 60 minutes after drinking, even though plasma ethanol levels continued to increase.

DISCUSSION

In the present study, subjective reports of self-perceived euphoria occurred between 10 and 15 minutes after drinking ethanol and were accompanied by a significant increase in EEG alpha power and increased plasma levels of ACTH. These data indicate that major physiological and behavioral concomitants of ethanol intoxication occur at relatively low blood ethanol levels (approximately 32 mg/dl) during the ascending phase of the blood ethanol curve. Previous studies have noted that ethanol intake is associated with activation of the hypothalamic-pituitary-adrenal axis (Mendelson and Stein, 1966; Noth and Walter, 1984), but we have been unable to locate any report that describes the initiation of such activation after such a short time course and low blood ethanol levels after ethanol intake

Enhanced secretion of ACTH at low blood ethanol levels could be the result of ethanol-induced stimulation of corticotropin-releasing factor (CRF). Although subsequent activation of the adrenal cortex after ethanol-related ACTH release could mediate changes in central nervous system function and behavior, ACTH and probably CRF itself may also directly affect neuronal function in regional portions of the central nervous system (Ehlers, 1986). It is also possible that low doses of ethanol may directly stimulate release of ACTH from pituitary corticotrophs (Redei et al., 1986).

The acute effects of ethanol on human EEG activity consists of increased voltage and decreased alpha frequency (Docter et al., 1966; Engel and Rosenbaum, 1945; Holmberg and Martens, 1955; Varga and Nagy, 1960). However, most of these studies have examined EEG effects that appear during the "peak" behavioral responses, which typically occur 30 to 75 minutes after drinking. Data obtained in this study and our previous study (Lukas et al., 1986c) focused on very early components of the ethanol response and found that neurophysiological and neuroendocrine measures covaried with ethanol-induced intoxication in normal persons. Abrupt increases in EEG alpha power have been associated with specific subjective mood states generally reported as pleasurable, floating and extremely relaxed (Brown, 1970; Lindsley, 1952; Matejcek, 1982; Wallace, 1970). These data suggest that the reinforcing properties of ethanol intoxication reflect these rapid changes in EEG activity and ACTH secretion. A previous study reported that acute oral administration of 40 mg of ACTH 4-9 analog to human subjects reduced alpha activity (Bonn et al., 1984, 1985). However, this study was conducted to assess selective attention to a dichotic listening task, which may have induced an alpha-suppressing alerting response.

These positive early effects of ethanol are probably transient and dose-dependent, as high ethanol doses and chronic ethanol abuse are followed by increased anxiety, dysphoria and depression (Alterman et al., 1975; McGuire et al., 1966; Mello and Mendelson, 1978). Yet, it is tempting to speculate that the early positive effects of ethanol may be especially salient for ethanol abusers. Ethanol abusers also have low amounts of spontaneous EEG alpha activity (Davis et al., 1941; Little and McAvoy, 1952) and many abnormal endocrine and physiological responses (e.g., impaired adrenocortical responses, regulation of arterial blood pressure) that are reversed or "normalized" after consumption of small amounts of ethanol (Kissin et al., 1959, 1960).

The paroxysmal short epochs of euphoria associated with concomitant neurophysiological and neuroendocrine responses during the ascending phase of the blood ethanol curve may serve as powerful reinforcers for perpetuation of drinking. The rising phase of the blood ethanol curve may produce effects that are comparable to the heroin "rush" and cocaine "high"-intense sensations of intoxication that persist for seconds or minutes and then rapidly disappear.

Recent studies have shown that adrenocortical steroids may enhance or depress neuronal activity (Majewska et al., 1986) and that these changes may covary with positive and negative fluctuations in mood (Gold et al., 1986). Based on these observations, it has been postulated that adrenocortical activation of short-term duration that induces an acute glucocorticoid response may facilitate occurrence of positive mood states, whereas long-term adrenocortical activation and associated high levels of glucocorticoids may cause dysphoria (Barnes, 1986). Data obtained in this study are consistent with the notion that ethanol-induced ACTH secretion during the ascending phase of the blood ethanol curve covaries with subjective reports of euphoria and alterations of electrical activity in the central nervous system. Although chronic ethanol abuse, which is associated with chronic adrenocortical activation, may increase risk for dysphoria, acute low-dose ethanol intake clearly induces euphoria. Thus, the biphasic dose-related effects of ethanol on mood may be mediated in part by the effects of ethanol on the hypothalamic-pituitary-adrenal axis.

ACUTE ETHANOL EFFECTS ON THE HYPOTHALAMIC-PITUITARY-GONADAL AXIS DURING BASAL VERSUS PERTURBATED CONDITIONS: SIGNIFICANCE FOR ETHANOL REINFORCEMENT

Acute alcohol administration to normal males studied under basal conditions was associated with a fall in plasma testosterone (T) levels followed by an increase in levels of luteinizing hormone (LH) (Mendelson et al., 1977) (Fig. 3). In contrast, acute administration of alcohol to men after stimulation of LH with gonadotropin releasing hormone (GnRH) resulted in a significant increase in plasma testosterone levels (Phipps et al., 1987) (Fig. 4). No changes in plasma estradiol (E_2) levels were observed when ethanol was acutely administered to women under basal conditions (Mendelson et al., 1981) (Fig. 5). However, acute alcohol administration to women after gonadotropin stimulation with naltrexone or naloxone resulted in significantly higher plasma E_2 levels (Mendelson et al., 1987; Teoh et al., 1988) (Fig. 6). Administration of ethanol to women during the menstrual cycle phase when plasma gonadotropin levels were increasing also enhanced plasma estradiol levels (Mendelson et al., 1988) (Fig. 7). Therefore, both men and women have an increase in plasma gonadal steroid levels after gonadotropin stimulation and concurrent alcohol intake.

The rapid increase in plasma E_2 in women and plasma testosterone in men following concurrent gonadotropin stimulation and alcohol administration could be the consequence of increased steroid production or decreased steroid metabolism. Metabolism of ethanol in the liver which decreases the NAD: NADH ratio (Forsander et al., 1958) may also reduce the rate of oxidation of estradiol to estrone in women, and androstenedione to testosterone in men, a shift in equilibrium that has been demonstrated for other 17- hydroxy/17-ketosteroid pairs in plasma and gonadal tissue (Cronholm and Sjovall, 1968; Cronholm et al., 1969; Murono and Fisher-Simpson, 1984, 1985).

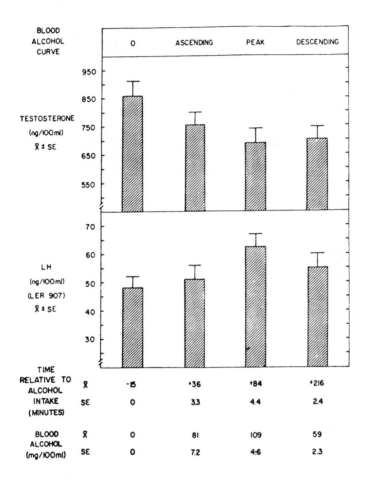

Figure 3. Plasma testosterone (T) and luteinizing (LH) hormone levels during the ascending, peak and descending phases of the blood alcohol curve for 16 normal adult males. Computation of plasma T and LH levels was carried out by obtaining the mean level for all values determined on the ascending, peak and descending phases of the blood alcohol curve. Reprinted with permission from American Society for Pharmacology and Experimental Therapeutics by Mendelson JH et al., (1977): Effects of acute alcohol intake on pituitary-gonadal hormones in normal human males. *J Pharmacol Exp Ther* 202:676-682.

242   Mendelson et al.

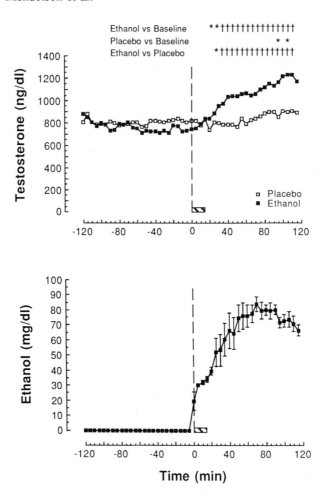

Figure 4. Mean plasma T levels in 6 subjects before and after administration of GnRH (500 μg iv at t = 0) and ethanol (0.695 g/kg po over 15-min period starting at t = 0, as indicated by black bar) or placebo (GnRH/ethanol ■; GnRH/placebo □), and mean plasma ethanol levels (±SEM) on days of ethanol administration. By ANOVA, statistically significant differences in T levels at the p<0.001 level were present for GnRH/ethanol vs. baseline, GnRH/placebo vs. baseline, and GnRH/ethanol vs. GnRH/placebo. By Dunnett's followup test, differences were p <0.01 for time points marked + and p<0.05 for time points marked X. This analysis is presented in the Fig. in lieu of standard error bars to enhance clarity. Reprinted with permission from Phipps et al., (1987): Acute ethanol administration enhances plasma testosterone levels following gonadotropin stimulation in men. *Psychoneuroendocrinology* 12:459-465.

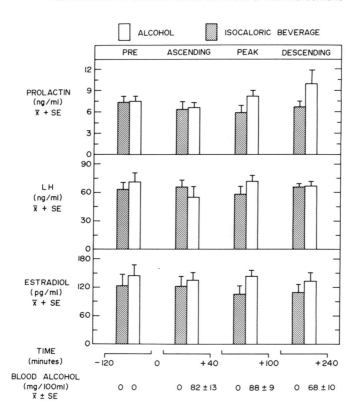

Figure 5.   Plasma prolactin, LH and estradiol levels during the ascending, peak and descending phases of the blood alcohol curve and after administration of isocaloric beverage for 6 normal females. Computation of plasma prolactin, LH and estradiol levels was carried out by obtaining the mean levels for all values determined on the ascending, peak and descending phases of the blood alcohol curve. Reprinted with permission from the American Society for Pharmacology and Experimental Therapeutics by Mendelson JH et al. (1981): Acute alcohol intake and pituitary gonadal hormones in normal human females. *J Pharmacol Exp Ther* 218:23-26.

Fig. 8 depicts ethanol dose-time effects on plasma testosterone and estradiol after gonadotropin (LH) stimulation. Gonadal steroid levels increase after gonadotropin stimulation under both ethanol and placebo conditions, but the increase is greater, occurs earlier and is sustained longer after alcohol intake. We postulate that this process may have either primary or secondary reinforcing properties, particularly if an increase in gonadal

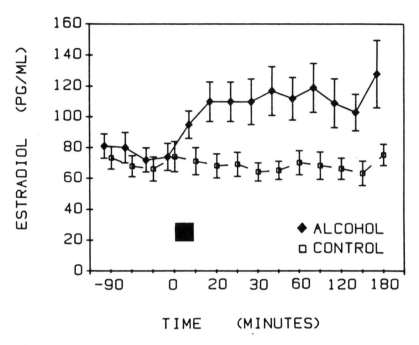

Figure 6. Effects of alcohol and placebo-control administration on plasma estradiol levels. Alcohol or placebo was administered concurrently with naloxone (5 mg) at 0 time. Reprinted with permission from Alcohol Research Documentation, Inc., Rutgers Center of Alcohol Studies, New Brunswick, NJ, by Mendelson JH et al. (1987): Alcohol effects on naloxone-stimulated luteinizing hormone, prolactin and estradiol in women. *J Stud Alcohol* 48:287-294.

steroids facilitates expression of either sexual or aggressive behavior in situations where the imbiber would consider such behaviors appropriate. We also postulate that cumulative dose time effects of this process would result in decrements in plasma gonadal steroids below basal levels as a consequence of chronic alcohol effects and evolution of ethanol tolerance. Significant decrements in plasma gonadal steroid levels in men and women might result in impotence and infertility respectively. Such adverse consequences of chronic alcohol abuse on reproductive function have been observed frequently in men and women who have become dependent on alcohol. Thus, alcohol-related changes in mood and behavior, which may be modulated by increased levels of gonadal steroids, would initially enhance for some the reinforcing properties of alcohol. But as a consequence of chronic alcohol abuse, such reinforcement would not only diminish but will ultimately fail to occur. It is also possible that some persons may perpetuate and increase alcohol consumption in order to recapitulate the initial reinforcing properties of acute ethanol-induced changes in plasma levels of gonadal steroids.

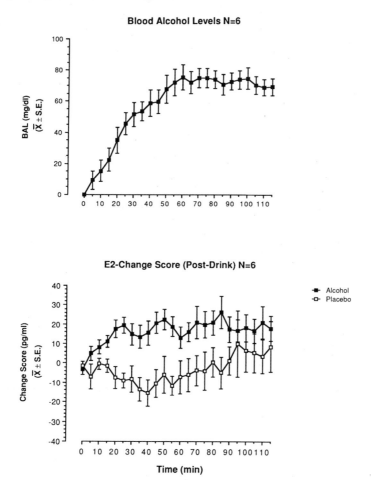

Figure 7.   Blood alcohol levels and E_2 change scores for 6 subjects administered ethanol (0.695 g/kg) and 6 subjects administered ethanol placebo. ■ Alcohol; □ Placebo. Reprinted with permission of Springer-Verlag, New York, from JH Mendelson et al., (1988): Acute alcohol effects on plasma estradiol levels in women. *Psychopharmacology* 94:464-467.

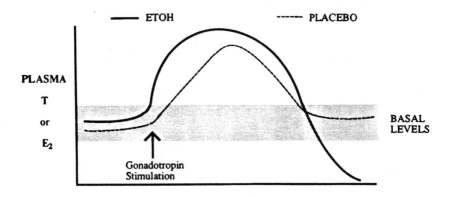

DOSE-TIME EFFECT

Fig. 8. A schematic depiction of dose time effects of ethanol and placebo on plasma levels of testosterone or E_2 after gonadotropin stimulation.

ACKNOWLEDGMENTS

These studies were supported in part by grants: DA 4RG 010, DA 00064, DA 00101 from the National Institute on Drug Abuse; AA 06252, AA 04368 from the National Institute on Alcohol Abuse and Alcoholism; and grants from Joseph E. Seagrams and Sons and Heublein, Inc.

We thank the following journals for permission to reprint portions of previously published papers in this chapter: Journal of Pharmacology and Experimental Therapeutics, Psychoneuroendocrinology, Journal of Studies on Alcohol, Psychopharmacology, and Biological Psychiatry.

REFERENCES

Alterman AL, Gottheil C, Crawford DH (1975): Mood changes in an alcoholism treatment program based on drinking decisions. *Am J Psychiatry* 132:1032-1037

Barnes DM (1986): Steroids may influence changes in mood. *Science* 232:1344-1345

Bonn J, Fehm-Wolfsdorf G, Schiebe M, Birbaumer N, Fehm HL, Voight KH (1985): An ACTH 4-9 analog impairs selective attention in man. *Life Sci*

36:2117-2125

Bonn J, Fehm-Wolfsdorf G, Schiebe M, Rockstroh B, Fehm HL, Voight KH (1984): Dishabituating effects of an ACTH 4-9 analog in a vigilance task. *Pharmacol Biochem Behav* 21:513-519

Brown BB (1970): Recognition of aspects of consciousness through association with EEG alpha activity represented by a light signal. *Psychophysiol* 6:442-452

Cicero TJ (1980): Common mechanisms underlying the effects of ethanol and narcotics on neuroendocrine function. In: *Advances in Substance Abuse, Behavioral and Biological Research, vol. 1.* NK Mello, ed. Greenwich, Conn: JAI Press, Inc, pp 201-254

Cicero TJ (1981): Neuroendocrinological effects of alcohol. *Ann Rev Med* 32:123-142

Cronholm T, Sjovall J (1968): Effect of ethanol on the concentrations of solvolyzable plasma steroids. *Biochem Biophys Acta* 152:233-236

Cronholm T, Sjovall J, Sjovall K (1969): Ethanol induced increase of the ratio between hydroxy-and ketosteroids in human pregnancy plasma. *Steroids* 13:671-678

Davis PA, Gibbs FA, Davis H, Jetter WW, Trowbridge LS (1941): Effects of alcohol upon electroencephalogram. *Q J Stud Alcohol* 1:626-637

Docter RF, Naitoh P, Smith JC (1966): Electroencephalographic changes and vigilance behavior during experimentally induced intoxication with alcoholic subjects. *Psychosom Med* 28:605-615

Ehlers CL (1986): EEG stability following corticotropin releasing factor in rats. *Psychoneuroendocrinology* 11:121-125

Engel GL, Rosenbaum M (1945): Delirium: electroencephalographic changes associated with acute alcoholic intoxication. *Arch Neurol Psychiatry* 53:44-50

Forsander O, Raiha N, Sumalainen H (1958): Alkohol oxydation und bildung von acetoacetat in normaler und glykogenarmer intakter rattenleber. Hoppe Seyler. *Z Physiol Chem* 312:243-248

Gold PW, Loriaux DL, Roy A, Kling MA, Calabrese JR, Kellner CH, Nieman LK, Post RM, Pickar D, Gallucci W, Augerinos P, Paul S, Oldfield EH, Cutler GB, Chrousos GP (1986): Responses to corticotropin-releasing hormone in the hypercortisolism of depression and Cushing's disease: pathophysiologic and diagnostic implications. *N Eng J Med* 314:1329-1335

Goldberg L (1943): Quantitative studies on alcohol tolerance in man. *Acta Physiol Scand* 5(Suppl. 16):1-128

Holmberg G, Martens S (1955): Electroencephalographic changes in man correlated with blood alcohol concentration and some other conditions following standardized ingestion of alcohol. *Q J Stud Alcohol* 16:411-424

Jasper HH (1958): The 10-20 electrode system of the International Federation. *Electroenceph Clin Neurophysiol* 10:371-375

Jones BM (1973): Memory impairment on the ascending and descending limbs of the blood alcohol curve. *J Abnorm Psychol* 82:24-32

Kissin B, Schenker V, Schenker A (1959): The acute effects of ethyl alcohol and chlorpromazine on certain physiological functions in alcoholics. *Q J Stud Alcohol* 20:480-492

Kissin B, Schenker V, Schenker AC (1960): The acute effect of ethanol ingestion on plasma and urinary 17-hydroxycorticoids in alcoholic subjects. *Am J Med Sci* 239:690-705

Lindsley D (1952): Psychological phenomena and the electroencephalogram. *Electroenceph Clin Neurophysiol* 4:443-456

Little SC, McAvoy M (1952): Electroencephalographic studies in alcoholism. *Q J Stud Alcohol* 13:9-15

Lukas SE, Mendelson JH (1988): Electroencephalographic activity and plasma ACTH during ethanol-induced euphoria. *Biol Psychiatry* 23:141-148

Lukas SE, Mendelson JH, Benedikt RA (1986a): Instrumental analysis of ethanol-induced intoxication in human males. *Psychopharmacol* 89:8-13

Lukas SE, Mendelson JH, Benedikt RA, Jones B (1986b): EEG alpha activity increases during transient episodes of ethanol-induced euphoria. *Pharmacol Biochem Behav* 25:889-895, 1986b.

Lukas SE, Mendelson JH, Benedikt RA, Jones B (1986c): EEG, physiologic and behavioral effects of ethanol administration. In: *Problems of Drug Dependence*, Harris LS, ed. 1985, NIDA Research Monograph No. 67. Washington, D.C.: U.S. Government Printing Office, pp 209-214

Majewska MD, Harrison NL, Schwartz RD, Barker JL, Paul SM (1986): Steroid hormone metabolites are barbiturate-like modulators of the GABA receptor. *Science* 232:1004-1007

Matejcek M (1982): Vigilance and the EEG: Psychological, physiological and pharmacological aspects. In: *EEG in Drug Research*. WM Hermann, ed. Stuttgart: Gustav Fischer, pp 405-508

Matousek M, Petersen I (1983): A method of assessing alertness fluctuations from EEG spectra. *Electroenceph Clin Neurophysiol* 55:108-113

McGuire MT, Mendelson JH, Stein S (1966): Comparative psychosocial studies of alcoholic and non-alcoholic subjects undergoing experimentally induced ethanol intoxication. *Psychosom Med* 28:13-26

Mello NK (1972): Behavioral studies of alcoholism. In: *The Biology of Alcoholism, vol. II, Physiology and Behavior*. Kissin B, Begleiter H, eds. New York: Plenum Press, pp 219-291

Mello NK (1988): Effects of alcohol abuse on reproductive function in women. In: *Recent Developments in Alcoholism, vol. 6*. Galanter M, ed. New York: Plenum Publishing Corp, pp 253-276

Mello NK, Mendelson JH (1978): Alcohol and human behavior. In: *Handbook of Psychopharmacology, Section III, Chemistry, Pharmacology and Human Use*, Iversen LL, Iversen SD, and Snyder, SH, eds. New York: Plenum Press, pp 235-317

Mello NK, Mendelson JH, Teoh S (1989): Neuroendocrine consequences of alcohol abuse in women. In: *Prenatal Abuse of Licit and Illicit Drugs*. Hutchings DE, ed. New York: Ann NY Acad Sci 562:211-240

Mendelson JH (1964): Experimentally induced chronic intoxication and withdrawal in alcoholics. *Q J Stud Alcohol*, Suppl. 2

Mendelson JH (1970): Biological concomitants of alcoholism. *N Engl J Med* 283:24-32

Mendelson JH, Lukas SE, Mello NK, Amass L, Ellingboe J, Skupny A (1988): Acute alcohol effects on plasma estradiol levels in women. *Psychopharmacol* 94:464-467

Mendelson JH, McGuire M, Mello NK (1984): A new device for administering placebo alcohol. *Alcohol* 1:417-419

Mendelson JH, Mello NK, Cristofaro P, Ellingboe J, Skupny A, Palmieri SL, Benedikt R, Schiff I (1987): Alcohol effects on naloxone-stimulated luteinizing hormone, prolactin and estradiol in women. *J Stud Alcohol* 48:287-294

Mendelson JH, Mello NK, Ellingboe J (1977): Effects of acute alcohol intake on pituitary gonadal hormones in normal males. *J Pharmacol Exp Ther* 202:676-682

Mendelson JH, Mello NK, Ellingboe J (1981): Acute alcohol intake and pituitary gonadal hormones in normal human females. *J Pharmacol Exp Ther* 218:23-26

Mendelson JH, Stein S (1966): Serum cortisol levels in alcoholic and nonalcoholic subjects during experimentally induced ethanol intoxication. *Psychosom Med* 28:616-626

Murono EP, Fisher-Simpson V (1984): Ethanol directly increases dihydrotestosterone conversion to 5α-androstan-3β, 17β-diol and 5α-androstan-3α, 17β-diol in rat leydig cells. *Biochem Biophys Res Commun* 121:558-565

Murono EP, Fisher-Simpson V (1985): Ethanol directly stimulates dihydrotestosterone conversion to 5α-androstan-3α, 17β-diol and 5α-androstan-3β, 17β-diol in rat liver. *Life Sci* 36:1117-1124

Nathan PE, Titler NA, Lowenstein LM, Solomon P, Rossi AM (1970): Behavioral analysis of chronic alcoholism. Interaction of alcohol and human contact. *Arch Gen Psychiatry* 22:419-430

Noth RH, Walter Jr RM (1984): The effects of alcohol on the endocrine system. *Med Clin North Am* 68:133-146

Otto E (1967): The effect of instructions influencing the level of alertness of the EEG activity. In: *Mechanisms of Orienting Reaction in Man*. Nedecky I, ed. Bratislava: Slovak Academy of Sciences Publishing House, pp 351-365

Phipps WR, Lukas SE, Mendelson JH, Ellingboe J, Palmieri SL, Schiff I (1987): Acute ethanol administration enhances plasma testosterone levels following gonadotropin stimulation in men. *Psychoneuroendocrinol* 12:459-465

Redei E, Branch B, Taylor AN (1986): Abstracts of the First International Congress of Neuroendocrinology 293:98

Teoh SK, Mendelson JH, Mello NK, Skupny A (1988): Alcohol effects on naltrexone-induced stimulation of pituitary, adrenal and gonadal hormones during the early follicular phase of the menstrual cycle. *J Clin Endocrinol Metab* 66:1181-1186

Tallarida RJ, Murray RB (1981): *Manual of Pharmacologic Calculations*. New York: Springer-Verlag

Van Thiel DH, Gavaler JS, Cobb CF, Chiao Y-B (1982): Effects of ethanol upon the hypothalamic pituitary gonadal axis. In: *The Endocrines and the Liver*. Langer M, Chiandussi L, Chopra IJ, and Martini L, eds. New York: Academic Press, pp117-134

Van Thiel DH, Tarter RE, Rosenblum E, Gavaler JS (1988): Ethanol, its metabolism and gonadal effects: does sex make a difference? In: *Advances in Alcohol and Substance Abuse: Alcohol Research from Bench to Bedside*. Stimmel B, ed. New York: Haworth Press pp 131-169

Varga B, Nagy T (1960): Analysis of alpha-rhythms in the electroencephalogram of alcoholics. *Electroenceph Clin Neurophysiol* 12:933

Wallace RK (1970): Physiological effects of transcendental meditation. *Science* 167:1751-1754

Alcohol Reinforcement:
Biobehavioral and Clinical Considerations

Roger E. Meyer and Zelig Dolinsky

When compared with stimulants, opioids, and barbiturates (Schuster and Thompson, 1969; Schuster and Villareal, 1968; Winger et al., 1983; Yanagita et al., 1969) in intravenous self-administration paradigms in monkeys and rats, ethanol is a relatively weak reinforcer. The delay in reinforcement associated with oral self-administration of ethanol further inhibits its reinforcing efficacy. A relatively prolonged period of exposure to frequent high doses of ethanol is necessary for the development of alcohol dependence in humans. In contrast, in vulnerable individuals, intravenous opiate self-administration, and intravenously self-administered or smoked cocaine are associated with the rapid development of dependence. The risk of developing alcohol dependence is strongly influenced by factors in the individual (e.g., genetics, temperament, psychopathology) and the environment (e.g., culture).

Over the past 25 years a number of animal models of alcohol consumption have been developed that were designed to model human alcoholism. There is general consensus that no animal model *fully* satifies all of the criteria for an animal model of alcoholism. However, it is also clear that not all of these criteria need to be met for an animal model to be useful (Cicero, 1979). These models can provide a framework to clarify the biological and behavioral determinants of alcohol consumption. Two important observations can be noted from animal ethanol self-administration literature: (1) ethanol consumption can be significantly affected by schedules of reinforcement and/or association with other reinforcers, and (2) ethanol consumption is significantly affected by pharmacogenetic factors (Symposium, 1988). The initiation and maintenance of oral ethanol self-administration is a key goal for alcoholism that must be met by an animal model. In addition, it is important to demonstrate that oral ingestion is reinforcing on the basis of the pharmocological effects of ethanol, and not as a function of its nutrient value.

Behavioral paradigms for the induction of alcohol consumption include schedule-induced polydipsia (Falk et al., 1972) the limited access paradigm (Gill et al., 1986) and the sucrose or saccharine fading technique (Samson, 1986). Using the technique of schedule-induced polydipsia, rats will regularly consume sufficient quantities of ethanol over a 3-month period to develop physical dependence. Whereas the presence of physical dependence is not sufficient to maintain heavy drinking behavior, schedule-induced ethanol drinking can result in high blood ethanol levels over many months (Falk and Tang, 1988). This technique has been criticized as a model for alcoholism because the schedule-induced polydipsia is not specific to ethanol (it will also yield high levels of water consumption).

The limited access paradigm exposes rats to ethanol for a limited anount of time in a novel environment. Animals consume ethanol over a 20-minute period during their light cycle, resulting in blood alcohol concentrations (BAC) $\geq$ 80 mg/% (Gill et al., 1986). This BAC produces alcohol-related behavioral effects. The limited access paradigm does not yield increased intake of water. However, animals do not develop physical dependence because of limited daily exposure and the relatively modest blood levels of ethanol. The presence of withdrawal symptoms is one of the specific characteristics of the alcohol dependence syndrome (Edwards and Gross, 1976).

The final behavioral paradigm, the sucrose or saccharine fading technique, generally uses operant techniques and pairs sweet taste with ethanol consumption until a stable pattern of high consumption has been attained with a 10% ethanol solution. The sweet taste is gradually withdrawn, but the high levels of ethanol consumption continues. Food deprivation is not required to maintain high levels of ethanol self-administration, suggesting that reinforcement in this paradigm is associated with the pharmacological effects of ethanol (or the conditioned expectation of sweetness). As Samson has described the rationale for this technique, it serves to overcome ethanol taste aversion and it results in pharmacologically significant levels of ethanol consumption (Samson, 1986). Taken together, the three paradigms suggest that the association of ethanol consumption with salient reinforcers[1] (e.g., food, novelty, taste) causes initiation of increased ethanol consumption, which may result in the establishment of stable patterns of ethanol consumption over time. These data seem remarkably symmetrical with Kornetsky's report on the effects of ethanol on brain stimulation reward (BSR). As described elsewhere in this volume, Kornetsky reports that the threshold for electrical brain stimulation is decreased in rats after 2.5 months of ethanol self-administration, but not in yoked control animals receiving ethanol via intragastric administration. These results suggest that self-administration of ethanol is an important factor mediating its reinforcing properties. Gardner (personal communication) also demonstrated a decrease in electrical brain stimulation reward threshold only in animals trained to self-administer ethanol as compared to animals receiving ethanol intragastrically. These results should be contrasted with the work of Lewis in this volume who reported low-dose effects of ethanol on brain stimulation reward. His studies suggest that ethanol is reinforcing in dosages that produce predominantly stimulant effects, whereas it is not reinforcing at high doses. Lewis' data appear to differ from the work of Kornetsky and of Gardner since self-administration was not required to establish reinforcement effects. Nonetheless, the observation of decreased brain reward thresholds with ethanol administration in three laboratories, using different paradigms and routes of ethanol administration, suggests that ethanol interacts with brain pathways known to be involved with reinforcement. These pathways involve the mesolimbic dopamine system, which appears to play the major role in brain stimulation reward.

The effects of ethanol on brain stimulation reward threshold are more variable and less robust than has been observed with stimulants and opiates (Kornetsky, 1985; Wise, 1980). Koob and Bloom (1988) suggest that multiple neurotransmitter systems may be responsible for the reinforcing properties of ethanol. These neurotransmitter systems include opioid peptides, dopamine, serotonin, norepinephrine and gamma-aminobutyric acid (GABA). Since alcoholics report various reasons for drinking (including anxiolysis), and since the development of alcohol dependence significantly enhances the reinforcing potency of ethanol, it is likely that factors including temperament, environment, pharmacogentics, and chronic alcohol administration need to be considered in the developing literature on

---

[1] Hubbel, et al. were able to induce ethanol consumption by pairing it with morphine injections (Hubbell et al., 1986).

the neurobiology of ethanol reinforcement. Efforts to apply brain stimulation reward methodology to animals that differ in ethanol preference on the basis of pharmacogenetic factors represent a logical next step in the work described by Kornetsky and by Lewis in this volume.

Selective breeding of lines of rats that differ in their ethanol drinking behavior has led to the development of alcohol accepting (AA) and alcohol non-accepting (ANA) rats (Eriksson, 1971), preferring (P) and non-preferring (NP) rats (Li et al., 1988) and more recently, high alcohol drinking (HAD) and low alcohol drinking (LAD) lines (Li, this volume). The P rats will drink a 10% ethanol solution in a free-choice situation; they will bar press for an ethanol reward in a traditonal operant paradigm; they will consume sufficient amounts of ethanol to display signs of physical dependence and they will self-administer ethanol intragastrically (Waller et al., 1984). As described in the article by Waller et al. (1984), a variety of lines of evidence now support the general premise that ethanol is reinforcing in these animals, apart from its caloric value. P rats have lower levels of serotonin (5-HT) in several central nervous system (CNS) regions and lower levels of both dopamine (DA) and 5-HT in the nucleus accumbens compared with rats of the NP line (Li et al., 1988). Although the meaning of these differences in relation to ethanol reinforcement is not known, there has been an increasing interest in the role which the serotonin (5-HT) system plays in influencing alcohol intake. A number of investigators have reported that 5-HT reuptake inhibitors decrease alcohol intake in rats and heavy drinking (but non-dependent) humans (Amit et al., 1985; Kranzler and Orrok, 1989; Naranjo et al., 1984; Naranjo et al., 1987). It is possible that P rats, with a relative deficiency of 5-HT, do not experience the aversive effects of ethanol, or quickly develop tolerance to the aversive effects. In sum, the reinforcing effects are greater in the P rats than in the NP rats. Likewise, 5-HT reuptake inhibitors may result in decreased alcohol consumption not because 5-HT mediates craving or reinforcement per se, but because the aversive properties of ethanol become more pronounced in the presence of higher levels of 5-HT. Parenthetically, it is also of interest that alcohol consumption decreases 5-HT levels (Murphy et al., 1988). This could contribute to the development of tolerance to the aversive properties of ethanol over time.

There are contradictory reports regarding the possibility of inducing alcohol preference drinking in NP animals. George (1988) recently reported that he was unable to establish ethanol as a reinforcer in NP animals, whereas Samson has reported that NP rats can be trained to self-administer ethanol using the sucrose fading technique (Samson et al., 1988). Despite Samson's report, it would appear that there are substantial pharmacogenetic differences in the reinforcing potency of ethanol in rodents and presumably other species. At this juncture, genetic studies of biological and behavioral aspects of ethanol reinforcement represent one of the most promising approaches to the biology of alcohol dependence. A variety of methodologies are being applied to this field of inquiry. Drug discrimination paradigms (Signs and Schecter, 1987), pharmacological perturbation of specific neurotransmitters and/or ion channels (Engel et al., 1988; Gill et al., 1986; Koob et al., 1988; Pfeffer and Samson, 1987; Weiss et al., in press), *in vivo* receptor binding (Vavrousek-Jakuba et al., 1989), *in vivo* brain dialysis (DiChiara and Imperato, 1988), single cell electrophysiology (Siggins et al., 1987), as well as brain stimulation reward, are being used in efforts to identify the biological changes involved in alcohol intoxication, tolerance, reinforcement, and dependence at the molecular, cellular, and neuronal network level. At this stage, findings are contradictory (e.g., narcotic antagonists have been reported to decrease (Myers et al., 1986) and to have no effect (Weiss et al., in press) on alcohol consumption). The availability of a number of relevant genetic and behavioral animal models of alcohol consumption, in combination with new technologies (including molecular genetics), should clarify the biological basis of alcohol reinforcement and dependence.

CLINICAL CONSIDERATIONS

The chapters by Mendelson and by Lukas in this volume suggest the feasibility of measuring biological correlates of alcohol reinforcement in human subjects. Their work involves examining the EEG, subjective and neuroendocrine effects associated with low to moderate doses of ethanol. They have reported an association between increased CNS alpha activity, and the euphoric effects of ethanol and increases in adrenocorticotropic hormone (ACTH) within 15 minutes after ethanol ingestion. At this time the results are intriguing but only demonstrate associations between these variables. A critical question concerns whether the associations are causative, and not simply related. In addition, future work should investigate the mechanisms by which alterations in ACTH may influence the perceptions of euphoria. Their work raises an intriguing question. Is ethanol reinforcing in all human beings; and is it always reinforcing via the same biological mechanism? These issues, related to the underlying biological mechanisms for reinforcement, have been discussed above in relation to the basic animal studies where genetic variability can be considered.

In human research, Cloninger and his colleagues (1988) have postulated a heritable vulnerability to alcoholism based on genetically-determined traits of temperament. He has postulated that specific neurochemical mechanisms are associated with these traits (Cloninger, 1987). He has described two subtypes of alcoholism: type II alcoholics are males with a paternal family history of alcoholism, who may be less severely alcohol dependent than other types of familial alcoholics. Temperamentally, they score high on measures of novelty seeking and low on measures of reward dependence and harm avoidance. Cloninger has postulated that these individuals' traits of temperament derive from dopaminergic function (Cloninger, 1987). They appear to seek alcohol's hedonic efects when they drink. In contrast, type I alcoholics may be male or female offspring, where alcoholism may be in the family of the mother or the father. The severity of alcohol dependence is strongly influenced in these individuals by environmental factors, particularly socioeconomic status. Cloninger postulates that alcohol's anxiolytic properties will influence the development of alcohol dependence in these individuals. It would be of interest to apply Cloninger's model to studies in children of alcoholics in the Mendelson and Lucas paradigms. It is of interest that Cloninger's model does not posit vulnerability on the basis of sensitivity or response to ethanol. Rather, vulnerability resides in personality traits that are inherited within cultures where ethanol is generally available. In a parallel with Cloninger's work, early work by Beecher (1959) examined the reinforcing effects of morphine in groups of normal subjects who differed along certain personality dimensions. More "neurotic" individuals found morphine more pleasurable than did less disturbed individuals.

Begleiter et al. (1984) have identified an electrophysiological marker as an indicator of risk in sons of alcoholics. Approximately one out of three sons with alcoholic fathers have decreased P300 amplitude and increased P300 latency. P300 has been associated with orientation to novel and task-relevant stimuli. It might also be of interest to study individuals who show this biological marker (P300 decrement) in the specific paradigms developed by Mendelson and by Lukas. The Lukas and Mendelson paradigms may be useful in the context of assessing the differential euphoric properties of ethanol in FH+ and negative family history (FH−) individuals, as well as in known alcoholics. Those FH+ individuals whose response pattern most clearly resembles the alcoholic individual's might be those subjects at greatest risk. However, additional research is necessary to establish the relevance of reinforcement measures that Lukas and Mendelson are assessing concerning their importance in influencing the development of alcohol dependence. The Lukas and Mendelson paradigms demonstrate euphoric effects of acute low doses of ethanol in nondependent individuals. This is in contrast to the relatively long period of time necessary for the development of dependence. It raises the possibility that different mechanisms are involved in the acute euphoric vs. dependence producing effects of ethanol.

Schuckit (1984; Schuckit et al., 1987a,b) has described relative alcohol insensitivity in sons of alcoholic persons compared with controls across a variety of subjective, psychomotor, and neuroendocrine parameters. Lukas et al. (1988) have demonstrated similar findings in daughters of alcoholic parents. It would be of interest to study the relationship between alcohol insensitivity and its reinforcing potency in sons of alcoholic parents (compared with controls). The animal model literature, although limited, is divided on this issue (Crabbe, 1983; George, 1988; Waller et al., 1983). The critical question regarding the establishment of ethanol as a reinforcer in human beings concerns the evolution of its reinforcing potency with the development of alcohol dependence. Is there a neurobiological basis for craving and loss of control, or are these merely epiphenomena that are best explained on the basis of schedules of reinforcement? Recent work in our psychophysiology and neuroendocrine laboratories has focused on the relationship between craving and a number of psychophysiological and biochemical/neuroendocrine factors in various samples of subjects, including alcoholic persons and individuals with and without a family history (father) who are alcoholic. Patterns of responding to alcohol containing beverages in FH+ individuals are being examined relative to responses observed in known alcohol-dependent patients. This approach can be used to identify FH+ subjects who may be at greatest risk for developing alcoholism. This work follows from preliminary studies on the psychophysiological and neuroendocrine responses of alcoholic (vs. control) subjects to alcohol-related stimuli and beverage consumption (Dolinsky et al., 1987; Kaplan et al., 1983; Kaplan et al., 1984; Kaplan et al., 1985; Kaplan et al., 1988; Meyer and Dolinsky, 1990). In these studies, alcohol-dependent subjects can be clearly differentiated from control subjects on the basis of their biological and subjective responses.

The important studies of Mendelson and Mello (Mello and Mendelson, 1970; Mendelson and Mello, 1966), using human operant methodology, suggested strongly that alcoholic persons did not drink to avoid withdrawal symptoms. They also failed to find evidence of "loss of control," reporting that drinking behavior was, like any other operant, controlled by its consequences. In contrast, Funderburk and Allen (1977) used operant methodology (a progressive ratio task) to demonstrate that alcoholic persons found it more difficult to delay additional drinks if they had been recently withdrawn from ethanol. Porjesz and Begleiter (1985) have demonstrated electrophysiological evidence of protracted abstinence in detoxified alcoholic individuals and in alcohol-addicted rats and monkeys (Begleiter et al., 1980). Their data in monkeys suggest that the acute and subacute period after alcohol withdrawal is characterized by CNS hyperexcitability; this is followed by a period of latent hyperexcitability that can be triggered by ethanol administration (Begleiter et al., 1980). If this is also true in dependent human alcoholics, the effects of low doses of ethanol would appear to be quite different in detoxified alcoholic vs. non-alcoholic subjects.

A number of investigators have reported that alcoholics manifest autonomic arousal when presented with an alcohol-related stimulus (Kaplan et al., 1983; Kaplan et al., 1984; Laberg, 1986; Ludwig and Wikler, 1976; Monti et al., 1987). Most have reported that the autonomic arousal is associated with an increased desire to drink. Our group has suggested that there are other CNS correlates of craving that may be triggered by an alcohol stimulus or actual consumption of a beverage in these subjects (Dolinsky et al., 1987; Meyer and Dolinsky, 1990). It is also of interest that more dependent drinkers (vs. control subjects) find placebo beverage reinforcing in double-blind studies in which they have been told that they would receive either real beer or a placebo (Kaplan et al., 1983). Future research should focus on studying recently detoxified alcoholic subjects in the Mendelson and Lukas paradigms where alcohol and placebo are administered in a balanced placebo design (Marlatt and Rohsenow, 1980). The question of conditioned reinforcement can be addressed in such a paradigm under conditions when subjects are told that they will receive an alcoholic beverage when in fact they receive a placebo.[2]

CONCLUSIONS AND SUMMARY

It is likely that the reinforcing effects of ethanol probably are mediated through several neural subtrates that involve the euphoric, anxiolytic, cognitive, and aversive properties of ethanol. The development of alcohol dependence probably results in an increase in the reinforcing potency of ethanol, as well as possible alterations in mechanisms of appetite and/or satiation. Gaining an understanding of how these factors interact requires animal models of alcohol drinking, including pharmocogenetic and behavioral paradigms. The relationship between the acute and chronic reinforcing effects of ethanol and the neural mechanisms responsible for the development of dependence can be investigated using a variety of new and established methods in neurobiology, which permit biobehavioral correlations in *in vivo* studies. The results generated by these animal studies can be combined with data from human studies to enhance our knowledge about the actions of ethanol in alcohol-dependent individuals, as well as individuals at risk (e.g., FH+). Such research will be critical in developing pharmacological interventions for alcohol-dependent individuals, (Meyer, 1989). These interventions may be aimed at reducing or altering the direct reinforcing qualities of ethanol that subsequently motivate individuals to continue drinking. From a prevention point of view, this research could lead to the identification of risk factors in human beings that predispose them to the development of alcohol dependence. The challenge to researchers will continue to be to clarify how a widely available (but weak reinforcer) such as ethanol becomes a more potent reinforcer (over time) in vulnerable individuals.

---

[2] Human subject issues: In such studies, subjects are routinely debriefed to clarify which condition they were in. In addition, the National Advisory Council on Alcohol Abuse and Alcoholism recently issued guidelines that spell out the conditions under which alcohol can be administered to alcoholic individuals (Recommended Council Guidelines, June, 1989).

ACKNOWLEDGMENTS

This chapter was supported by the National Institute on Alcohol Abuse and Alcoholism grant 5 P50 AA03510.

REFERENCES

Amit Z, Brown Z, Sutherland A, Rockman G, Gill K, Selvaggi N (1985): Reduction in alcohol intake in humans as a function of treatment with zimelidine: implications for treatment. In: *Research Advances in New Psychopharmocological Treatments for Alcoholism.* Naranjo CA, Sellers EM, eds. Amsterdam: Elsevier, pp 189-198

Beecher HK (1959): Measurement of subjective responses. In: *Quantitative Effects of Drugs.* Beecher HK, ed. London: Oxford University Press, pp 321-334

Begleiter H, DeNoble V, Porjesz B (1980): Protracted brain dysfunction after alcohol withdrawal in monkeys. In: *Biological Effects of Alcohol.* Begleiter H, ed. New York: Plenum Press, pp 231-249

Begleiter H, Porjesz B, Bihari B, Kissin B (1984): Event-related brain potentials in boys at risk for alcoholism. *Science* 225:1493-1496

Cicero TJ (1979): A critique of animal analogues of alcoholism. In: *Biochemistry and Pharmacology of Ethanol, vol. 2.* Majchrowicz E, Noble EP, eds. New York: Plenum Press, pp 533-560

Cloninger CR (1987): Neurogenetic adaptive mechanisms in alcoholism. *Science* 236:410-416

Cloninger CR, Sigvardsson S, Bohman M (1988): Childhood personality predicts alcohol abuse in young adults. *Alcohol Clin Exp Res* 12:494-505

Crabbe JC (1983): Sensitivity to ethanol in inbred mice: genotypic correlations among several behavioral responses. *Behav Neurosci* 97:280-289

DiChiara G, Imperato A (1988): Drugs abused by humans preferentially increase synaptic dopamine concentrations in the mesolimbic system of freely moving rats. *Proc Nat Acad Sci* 85:5274-5278

Dolinsky ZS, Morse DE, Kaplan RF, Meyer RE, Corry D, Pomerleau OF (1987): Psychophysiological and subjective reactivity to an alcohol placebo in male alcoholic patients. *Alcohol Clin Exp Res* 11:296-300

Edwards G, Gross MM (1976): Alcohol dependence: provisional description of a clinical syndrome. *Br Med J* 1:1058-1061

Engel JA, Fahlke C, Hulthe P, Hard E, Johannessen K, Snape B, Svensson L (1988): Biochemical and behavioral evidence for an interaction between ethanol and calcium channel antagonists. *J Neural Transm* 74:181-193

Eriksson K (1971): Rat strains specially selected for their voluntary alcohol consumption. *Ann Med Exp Biol Fenn* 49:67-72

Falk JL, Samson HH, Winger G (1972): Behavioral maintenance of high concentrations of blood ethanol and physical dependence in the rat. *Science* 177:811-813

Falk JL, Tang M (1988): What schedule-induced polydipsia can tell us about alcoholism. *Alcohol Clin Exp Res* 12(5): 577-586

Funderburk FR, Allen RP (1977): Alcoholics disposition to drink: effects of abstinence and heavy drinking. *J Stud Alcohol* 38:410-425

George FR (1988): Genetic tools in the study of self administration. *Alcohol Clin Exp Res* 12:586-590

Gill K, France C, Amit Z (1986): Voluntary ethanol consumption in rats: an examination of blood/brain ethanol levels and behavior. *Alcohol Clin Exp Res* 10(4):457-462

Hubbell CL, Czirr SA, Hunter GA, Beaman CM, LeCann NC, Reed LD (1986): Consumption of an ethanol solution is potentiated by morphine and attenuated by naloxone persistently across repeated daily administrations. *Alcohol* 3:39-54

Kaplan RF, Hesselbrock VM, O'Connor S, DePalma N (1988): Behavioral and EEG responses to alcohol in nonalcoholic men with a family history of alcoholism. *Prog Neuropsychopharmacol Biol Psychiatry* 12:873-885

Kaplan RF, Meyer RE, Stroebel CF (1983): Alcohol dependence and responsivity to an ethanol stimulus as predictors of alcohol consumption. *Br J Addict* 78:259-267

Kaplan RF, Meyer RE, Virgillio LM (1984): Physiological reactivity to alcohol cues and the awareness of an alcohol effect in a double blind placebo design. *Br J Addict* 79:439-442

Kaplan RF, Cooney NL, Baker LH, Gillespie RA, Meyer RE, Pomerleau OF (1985): Reactivity to alcohol related cues: physiological and subjective responses in alcoholics and nonproblem drinkers. *J Stud Alcohol* 46:267-272

Koob G, et al. (1988): Picrotoxin receptor ligand blocks antipunishment effects of alcohol. *Alcohol* 5:437-443

Koob GF, Bloom FE (1988): Cellular and molecular mechanisms of drug dependence. *Science* 242:715-723

Kornetsky C (1985): Brain stimulation reward: a model for the neuronal basis for drug induced euphoria. In: *Neuroscience Methods In Drug Abuse Research*. Brown RM, Freedman DP, Nimit Y, eds. Washington, DC: NIDA Research Monograph 62, Superintendent of Documents, U.S. Government Printing Office, pp 30-50

Kranzler HR, Orrok B (1989): The pharmacotherapy of alcoholism. In: *Review of Psychiatry, vol. 8*. Tasman A, Hales RE, Frances AJ, eds. Washington, DC: American Psychiatric Press Inc., pp 359-379

Laberg JC, (1986): Alcohol and expectancies: subjective psychophysiological and behavioral responses to alcohol stimuli in severely, moderately and non-dependent drinkers. *Br J Addict* 81:797-808

Li T-K, Lumeng GL, McBride WJ (1988): Pharmacology of alcohol preference in rodents. *Adv Alcohol Subst Abuse* 7:73-86

Ludwig AM, Wickler A (1976): Craving and relapse to drink. *Q J Stud Alcohol* 35:108-130

Lukas SE, Greewald NE, Mendelson JH (1988): Alcohol induced changes in body sway in women at risk for alcoholism: a pilot study. *J Stud Alcohol* 49:346-356

Marlatt GA, Rohsenow DR (1980): Cognitive processes in alcohol use: expectancy and the balanced-placebo design. In: *Advances in Substance Abuse, vol. 1.* Mello NK, ed. Greenwich, Conn: JAI Press, pp 159-199

Mello NK, Mendelson JH (1970): Experimentally induced intoxication in alcoholics: a comparison between programmed and spontaneous drinking. *J Pharmacol Exp Ther* 173:101-116

Mendelson JH, Mello NK (1966): Experimental analysis of drinking behavior of chronic alcoholics. *Ann NY Acad Sci* 133:828-845

Meyer RE, Dolinsky ZS (1990): Ethanol beverage anticipation: effects on plasma testosterone and luteinizing hormone levels. *J Stud Alcohol* 51:350-355

Meyer RE (1989): Prospects for a rational pharmacotherapy of alcoholism. *J Clin Psychiatry* 50(11):403-412

Monti PM, Binkhoff JA, Abrams DB, Zwicki WR, Nirenberg RD, Liepman MR (1987): Reactivity of alcoholics and nonalcoholics to drinking cues. *J Abnorm Psychol* 96:122-126

Murphy JM, McBride WJ, Gatto GJ, Lumen GL, Li T-K (1988): Effects of acute ethanol administration on monoamine and metabolite content in four brain regions of ethanol tolerant and nontolerant alcohol preferring rats. *Biochem Behav* 29:169-174

Myers RD, Borg S, Mossberg R (1986): Antagonism by naltrexone of voluntary alcohol selection in the chronically drinking macaque monkey. *Alcohol* Nov-Dec 3(6):383-388

Naranjo CA, Sellers EM, Roach CA, Woodley DV, Kadlec K, Sykora K (1984): Zimelidine-induced variations in alcohol intake by nondepressed heavy drinkers. *Clin Pharmacol Ther* 35:374-381

Naranjo CA, Sellers EM, Sullivan JT, Sanchez-Craig M, Sykora K (1987): The serotonin uptake inhibitor citalopram attenutes ethanol intake. *Clin Pharmacol Ther* 41(3):266-274

Pfeffer A, Samson H (1987): Apomorphine effects of ethanol reinforcement in free feeding rats. *Pharmacol Biochem Behav* 29:343-350

Porjesz B, Begleiter H (1985): Human brain electrophysiology and alcoholism. In: *Alcohol and the Brain: Chronic Effects*. Tarter RE, Van Thiel DH, eds. New York: Plenum Press, pp139-182 Recommended Council Guidelines on Alcohol Administration in Human Experimentation. Prepared by the National Advisory Council on Alcohol abuse and Alcoholism. Revised June 1989

Samson HH (1986): Initiation of ethanol reinforcement using a sucrose-substitution procedure in food-and water-sated rats. *Alcohol Clin Exp Res* 10(4):436-442

Samson HH, Tolliver GA, Lumeng L, Li T-K (1988): Ethanol reinforcement in the alcohol non-preferring (NP) rat: initiation using behavioral techniques without food restriction. *Alcohol Clin Exp Res* 13:378-385

Schuckit MA (1984): Subjective responses to alcohol in sons of alcoholics and controlled subjects. *Arch Gen Psychiatry* 41:879-884

Schuckit MA, Gold MS, Risch C (1987a): Serum prolactin levels in sons of alcoholics and control subjects. *Am J Psychiatry* 144:854-859

Schuckit MA, Gold MS, Risch C (1987b): Plasma cortisol levels following ethanol in sons of alcoholics and controls. *Arch Gen Psychiatry* 144:42-945

Schuster CR, Thompson T (1969): Self-administration of and behavioral dependence on drugs. *Ann Rev Pharmacol* 9:483-502

Schuster CR, Villareal JE (1968): The experimental analysis of opioid dependence. In: *Psychopharmacology: A Review of Progress*. Efron DH, ed. Washington, DC: Public Health Service Publ, U.S. Government Printing Office, pp 811-828

Siggins GR, Bloom FE, French ED, Madamba SG, Mancillas J, Pittman QJ, Rogers J (1987): Electrophysiology of ethanol on central neurons. *Ann NY Acad Sci* 492:350-366

Signs SA, Schecter MD (1987): The role of dopamine and serotonin receptors in the mediation of the ethanol introceptive cue. *Pharmacol Biochem Behav* 30:55-64

Vavrousek-Jakuba, Dolinsky ZS, Shoemaker WJ (1989): *In vivo* opiate receptor binding in rats offered limited access to ethanol and other fluids of varying palatability. *Alcohol Clin Exp Res* 13(2):305 abstract 18N

Waller MB, McBride WJ, Lumeng L, Li T-K (1983): Initial sensitivity and acute tolerance to ethanol in the PNP lines of rats. *Pharmacol Biochem Behav* 9:683-686

Waller MB, McBride WJ, Gatto GJ, Lumeng L, Li T-K (1984): Intragastric self-infusion of ethanol of the P and NP (alcohol preferring and non-preferring) lines of rats. *Science* 225:78-80

Weiss F, Mitchiner M, Bloom FE, Koob GF (1990): Free-choice responding for ethanol vs. water in alcohol preferring-and unselected wistar rats is differentially modified by naloxone, bromocriptine and methylsergide. *Psychopharmacol* 101:178-186

Winger G, Young AM, Woods JH (1983): Ethanol as a reinforcer: comparison with other drugs, In: *The Biology of Alcoholism: The Pathogenesis of Alcoholism-Biological Factors, vol. 7.* Kissen B, Begleiter H, eds. New York: Plenum Press, pp 107-132

Wise R (1980): Actions of drugs of abuse on brain reward systems. *Pharmacol Biochem Behav* 13(1):213-224

Yanagita T, Kiyoshi A, Takahashi S, Ishida K (1969): Self-administration of barbiturates, alcohol (intragastric) and CNS stimulants (intravenous) in monkeys. *NAS-NRC Committee on Problems of Drug Dependence*, Palo Alto, CA, pp 6039-6051

Subject Index

Acetaldehyde, 108-109, 133
Acetylcholine (ACh), 11, 27, 42, 79, 96
Adenylate cyclase (AC), 8
Adrenocorticotropic hormone (ACTH),
  234-245, 255-256
Alcohol:
  alcoholism and, 9, 107, 114, 256
  anesthesia and, 1-14, 22, 28, 77-89
  animal studies. *See* Animal studies
  behavior studies, 107-120
  blood concentrations. *See* Blood
    alcohol concentrations
  brain stimulation reward and, 163-175,
    179-196, 253
  dependence studies, 251-252
  depression and, 3, 11, 179, 193, 239
  flush reaction and, 108-109
  human studies, 203-294
  metabolism of, 108
  molecular sites of action, 21-42
  neuronal proteins and, 6-9
  reinforcement and, 233-245, 251-259
  self-administration of, 125-151,
    179-196
  tolerance studies, 3, 145, 254
  See also specific studies, types
Alcohol dehydrogenase (ADH), 108-109
Aldehyde condensation, 133
Aldehyde dehydrogenase (ALDH),
  108-112, 117

Alkanols, 82
Alpha brain waves, 213-225, 239, 255
Amino acid sequencing, 109
D-2-amino-5-phosphonovaleric acid
  (2-APV), 95
Amphetamine, 143, 180
Amygdala, 194
Androstenedione, 240
Anesthetics, 1-14, 22, 28, 77-89
Angiotensin, 126, 149-150
Animal studies, 10
  blood alcohol concentrations.
    See Blood alcohol concentration
  ethanol self-administration, 125-151,
    179-196
  genetic studies, 113-116
  human studies and, 259
  hybridization studies, 65, 119
  rat lines and. *See* Rat studies
  See also specific studies
Antabuse, 109
Anticonflict paradigm, 58
Anticonvulsant effects, 60
Anxiety states, 163, 179-196, 202, 239
Anxiolytic agents, 125, 163, 179
Apomorphine, 144
Asian population studies, 112-113
Autonomic nervous system, 258
Autosomal recessive gene, 109

Barbiturates, 49, 51, 78, 224, 251.
    See also specific agents
Bay K 8644, 34
B-carboline, 55
BEAM. *See* Brain electrical activity
    mapping system
Behavior studies, 58, 107-120, 211-213,
    222, 236, 251-259
Benzodiazepines, 13, 26, 49, 51, 55, 61,
    95, 195.
    See also specific agents
Beta brain waves, 223
Beta-endorphin, 134
Bicuculline, 52, 60
Biobehavioral studies, 251-259
Biofeedback techniques, 224
Blood alcohol concentrations (BACs):
    assay of, 206-207
    brain stimulation reward and, 127,
        150, 163-175, 179-196, 253
    schedule-induced drinking and,
        252-253
    voluntary drinking and, 114, 130-131
    withdrawal procedures, 234-235
Bragg's Law , 32-33
Brain:
    alpha waves, 213-225, 239, 255
    beta waves, 223
    electroencephalogram (EEG) and, 11,
        201-226, 234-245, 255-256
    Electrical Activity Mapping (BEAM)
        system, 207-209, 225-226
    dialysis and, 255
    halothane and, 87
    re-dox systems and, 3
    physiology of, 201-226
Significant Probability Mapping (SPM)
    techniques, 209, 220, 225-226

stimulation reward (BSR), 127, 150,
    163-175, 179-196, 253
theta waves, 213-221
topographic mapping, 201-202, 207,
    225
    See also specific regions
Bromocriptine, 141-145
BSR. *See* Brain stimulation reward
Butanol, 5

Calcium channels, 23-27, 96-97
3-carboethoxy-b-carboline, 85
Carbolines, 55, 85-86
Cardiac sarcolemma lipids (CSL), 34
Catecholamines, 9, 11, 96, 125, 140, 174,
    253.
    See also specific agents
Central nervous system, 1, 21.
    See also specific organs
Cerebellum, 10-13, 25
Cerebral cortex, 50, 146, 224
Charles River rats, 173
Chinese population studies, 112-113
P-chloramphetamine, 145
Chloride channels, 24-27, 49, 70
Chlorimipramine, 145
Chlormethiazole, 82
Cholesterol concentration, 37-38
Clonidine, 52
Cocaine, 141, 143, 163, 194-195, 222,
    239
Computerized analysis, 201
Continuous reinforcement (CRF) sched-
    ule, 164-165
Corpus striatum, 146
Corticotrophin-releasing factor (CRF),
    234-245

Dehydroepiandrosterone (DHA), 4
Denervation treatments, 144
Dependence studies, 251-252
Depression, 3, 11, 179, 193, 239
DHP. See Dihydropyridine
Diazepam, 95
Differential scanning calorimeter, 22,
    31-33
Digitized image reproduction, 226
Dihydropyridine (DHP), 22-23, 26, 34-36,
    40-41, 100
Dihydroxyphenylacetic acid (DOPAC),
    172
Dihydroxytryptamine (DHT), 145
Dimyristoyllecithin (DML), 29
Disulfiram, 109
DNA, marker studies, 116-118
Dopamine (DA):
    brain stimulation reward and, 150,
        165, 171-173, 253-254
    mesolimbic system and, 139-145,
        192-193
    neurochemical assays of, 114-116
    release of, 8, 97
Drug disrimination techniques, 99, 255
Drug-induced reinforcement, 125,
    222-223
Drug partition coefficients, 36-38
Drug-receptor interactions, 21-42
Dysphoria, 202, 239

Electroencephalograms (EEGs), 11,
    201-226, 234-245, 255-256
Electromyography, 224
Electron resonance studies, 21-22, 28
Electrophoresis, 109
Electrophysiological studies, 50, 201-226,
    256-257

Endogenous opioids, 135
Endorphins, 134
Enflurane, 79, 81
Enkephalins, 174
Environmental factors, 107
Epileptiform seizure activity, 94, 99
Estradiol (E2) levels, 240-245
Ethanol:
    acute effects of, 21-42, 231-240
    anticonvulsant effects of, 60
    cerebellar function and, 10-13, 25
    chronic administration of, 21-42
    contingent vs. noncontingent
        administration, 191-192
    dopamine and. See Dopamine
    electrophysiological studies, 50,
        201-226, 256-257
    euphoria and, 125, 163, 179, 195,
        202, 212, 215, 237
    GABA and. See Gamma
        aminobutyric acid
    human studies, 203-294
    hyperthermia and, 6
    intoxication and. See Intoxication
    ion channel receptors and, 9
    metabolism of, 108
    motor effects of, 140, 181
    opioids and, 125, 133-139, 251, 253
    pharmacogenetic factors and, 251
    plasma concentrations, 206, 214,
        236-238
    reinforcement and, 240-245
    reward and, 141, 179-196, 251-259
    second messenger regulation, 8-9
    self-administration studies, 125-151,
        179-196
    withdrawal syndrome, 38, 49, 61, 101,
        108, 252, 258

See also Alcohol; *specific studies*
Ether, 82
Euphoric effects:
    alcohol abuse and, 125, 163
    drug-induced, 179, 195
    EEG studies, 202, 215, 237
    multiple paroxysmal, 212

Fenfluramine, 145
FG-7142, 49
Firefly luciferase, 78
Fixed-ratio (FR) schedule, 129, 164-165
Flame ionization detector, 207
Flumazenil, 24, 32, 49, 55-60, 83, 85
Flunitrazepam, 63
Fluorescence studies, 22-23, 95
Fluoxetine, 145-146, 149
Flurazepam, 95
Forebrain, 165, 184-186
Fourier analysis, 33, 201, 208
FRAP technique, 23
Freeze fracture studies, 22
Frontal brain lobes, 194, 218

GABA. *See* Gamma aminobutyric acid
Gamma aminobutyric acid (GABA)
    chloride channels and, 24-27
    receptor complex, 7, 77-89
    synaptic transmission of, 12-13, 253
    terminals of, 116
Gel chromatography, 119, 206-207
General anesthesia, 77
Genetic studies, 77, 107, 109, 225, 251, 255
Glutamate receptors, 12, 96
Glycine, 10, 79, 97-98

Gonadotropin levels, 240-245
Guanine nucleotide binding proteins (G-proteins), 7, 93
Guanosine monophosphate (GMP), 96
Guanosine triphosphate (GTP), 8

Hair-root analysis, 112
Haloperidol, 52, 141
Halothane, 77-81, 87
Heroin, 195, 239
High-alcohol drinking (HAD) rats, 114-11 149-150, 254
Hippocampus, 11, 24, 50, 146, 194
Holeboard test, 59
Home cage drinking, 127
Homotetrameric proteins, 110
Horizontal wire tests, 59
Human studies, 77, 107, 109, 203-294. *See also specific studies*
Hybridization studies, 65, 119
5-hydroxyindoleacetic acid (5-HIAA), 146
Hyperthermia, 6
Hypothalamus, 146, 165, 184, 233-245

Imidazobenzodiazepine, 24, 29, 32, 34-36 41
Immunocytochemical studies, 114
Inhalation anesthetics, 77-89
Inositol, 26
Instrumental self-reports, 211, 213
Interresponse interval (IRI), 165
Intoxication:
    acute ethanol, 2-3
    behavioral signs of, 131
    opioids, 125, 133-139, 251-253

self-reports of, 210-213
sensations of, 239
subjective reports of, 235-238
verbal reports of, 210
See also specific studies
Intracranial self-stimulation, 180
Intraperitoneal administration, 184-186
In vitro studies, 51-58, 259
Ion channels, 7, 9, 11, 21, 49-70

Japanese population studies, 110-112

Kainate, 94-95
Ketamine, 5

Lamellar neutron diffraction, 31
Lateral hypothalamus (LH), 165, 184
Light sarcoplasmic reticulum, 36-38
Lipids, 1-14, 57, 77
Lipophilic drugs, 27
Liver diseases, 112, 240
Local anesthetics, 22, 28
Lorentz correction factor, 33
Low-alcohol drinking (LAD) rats,
    114-116, 254
Luciferase, 78
Luteinizing hormone (LH), 240-245
Lymphoma cells, 8

Majchrowicz behavioral rating scale, 58
Medial forebrain bundle (MFB), 186
Meditation, transcendental, 222
Men, acute ethanol effects, 234-240
Mesencephalic ventral noradrenergic
    bundle, 165
Mesolimbic dopamine system, 139, 145,
    192-193
Metenkephalin, 134

Methoxyflurane, 81, 84, 85
Methysergide, 147, 149
Meyer-Overton rule, 1, 5
Microcomputer system, 226
Midbrain, 9-10
MK-801, 100
Molecular biology techniques, 107,
    114-120
Monoclonal antibodies, 40
Mood states, 202, 220, 233-234
Morphine, 163, 182-183
Motor effects, ethanol and, 140, 181
Muscarinic receptors, 42
Muscimol, 50, 54, 60-65, 80

Naloxone, 133-138
Neural membranes, 31-33, 36-38
Neurotransmitter systems, 3, 7, 253.
    See also specific chemicals
Neutron diffraction studies, 23-24, 29
Nitrandipine, 26-27
N-Methyl D-Aspartic Acid (NMDA), 12,
    93-102
Nonpreferring (NP) rats, 141, 254
Nonverbal instrumental device, 203-205
Norepinephrine, 11, 96, 140, 174, 253
Northern analysis, 65
N6-Phenylisopropyladenosine (N6-PIA),
    8
Nuclear magnetic resonance, 22, 86
Nucleus accumbens (NA), 172-173, 194

Occipital brain lobes, 218
Olivary complex, 10
Opioids, 125, 133-139, 251, 253

Parallelism tests, 237
Parietal brain lobes, 218

Partition coefficient measurements, 33-34
P-chlorophenylalanine (PCPA), 145
Pentobarbital, 50, 52, 58, 63, 81-82, 180
Pharmacogenetic factors, 251
Phencyclidine (PCD), 94-95, 97-98
Phenoxybenzamine, 52
Phosphatidylinositol fraction, 2, 94
Photoaffinity labeling experiments, 28
Picrotoxin, 26, 52, 60, 79, 98
Pimozide, 140-141
Pituitary corticotrophins, 234-245
Placebo responses, 212, 236-237
Plasma ethanol concentrations, 206, 214, 236-238
Plasma gonadal steroids, 240-245
Plasma membranes, 1-14
    bilayer pathway and, 22
    lipids and, 77
    molecular interactions of, 21-23
    partition coefficents and, 34
    proteins and, 78
Pleasureable states, 222
Polydipsia, 252
Polygraphic recordings, 206-208
Polymerase chain reaction (PCR), 110
Pontine brain region, 9-10
Population studies, 109-113.
    See also specific groups
Post-reinforcement pauses (PRP), 165
Prandial models, 127
Preferring (P) rats, 132, 141, 144, 149, 254
Prolactin levels, 243
Propranolol, 28, 31, 52
Psychomotor stimulation, 21, 181
Psychostimulant drugs, 125, 143
Purkinje cells, 10, 50

Quantitative trait loci (QTLs), 119
Quisqualate, 94-95

Radioligand binding studies, 63
Rat studies:
    accepting (AA) rates, 254
    Charles River rats, 173
    high alcohol drinking (HAD), 114-116, 149-150, 254
    low alcohol drinking (LAD), 114-116, 254
    non-preferring (NP) rats, 141, 254
    prandial models, 127
    preferring (P) rats, 132, 141, 144, 149, 254
    recombinant strains, 117
    selective breding of, 113-118
    Sprague-Dawley rats, 173
    Wistar rats, 130-132, 144
    wheel-running behavior, 59
Receptor molecules, 7, 21, 49-70
Recombinant inbred (RI) strains, 117
Restriction fragment length polymorphism (RFLP), 118
Ro 15-1788 (Flumazenil), 24, 32, 49, 55-60, 83, 85

Schedule-induced polydipsia technique, 127
Scheffe F test, 219
Second messenger regulation, 8-9
Self-administration studies, 125-151, 179-196
Sensorimotor cortex, 223
Serotonin (5-HT):
    animal studies, 114, 116
    hippocampus and, 11

hypothalamus and, 174
olivary complex and, 10-11, 145-150
reward and, 253-254
Significant probability mapping (SPM) techniques, 209, 220, 225-226
Social drinking behavior, 181, 220, 233
Spectral analysis studies, 201, 234-245
Spermine, 94
Spinal cord, 50
SPM techniques. *See* Significant probability mapping
Spontaneous electromyographic activity, 224
Sprague-Dawley rats, 173
Stamatoff-Krimm algorithm, 33
Starch gel electrophoresis, 109
Steroid levels, 240-245
Strychnine, 52
Subjective state assessments, 203-205, 235-238
Subtractive hybridization probing techniques, 119
Synaptoneurosomes, 21-42, 79

Taste adulteration models, 126, 128
T-Butylbicyclophosphorothionate (TBPS), 81
Temporal brain lobes, 218
Testosterone (T) levels, 240-245
Tetrahydroisoquinolines (TIQs), 133-139
Tetrodotoxin, 97
Thalamus, 146, 223
Theta brain waves, 213-221
Tolerance, alcohol and, 3, 145, 254

Topographic brain mapping, 201-202, 207, 225
Transcendental meditation, 222
Transcerebral dialysis technique, 172
Triple-test cross analysis, 117
Two-bottle water test, 128, 138

Variable numbers of tandem repeat (VNTR) sequences, 119
Ventral tegmental area (VTA), 186
Verapamil, 52
Verbal reports, of intoxication, 210
Visual inspection studies, 201
Vogel anticonflict paradigm, 58
Voluntary drinking, 190, 223

Wheel-running behavior, in rats, 59
Wistar rats, 130-132, 144
Withdrawal syndrome, 38, 49, 61, 101, 108, 252, 258

X-ray diffraction, 24, 28,

Zimelidine, 145